AF477221

Computer Fundamentals with Pharmacy Applications

Second Edition

Computer Fundamentals with Pharmacy Applications

Second Edition

Dr. N.K. Tiwari

Director, Thakral College of Technology,
Oriental Group of Institutes

Formerly Scientist,
M.P. Council of Science and Technology,
Bhopal, (M.P)

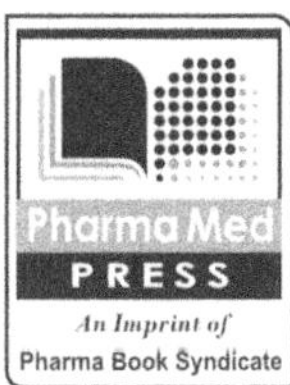

PharmaMed Press
An imprint of Pharma Book Syndicate

A unit of **BSP Books Pvt., Ltd.**

4-4-309/316, Giriraj Lane
Sultan Bazar, Hyderabad - 500 095.

Published by

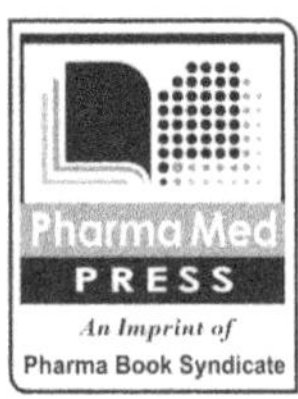

PharmaMed Press
An imprint of Pharma Book Syndicate

A unit of BSP Books Pvt., Ltd.

4-4-309/316, Giriraj Lane, Sultan Bazar, Hyderabad - 500 095.
Phone: 040-23445605, 23445688; Fax: 91+40-23445611
E-mail: info@pharmamedpress.com

ISBN : 978-93-52300-48-8 (HB)

Preface to Second Edition

The immense popularity of the first edition of this book by the faculty members and the students of various colleges has resulted in publishing the Second Edition, with the new chapters; now in all 15 chapters systematically organised for the better understanding of the subject in building strong fundamentals of computer and its applications.

Chapter 11 presents the concept of 'C' programming language. Chapter 13 deals with application of software.

It would be our pleasure for any suggestions and critics in improving the content of the book.

- Author

Preface to First Edition

Information Technology plays a vital role in all fields of activity. Pharmaceutical science also utilizes information technology for research & development and production management. In this regard the author feels that a book that gives fundamental idea of information technology and fulfils the students' needs according to the syllabus is a *sine qua non*.

The book provides a detailed yet easy-to-understand description of the subject. Each and every aspect is presented very clearly and explained logically. The book has 13 chapters systematically organized for the convenience of students. Chapter 1 provides an overview of computer and gives an introduction to various aspects of the computer and its application. It gives a brief introduction to information technology, computer and human being, characteristics and limitations of computer. Chapter 2 deals with history of the computer. It provides the early methods of calculations abacus, babbage analytical engine to modern computers.

Chapter 3 discusses various types of computers. It provides comparison of analog, hybrid, digital computers and classification based on size. Chapters 4 presents important discussion on various types of numbers systems. It provides various methods of conversion from one number system to another. Chapter 5 is devoted to the system concept. It provides the comparison of hardware and software. It further provides an introduction and function of various types of hardware used in computer system.

Chapter 6 is very important chapter. It presents fundamentals of operating system. It describes the need of operating systems, functions, types of operating system, booting process etc. The chapter also explains DOS and Unix commands. Chapter 7 gives the introduction to computer languages. Then it deals with various types of languages.

Chapter 8 presents the concept of programming first; next, it introduces task analysis, designing aspects, flowcharts, pseudo code etc. It also explains the concept of algorithm, data validation, debugging and testing methods. Chapter 9 provides the fundamentals of networking. It provides the concept of networking, types of networking transmission media, OSI reference model, etc.

Chapter 10 presents the concept of data structure. It provides stack, array, queue, lists, trees and graph theory. Chapter 11 presents the concept of BASIC programming language. Chapter 12 deals with computer graphics. It starts with types of computer graphics and proceeds to give an overview of application of graphics and graphic devices. Chapter 13 discusses various applications of computer in pharmaceutical and clinical studies.

I hope that the book will be helpful to the students in building strong fundamentals of computer and its applications.

I am grateful to the publishers, PharmaMed for careful processing of the manuscript both at the editorial and production stages. I would like to thank my mother Smt.Gyan Devi Tiwari for her blessings and love, which helped me at every stage in life. I am indebted to my wife Smt. Neeta Tiwari for her support and encouragement. I also express my gratitude to all my family members for continuous encouragement. I also give lovely gratitude to my children for cooperation and also express my gratitude to Shri B.S.Yadav, Chairman of IES Group of Institutes. Lastly, but not the least, I express my thanks to Smt. Sadhan Saxena and Shri Arjun Choudhary for assisting in DTP work.

- Author

Contents

Chapter 1

Introduction to Computers

Chapter 2

History of Computer

Chapter 3

Classification of Computers

Chapter 4

Number System

Chapter 5

The System Concept

Chapter 6

Fundamentals of Operating System

Chapter 7

Computer Languages

Chapter 8

Concept of Programming

Chapter 9

Networks

Chapter 10

Data Structure

Chapter 11

Programming Language 'C'

Chapter 12

BASIC Programming Language

Chapter 13

Application Software

Chapter 14

Introduction to Computer Graphics

Chapter 15

Applications of Computers in
Pharmaceutical and Clinical Studies

CHAPTER 1

Introduction to Computers

1.1 Introduction

Today computers have an important and widespread influence on our society. Every educated person should study the basic disciplines of computer operation and its applications. A student must study the basics of computers. Wherever there are phenomena of interest to man, there can be a science to describe and explain those phenomena. Computer science is therefore the study of computers and the phenomena requiring their use. We can give a more specific definition of computer science after we describe a computer.

A computer is a device capable of accepting information or data, processing the information, and providing the results as an output. More specifically, a computer can be described as follows:

"Computer is a data processing machine that can perform substantial computation, including numerous, arithmetic or logic operations, without intervention by a human operator during the process" or it may be defined as a "device capable of solving problems by accepting data, performing described operations on the data, and supplying the results of these operations".

"A computer is a programmable, multiuse machine that accepts data – raw facts and figures – and processes or manipulates it into information that we can use, such as summaries or totals".

A visual representation or schematic diagram shows how the computer processes the information.

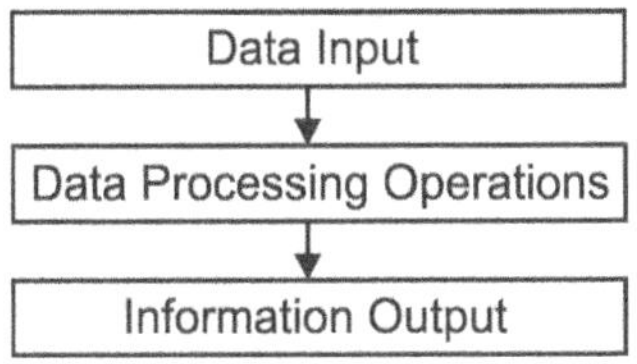

Fig. 1.1 Information processing system.

1.2   Information Processing and the Electronics Digital Computer

The electronic computer allows man to increase his productivity and permits him to do tasks he would be enabling to complete without computer. As we discussed above, the computer is a machine capable of :

- Accepting data
- Performing described operations on the data
- Providing the results of these operations.

Thus computer also permits man to improve his output permit of time, or productivity. We can say that the computer's two most important contributions as a tool are to increase :

1. Speed of the operation

2. Accuracy of the results.

Of course, when we consider these two factors, we realize that the computer enables us to accomplish tasks that we would probably never even attempt manually. For example, if the number of input data is greater than several millions and the time necessary to accomplish a task is more than fifty years, we would probably never attempt it, yet it is just tasks that we can require the computer to accomplish. The term electronic implies that the computer is powered by electrical and electronic devices rather than by mechanical ones or those affected by heat or air pressure. Here digital refers to discrete, non-continuous quantities, as contrasted with continuous quantities.

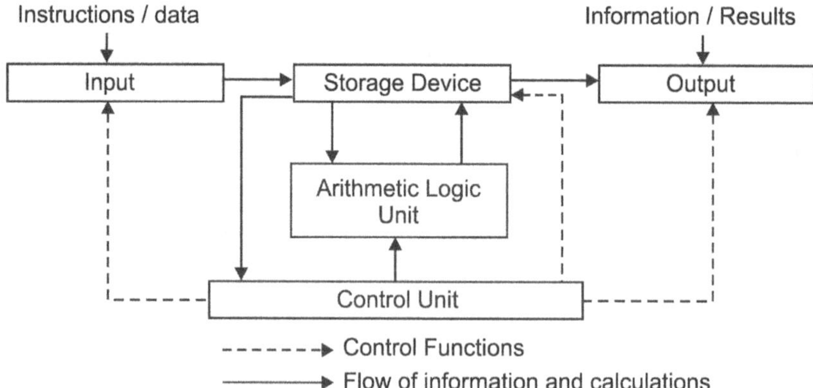

Fig. 1.2 Information processing on electronics digital computer.

Electronics digital computer is an information-processing device that accepts and processes data represented by discrete symbols. It is constructed primarily of electric or electronic devices.

We can use the computer to process the input data by sorting them, or by series of planned actions and operations. This may be illustrated by a common data processing operation which a person usually accomplishes manually, but which is increasing accomplished automatically by data processing service companies. These processing works require:

- Data input
- Storage and retrieval of data
- Arithmetic steps
- Output of result
- Control of all steps.

A computer follows a similar process. It is composed of five basic units :

Input unit — input data and instructions.

Storage or Memory unit — in which computer instructions and data as well as intermediate results are stored.

Arithmetic logic unit — in which mathematical operations can be performed and compare the numbers, results.

Output unit — provides the desired result in a suitable form.

Control unit — controls the data communication, operations and supervises overall operations of the computer.

The devices accomplish the functions of input, output and storages.

The arithmetic and control functions are accomplished by the control-processing unit locates with storage in the pattern.

1.3 Information Technology

Data communication, network and computer have brought a new technology, the Information Technology (IT). IT is the most powerful synthesis of computers and communications. The Information Technology mainly deals with customers, computers, costs and communication. Information is useful only if it is accurate, relevant, precise and provides timely information to the users. This would be possible, only when stored information is instantaneously retrievable at the time of need. Time will come when there will be only computer workstation around which we will receive data from some sources to do some processing with the data, convert it into information and forward it to some other person or workstation.

Computer has become an indispensable tool, helping to shape the society it serves. The banking industry is an integral part of the society and has grown phenomenally since last three decades with manifold rise in its transactions and area of activities. Thus the role and utility of the computer and Information Technology cannot be over emphasized.

1.4   Comparison of Computer with Human Being

Computer and Human

- Have Memory
- Capability of reading
- Perform arithmetic and logical calculation
- Manipulate symbols
- Make Comparisons.

Human

- Make processing based on results at a point
- Remember or read data from file
- Remember instructions for processing
- Write or speak out the output.

Computer

- Hold program instruction in internal storage
- Read data in machine readable form and store in the storage device
- Make processing possible by choosing instruction based on comparison or an examination result at a point
- Retrieve data from internal memory or secondary storage device
- Exhibits the results on an output device.

Table 1.1 Comparison between Human and Computer.

Character	Human	Computer
Speed of execution	Slow	Extremely fast
Continuous work	Poor	Excellent
Memory retrieval	Inaccurate	Accurate
Accuracy	Make errors	No errors
Follow instructions	Perfect / Imperfect	Consistency
Ability to innovate situation	Good	Lacking

1.5   Characteristics of Computers

The vital characteristics of the computers are as follows:

Speed

Computer works on electrical pulses, which travel at incredible speeds and because the computer is an electronic device, its internal speed is instantaneous. An arithmetic calculation can be performed in a thousandth, millionth, billionth things even in a trillionth seconds. It is capable of executing over ten thousand instructions in a second.

Milli. Sec. (ms) -   1/1000 of second

Micro. Sec (ms) - 1/1000000 of second

Nano sec (ms) -   1/1000000000 of second

Pic sec (ps) -   1/1000,000,000,00 of seconds.

Storage

This is very important character of the computer, which separates it from other machine. The basic unit of storage is bit (acronym of binary digit). The speed with which computer can perform, i.e. to input data and the instructions for processing, is humanly impossible. The storage space available in the central processing unit, being limited, large quantity of data and entire instructions of all the required programs cannot be stored in it. These are stored outside and read into the memory of CPU at the time of processing.

Bit   -   Smallest unit of storage

Byte -   8 Bits

KB   -   1024 bytes

MB   -   1024 KB

GB   -   1024 MB

Accuracy

Accuracy of the computers is consistently high. Errors in computing are due to machine failure, imprecise programming logic, inaccurate data, poorly designed systems. Precision is the degree of accuracy to which the computer gives the result. The precision of computers is phenomenal.

Versatility

Computers seem capable of performing almost any task, provided the task can be reduced to series of logical steps. It performs numeric and non-numeric tasks equally well. An algorithm, a step-by-step procedure, which applied to the problem, leads to solution. Programming is to convert this computer language to solve the problem.

Automation

Once a program is in the computers memory, CPU follows the instructions until it meets the last instruction. Once the process begins it would continue without human intervention until completion.

Diligence

Being a machine, a computer does not suffer from the human tracts of tiredness and lack of concentration. If five million calculations are to be performed, computer performs all these calculations with the same speed and accuracy.

1.6 Limitations of Computers

The computer also has certain limitations. It works at a very high speed and is extremely accurate. This very characteristic becomes its limitation when a mistake occurs because when a wrong instruction is fed, it excuses it with the same speed and accuracy that it would have executed with a right instruction. As a result, there is hardly any scope or time to recover. The computers understand only instructions and cannot distinguish between suspicious and genuine instructions. It does not possess intelligence and cannot take up even a simple action unless instructed to do so. It does not possess any morals and therefore can be easily misused in the hands of a wrong individual. However, the computers never make any mistake or error. Errors, whenever found in the computer-based on processing, are due to human errors.

1.7 Components of Computers

Computer is an electronic data processing machine. It is made up of various devices, which help you to interact, process it and output is the result. A computer system has three essential parts:

- Keyboard
- Central Processing Unit (CPU)
- Monitor.

Block Diagram of a Computer

As shown in the block diagram, the computer consists of three parts: Input device, CPU and output device. Keyboard, which is the input device, is connected to the central-processing unit. Central processing unit consists of three sections – memory, control unit and arithmetic logic unit.

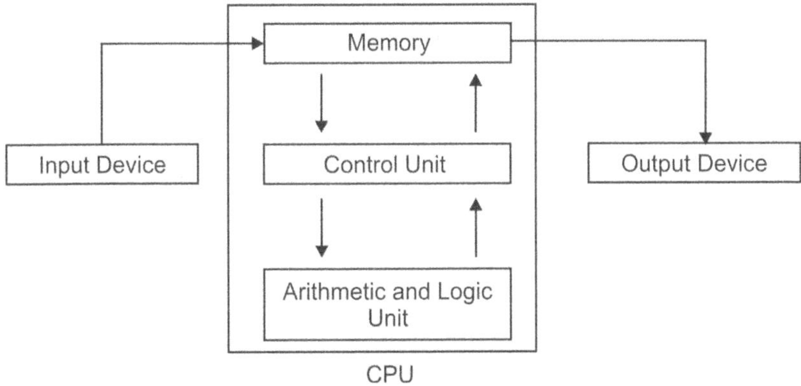

Fig. 1.3 Block diagram of computer

Keyboard

Programs and data are entered into a computer through a keyboard, which is attached to a microcomputer or the terminal of a mini or large computer. A keyboard is similar to the keyboard of a typewriter. It contains alphabets, digits, special characters and some control keys. When a key is pressed, an electronic signal is produced which is detected by an electronic circuit called keyboard encoder. A keyboard encoder may be special IC by an electronic circuit called keyboard encoder. A keyboard encoder may be special IC or a single chip microcomputer used as encoder. The function of an encoder is to detect which key has been pressed and send a binary code.

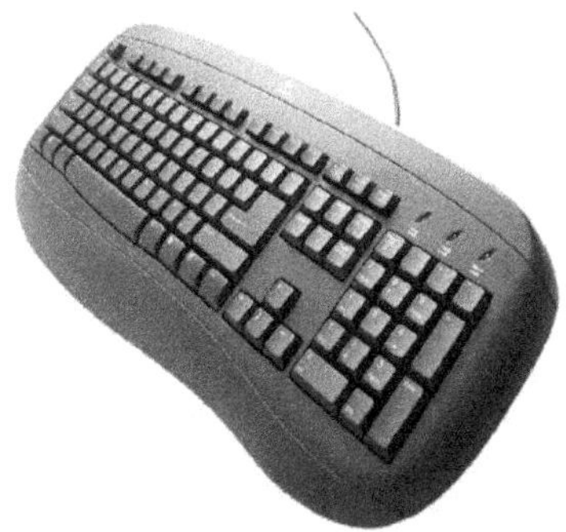

Central Processing Unit (CPU)

This is also called System unit, which is technically known as Microprocessor. CPU is the brain of computer. It is made of three units:

1. Control unit   2. Arithmetic logic unit   3. Memory

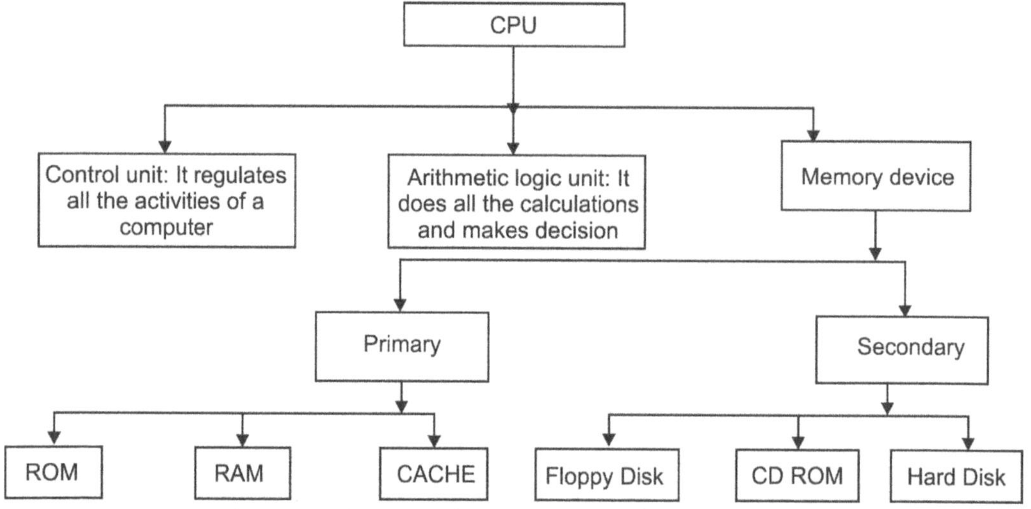

Fig. 1.4 Central Processing Unit with Different Devices.

- **Control unit**

  The control section of the CPU maintains and directs the operations of the entire system. It acts like the central nervous system for all the components, through it does not process any data.

- **Arithmetic Logic Unit (ALU)**

  The ALU processes the data entered. All types of processing, mathematical calculations, comparison, decision-making and processing of non-numeric information take place in ALU and data is once again moved to RAM.

- **Memory**

  Memory refers to the storage space in computer. Memory stores the data entered as well as the results given by the computer. Memory works on the application of binary system. The basic unit of memory is byte. Memory units can be divided into two sub-parts :

  (a) Primary storage

  (b) Secondary storage.

Monitor

Monitor is also called video display unit or CRT, are output devices. It accepts programming instructions and data as they are input and after it is processed, it displays. Sometimes a monitor is also referred to as a video display terminal (VDT).

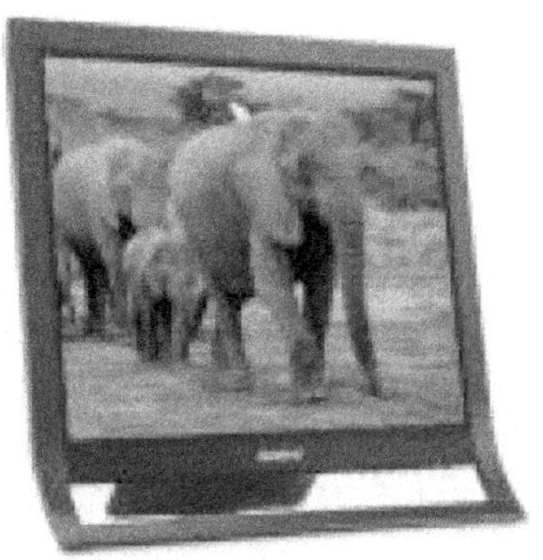

CHAPTER 2

History of Computer

In the first chapter, we understood what computer is. In this chapter we discuss the history of the computers and how this machine came into being over the years. The beginning of computers started for the development of a counting system. Therefore we start with the very early ages.

2.1 Early Methods of Calculation

Today we do all calculations, using computers. How were calculations done in olden days? The simplest calculating device was the finger. Even today we begin to learn calculations with the fingers but it has many limitations. You can only do simple additions and subtraction.

2.2 Abacus

In olden days, people learnt to do calculations by marking lines on the walls. This slowly developed into a device called the abacus.

The abacus was probably the first calculating device. It was invented over 3000 years ago and still used in some countries, including India. An abacus consists of a row of wires held in wooden frame, which have balls or beads strung on them. Calculations are done on an abacus by sliding the beads along the wires. An abacus in skilled hand can work almost as fast as an electronic calculator. There are three different kinds of abacus.

2.2.1 The Russian Abacus

It has ten beads on each wire. Beads on the first wire present single units, beads on the second wire 10s, beads, on the third wire 100s and so on. Calculations are done by sliding the beads along the wires.

The Russian Abacus is shown in the Fig 2.1 represents the number **1,24,00,23,070.**

2.2.2 The Chinese Abacus

In a Chinese Abacus, a beam is into two regions, known as heaven and earth, divides the frame. There are two beads on one side of the beam and five on the other. A bead in heaven was considered to have a value of five and a bead in earth a value of one.

Moving the beads away from or towards the beam did calculations. The bead has numerical value only when it is adjacent to the beam. The figure 2.2 shows a Chinese abacus presenting the number **1215235020.**

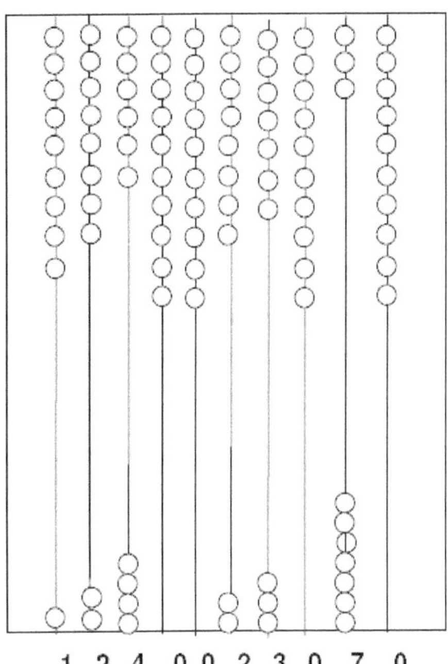

Fig. 2.1 Russian abacus.

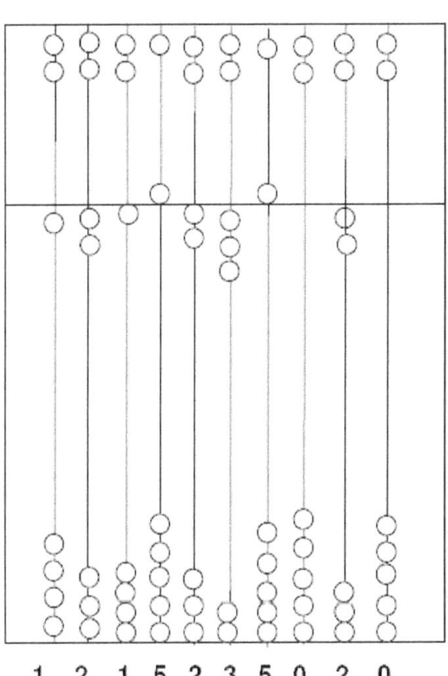

Fig. 2.2 Chinese abacus.

2.2.3 The Japanese Abacus

In a Japanese abacus, one bead is in the heaven side and 4 beads in the earth are placed for calculations. The value of the beads in heaven was considered to have a value of five and a bead in the earth, a value of one. This abacus is called SOROBAN. The Figure 2.3 shows a Japanese abacus presenting the number **1115235025**

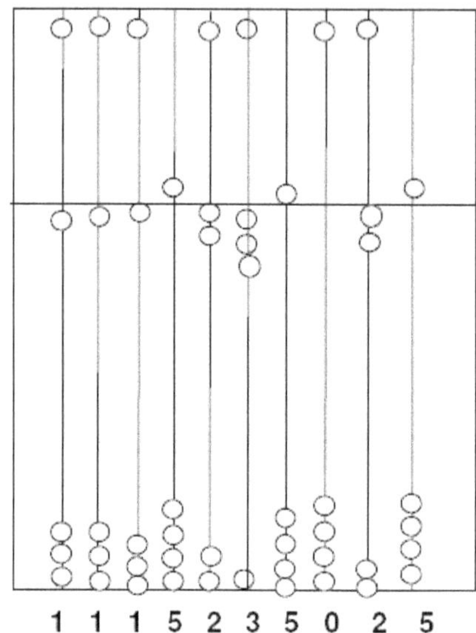

Fig. 2.3 Japanese abacus.

2.3 Napier's Bones

In the seventeenth century, John Napier, a mathematician from Scotland, did a considerable amount of work on calculations. He devised a set of even rods each having four faces, which were used as multiplication trolls. These rods were carved from bones and were called Napier's bones.

The rod have number marked on them in such a way that, by placing them side, products and quotients of large numbers can be obtained.

2.4 Pascal's Mechanical Calculating Machine

In 1642, Blaire Pascal, a French mathematician, invented the machine, dialing a series of numbered wheels and entered numbers. A series of toothed wheels transferred the movements to a dial, which showed the results. This machine also had limitation. It could be used for addition and subtraction only.

2.5 Leibnitz's Machine

1671, Goff pride Ven Leibnitz, a German mathematician, invented a calculating machine which could perform multiplications and divisions. This machine was an improved version of Pascal's machine.

2.6 Babbage Analytical Engine

In 1821, Charles Babbage designed a machine called the difference engine to calculate and print mathematical tables. Again in 1833-34 Babbage designed his analytical engine which was a programmed mechanical calculator.

The Analytical Engine had many features similar to modern computers. But it was too complicated to be built at that time. But for these ideas Charles Babbage is rightfully known as the FATHER OF COMPUTERS. Lady Ada Augusta developed ideas for Babbages machine. She is considered to be first programmer.

2.7 Hollerith's Card Machine

Herman Hollerith, an American statistician in 1887-1890 developed a punch card reading machine. He used punch cards as input and output devices. This machine was used for tabulating and calculating data.

This machine was also known as Tabulating machine. It was used in 1890 for census processing and proved to be very successful. Till recently punch cards were used in some computers.

2.8 The Analytical Engine by Babbage

It was a general purpose-computing device, which could be used for performing any mathematical operation automatically. It consisted of the following components.

The Store : A mechanical Memory unit consisting of sets of center wheels.

The Mill : An arithmetic unit which is capable of performing the four basic arithmetic operations.

Cards : There are basically two types of cards.

(a) *Operation Cards* : Selects one for arithmetic operations by activating the mill to perform the selected function.

(b) *Variable Cards:* Selects the memory locations to be used by the mill for a particular operation.

Output : Could be directed to a printer or a card punch device.

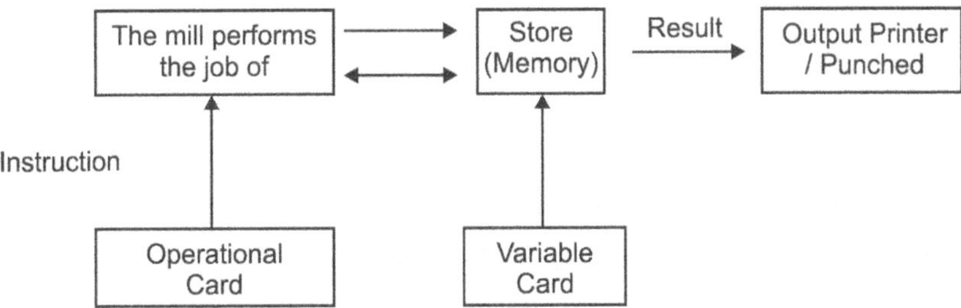

Fig. 2.4 Logical structure of Babbage's analytical engine.

2.9 Basic Features of Analytical Engine

- It was a general-purpose programmable machine.
- It had the provision of automatic sequence control, thus enabling programs to after its sequence of operations.
- The Prussian of sign checking of result assessed.
- Mechanism for changing or reversing of control card was permitted thus enabling execution of any desired instruction.

The Babbage machine is fundamentally the same as a modern computer. As a tribute to Charles Babbage his analytical engine was completed in the last decade and it is now on display at the Science Museum at London.

2.10   Prehistoric and Early Calculating Devices

When the electronic computer was introduced man has apparently always had a need to process data and calculate it. The history of computers and calculating devices in western civilisation reaches back a thousand years before the birth of Christ, when abacus was used.

2.11   First Electro Mechanical Computer

Howard Aiken, a Harvard professor with the help of some IBM engineers, developed the first electro mechanical computer "MARKET". This computer used Hollerith's punch cards. The principles of Charles Babbage were first time used practically in this computer.

This was huge machine, which occupied a large space. The inside of the machine had several miles of electrical wires, many electro-mechanical relays and mechanical counters for arithmetic calculations. With all these circuits the machine looked like a monster.

2.12   First Electronic Computer: ENIAC

ENIAC was the first general-purpose electronic computer, produced around 1943 for the US Army. It used 18,000 vacuum tubes, weighted 30 tons and occupied about 5000 square feet of space. It could perform 300 multiplications per second and was the fastest machine at the time of its development. In this machine, instructions were given by external plug boards or switches. The US Army used this computer until 1955.

2.13 EDSAC

Research work continued to make computers faster and smaller. John Van Nuemam, a mathematician, suggested that computers could be used not only for storing data calculations but could be used in development of program. In 1949, the first Electronic Delay Storage Automatic Calculator (EDSAC) was made and used at Cambridge University, London.

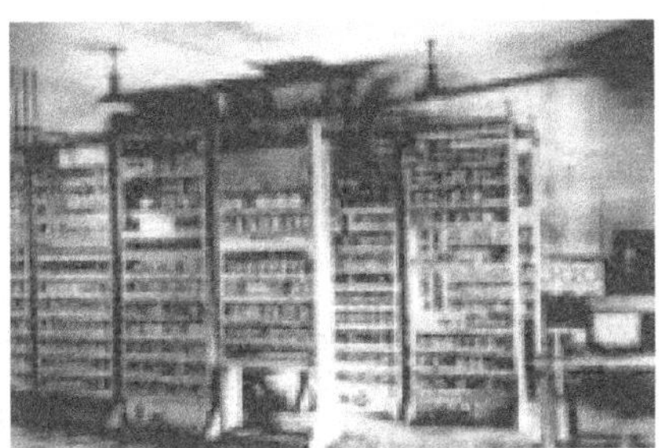

2.14 EDVAC

In 1949, Eckert and Mauchly developed the first stored program electronic computer and named it EDVAC. EDVAC stands for Electronic Discreet Variable Automatic Computer. This was the first commercial data processing machine used to store data and program instructions in its memory through the binary number system.

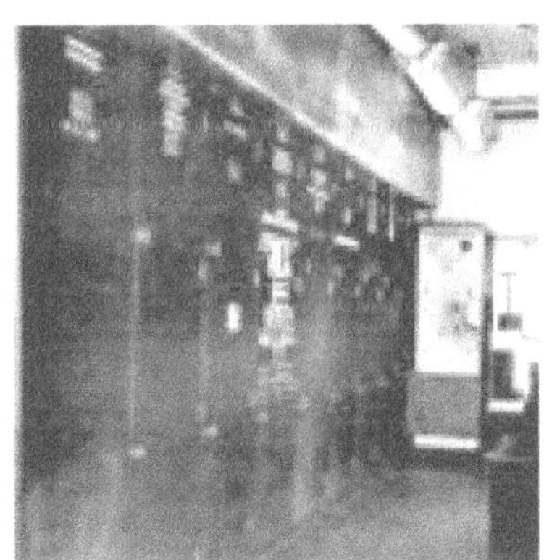

2.15 UNIVAC

Eckert and Mauchly developed Universal Automatic Computer in 1951 in their own company. In 1954 UNIVAC I was developed which was the computer used for business applications.

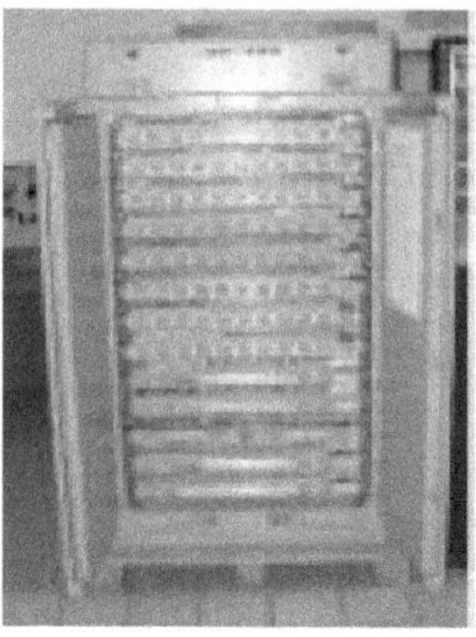

IBM 650

In the year 1955, Thomas Walton Jr., son of IBM's founder, was introduced this computer. This computer had a memory capacity of 2000 words. IBM 650 computer was widely accepted and became very popular which led IBM becoming the leader in computer production. The other computers produced by IBM were IBM 1401 and RAMAC 350.

2.16 From Vacuum Tube to Microprocessor

Computers used to be made from vacuum tubes. Then the small transistor came followed by integrated circuit (IC), circuits made from the common mineral silicon and followed by the micro processor.

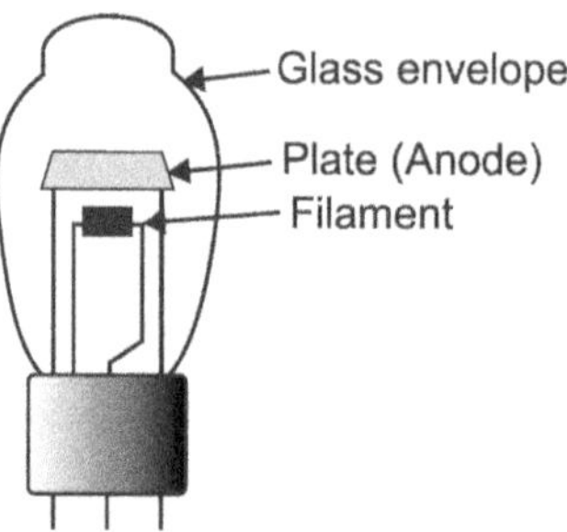

2.17 First Generation of Computer

The computers produced and used between 1940-1955 were called first generation of computers.

The first generation computers were characterized by vacuum tube (valve) circuitry. Hence, they were very large. They were placed in large air-conditioned rooms, had small internal storage and were relatively very slow. The first generation machines used punched paper tape, punched card, magnetic wire, magnetic tape and printers as input / output devices.

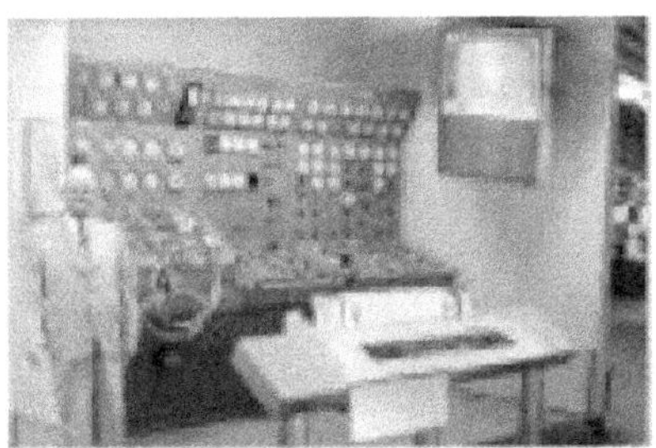

The trends, which were encountered during the era of first generation computers were :

- The first generation computer control was centralized in a single CPU, and all the operations required a direct intervention of the CPU.
- Use of finite-care main memory was started during this time.
- Concerts such as use of virtual memory and endure register started.
- Punched cards were used as input device.
- Magnetic tapes and magnetic drums were used as secondary memory.
- Binary coder or machine language was used as secondary memory.
- Towards the end, the use of symbolic language, which is now called assembly language started.
- Assembler was a program that translated assembly language program to machine language was made.
- Computer was accessible to only one programmer at a time.
- Advent of Von Neumann architecture.

2.18   Second Generation of Computer

The computer produced after 1955 are called second generation of computers. They had faster access and were more reliable than first generation of computers. Transistors replaced vacuum tubes of first generation in this period. By this time a wide range of input/output devices such as higher performance magnetic tapes, magnetic drums and early magnetic disks were available. During the second generation, computer languages such as FORTRAN and ALGOL were introduced.

The second generation of computers started with the advent of transistorized computers.

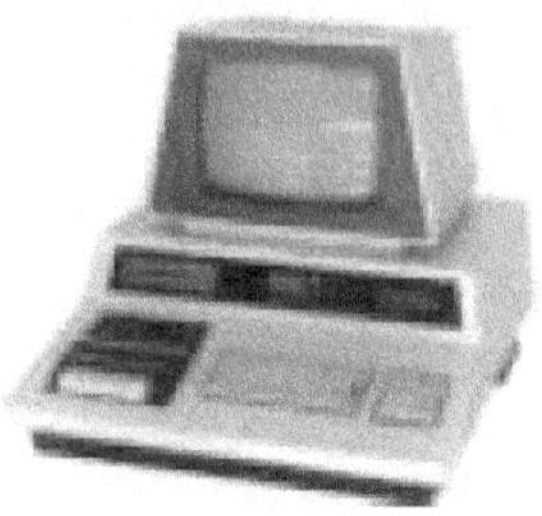

The generation of computers is basically differentiated by a fundamental hardware technology. Each new generation of computer is characterized by greater speed, large memory capacity and smaller size than the previous generation. Thus, second generation computers were more advanced in terms of arithmetic logic unit and control unit than their counterparts of first generation. Another feature of second generation was that by this time high-level languages were beginning to be used and the transmission for system software were starting.

The first of the IBM 7090 was delivered in 1959, which was followed by the CDC 1604, Philco 2000 and Remington Rand's UNIVAC LARC. Other widely used second generation computers were IBM 1620, IBM 1401 and IBM 7094.

2.19 Third Generation of Computer

IBM announced the third generation of computers in 1964 with its 360 line of computers. They used integrated circuits in the hardware. It also had the provision of facilities for time-sharing and multi programming. The speed and storage capacity of their computers were much higher than the previous generation computers and the size was much reduced.

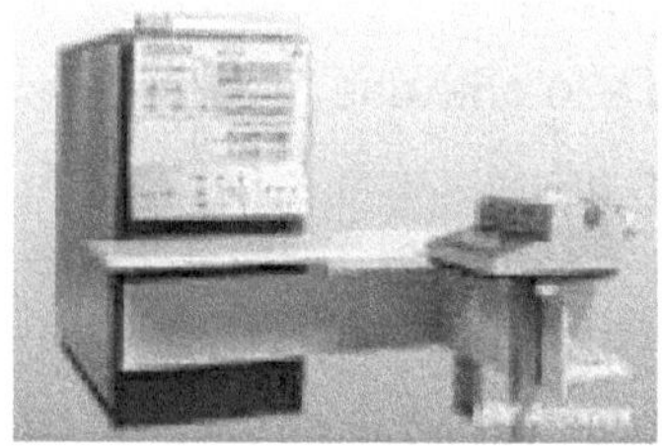

In the third generation of computer, more than one user could work with the computer at the same time, whereas the first and second generation of computer worked on a one-to-one basis. Almost all computers introduced after 1960 were said to be third generation computers. Most of the mainframe computers used in India till the early 1980s were third generation computers only.

In integrated circuits, components such as transistors, resistors and conductors are fabricated on a semi-conductor material such as silicon. Thus, a desired circuit can be fabricated in a tiny piece of silicon rather than assembling several discrete components into the same circuit. Hundreds or even thousands of transistors could be fabricated on a single wafer of silicon. In addition, these fabricated transistors can be connected with a process of metallisation from logic circuits on the same chip on which they have been produced.

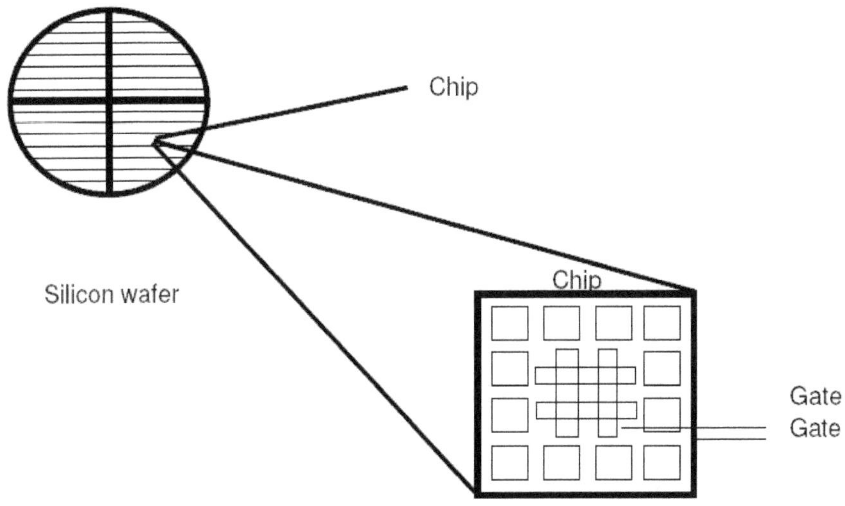

Fig. 2.5 Wafer, chip and gate.

Integrated circuits are constructed on a thin wafer of silicon which is divided into a matrix of small area. An identical circuit pattern is fabricated on each of their areas and the wafer is then broken into chips. Each of these chips consist several gates, which are made using transistors and a number of input and output connection points. Each of these chips then can be packaged separately In a housing to protect it. In addition, this housing provides a number of pins for connecting these chips with other circuits. The pins of these packages can be provided in two ways in two parallel rows with 0.1 inch spacing between two adjacent pins is each row.

This package is called dual in line package (DIP) (Fig.2.6 a).

In case more than hundred pins are required then pin grid array (PGA) is used, where pins are arranged in arrays of rows and columns, with spacing between two adjacent pins of 0.1 inch (Fig. 2.6 b).

Different circuits can be constructed on different wafers, all these packaged circuit chips then can be interconnected on a printed circuit board to produce several complier electronic circuits such as computers.

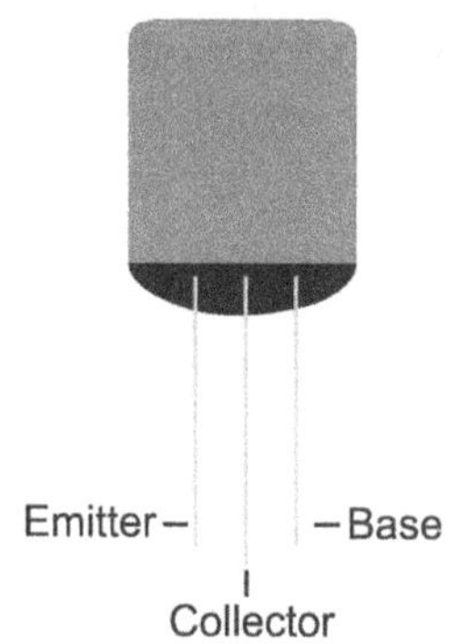

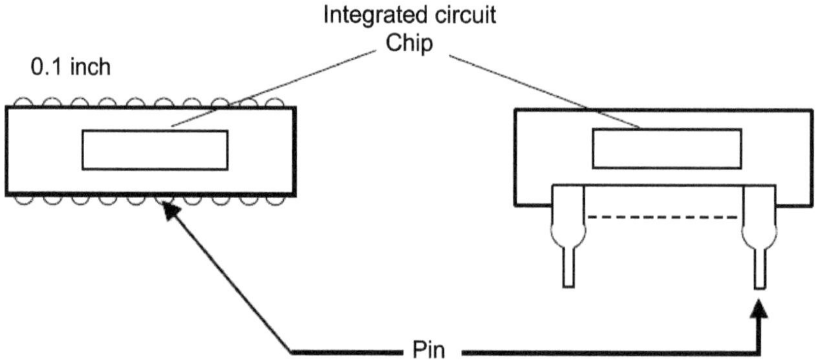

Fig. 2.6 (a) A 24 pin dual in line package (DIP).

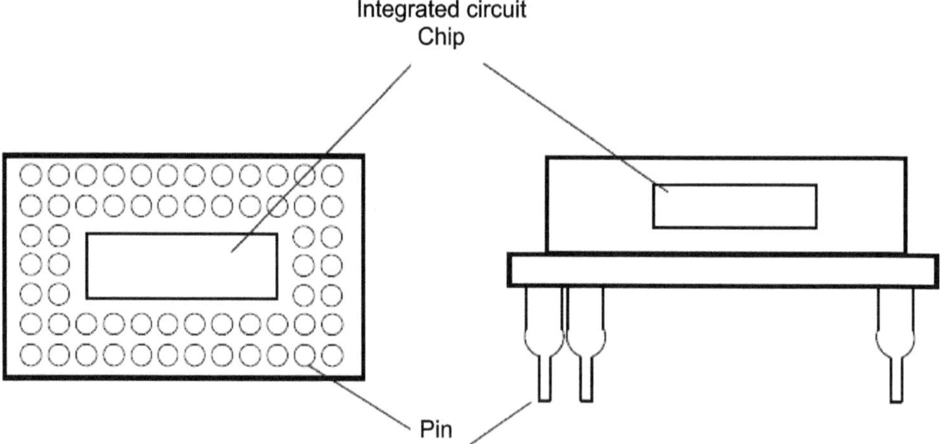

Fig. 2.6 (b) 144 Pin grid array (PGA) package.

Densely packed Integrated circuit has following advantage

- *Low cost :* The cost of a chip has remained almost constant while the chip density is ever increasing. It implies that the cost of computer logic and memory circuitry is reducing rapidly.
- *Fast Speed :* The more is density, the closer are the logic or memory elements, which implies shorter electrical paths and hence the higher operating speed.
- **Size Smaller**
- **Better portability**
- **Reduction in power and cooling requirements**
- **Reliability.**

Some of the examples of third generation computers are IBM system 360 family and DEC PDPI System. The third generation computers mainly used SSI chips. A family of computer consists of several models. Each model is assigned a model number, for example, the IBM system 360 family model 30, 40, 50, 65 and 75. As we go from lower model number to higher model number in this family, the memory capacity, processing speed and cost increase.

The main characteristics of the family are :

- The instructions set on a family are of similar type.
- The operating system used in family members is the same. In certain case some features can be added in the operating system for the higher members.
- The speed of execution of instruction increases from low-end family members to upper-end family members.
- The number of I/o ports interfaces increases as we move to higher members.
- Memory size increases as we move towards higher members.

The major developments, which took place in third generation, can be summarised as follows :

- IC circuits were starting to find their applications in the computer hardware replacing the discrete transistor circuits. This resulted in reduction in the cost and physical size of the computer.
- Semi-conductor memories were starting to augment finite core memory in main memory.
- The CPU design was made simple and more flexible using a technique called microprogramming.
- Certain new techniques were introduced to increase the effective speed of program execution. These techniques were pipelining and multi processing.
- The operating systems of computers were incorporated with the efficient method of sharing the facilities or resources such as processor and memory space, automatically.

2.20   Fourth Generation of Computer

The fourth generation computers were produced after 1970. The term fourth generation computer is used to designate microcomputers which use large-scale integrated circuits (LSI) and very large-scale integrated, had greater input / output capacity and system reliability.

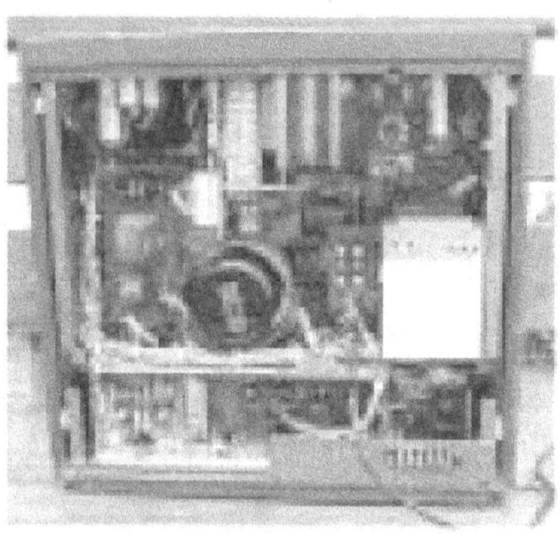

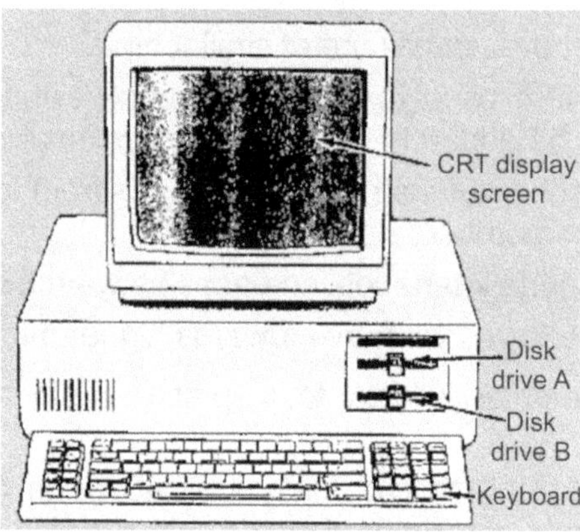

The most important criterion that can be used to separate them from third generation computers is that they have been designed work efficiently with the current generation of high-level languages.

Other developments that took place during 1975-1980 include: Package programs, word processing, voice response units and microprocessors. A microprocessor is a single "chip" which by itself can perform the control, arithmetic and logical functions of a computer. A microcomputer is a collection of a small number of memory chips and some input / output devices.

Semiconductor Memories

Initially the IC technology was used for constructing processor, but soon it was realised that same technology can be used for construction of memory. The first memory chip was constructed in 1970 and could hold 256 bits. The cost of this chip is high, but gradually the cost of semiconductor memory is going down. The memory capacity per chip has increased as 1K, 4K, 16K, 64K, 256K, and 1M bits.

Microprocessors

Keeping pace with electronics more and more components were fabricated on a single chip. Fewer chips were needed to construct a single processor. Intel in 1971 chirred the breakthrough of putting all the components on a single chip. The single chip processors are known as microprocessor. The Intel 4004 was the first microprocessor. It was a primitive microprocessor designed for a specific application. Intel 8080, which came in 1974, was the first general-purpose microprocessor. It was an 8-bit microprocessor. Motorola is another manufacturer in this field. At present 8, 64, 128 bit general-purpose microprocessors are available in the market. Figure 2.7 shows the families of INTEL & MOTOROLA microprocessor.

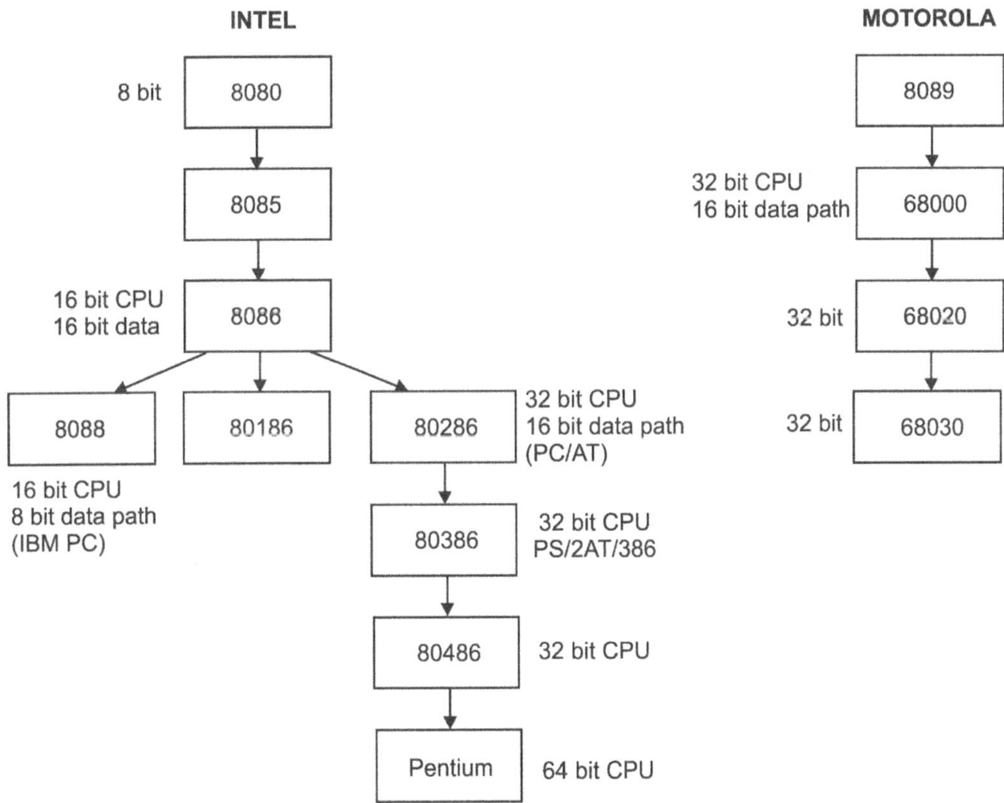

Fig. 2.7 Families of INTEL & MOTOROLA Microprocessor.

2.21   Fifth Generation of Computer

In October 1981, a conference of 300 computer scientists and engineers from fourteen countries was held in Japan to discuss the features of the fifth generation computers.

These machines will incorporate Artificial intelligence, which will not be far different from that of human intelligence. They will use stored reservoirs of knowledge to make expert judgment and decisions. They will process non-numerical information such as pictures and graphs.

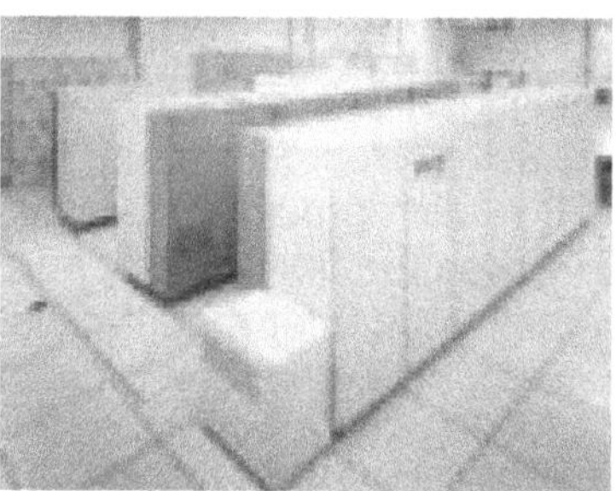

In these machines, intelligence will be greatly improved and the man-machine interface will be closes to the human systems. Progress on these has not been as fast as originally planned although same significant advances have been made.

Let us have a look at the major milestone, which led to present day computers.

3000 B.C.	-	The abacus- first computing device developed
1600 AD	-	Hindu-Arbic math become popular in Europe
1617	-	John Napier introduced Napier Bones
1642	-	Blaise Pascal developed 'Pascaline' the first mechanical computer.
1673	-	Hebniz's calculator developed
1801	-	Jacquard's punched card looms developed
1822	-	Charles Babbage invented difference engine
1832	-	Charles Babbage develops the principles of analytical engine. This was first world's programmable computer
1843	-	Lady Augusta Ada, the world first Programmer suggested the use of Binary data in computers
1847	-	George published his paper on book algebra – The basis of modern computation theory
1890	-	Herman Hollerith developed punched card based machine – Tabulator

1925	-	Vannevar Bush developed the first analog computer to solve differential equations
1941	-	Korard Zecc of Germany completes the world's first fully programmable digital computer named "Z-3"
1945	-	Korard Zecc develops 'Plankalkul' the first high-level language
1946	-	Jhan Presper Eskert and John W. Mucheley developed ENIAC, the world's first fully electronic general purpose programmable digital computer
1951	-	EDVAC, the first stored program computer developed.
1955	-	IBM introduces its first transistor-based calculator
1956	-	FORTRAN the first scientific computer programming language developed
1965	-	John G. Kameny developed BASIC language at Dartmouth College
1968	-	The Intel Corp. was founded
1971	-	The first microprocessor introduced
1977	-	Steven Jobs and Stephen Wozniak design and build the apple computer
1981	-	The first personal computer (PC) Introduced by IBM.

CHAPTER 3

Classification of Computers

3.1 Analog, Digital and Hybrid Computers

Computers, which are use today, are digital computers. They manipulate numbers. They operate on binary digits 0 and 1. They understand information composed of only 0s and 1s. In the case of alphabetic information, the alphabets are coded in binary digits. Computers do not operate on analog quantities directly. If any analog quantity is to be processed, it must be converted into digital quantity before processing. The output of a computer is also converted into analog quantity. The components, which convert alphanumeric characters to binary format and binary output to alphanumeric characters, are the essential parts of a digital computer.

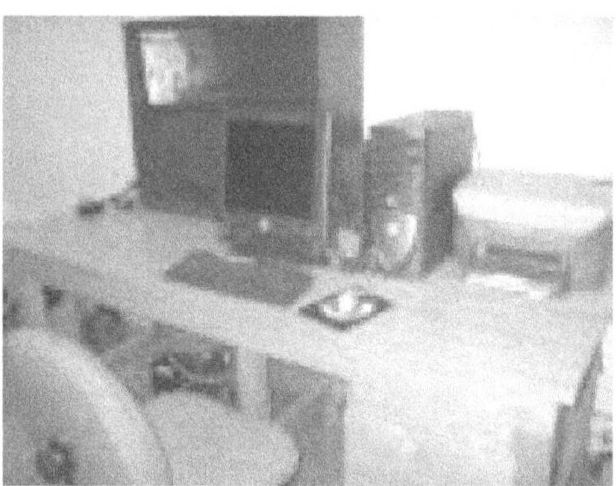

Digital computer

The computer, which can process analog quantities, is called analog computers. Today analog computers are rarely used. Earlier analog computers were used to simulate certain systems. They were used to solve differential equations.

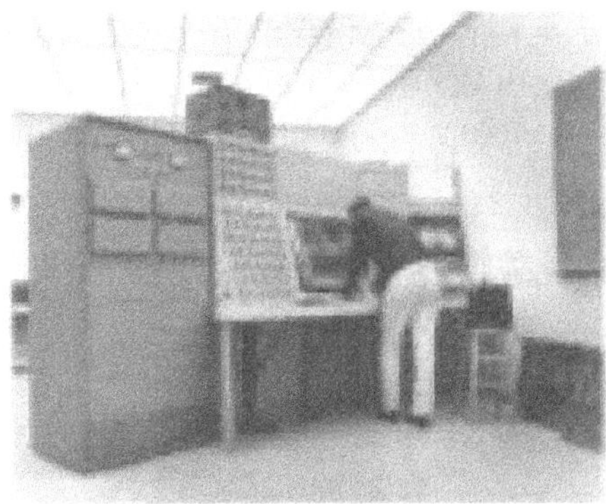

Analog computers

Hybrid computers are combination of digital and analog. Hybrid computer is mainly used in medical field.

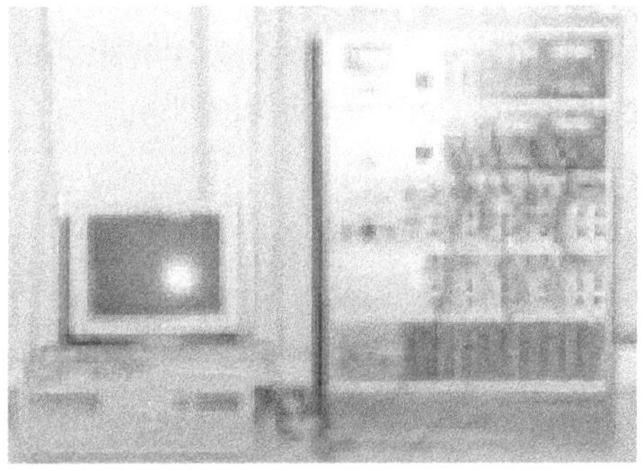

Hybrid computers

3.2 Classification of Computers Based on Size

Computers can be classified in various ways depending upon its size, memory capacity, processing speed etc. Here we are going to discuss the broadly accepted classification of computer. The criterion of this classification is as discussed above. Computers are classified into four categories.

1. Mainframe computers
2. Mini Computers
3. Micro Computers
4. Super Computers

3.2.1 Mainframe Computers

Mainframe computers are generally 32 bit machines or on the higher side. These are suited for organization to manage high volume applications. Few of popular mainframe series are MEDHA, SPERRY, DEC, IBM, HP, ICL etc. Mainframes are also used are just below super computers. In some ways mainframes are more powerful than super computers because they support more simultaneous programs. But super computers can execute a single program faster than mainframe.

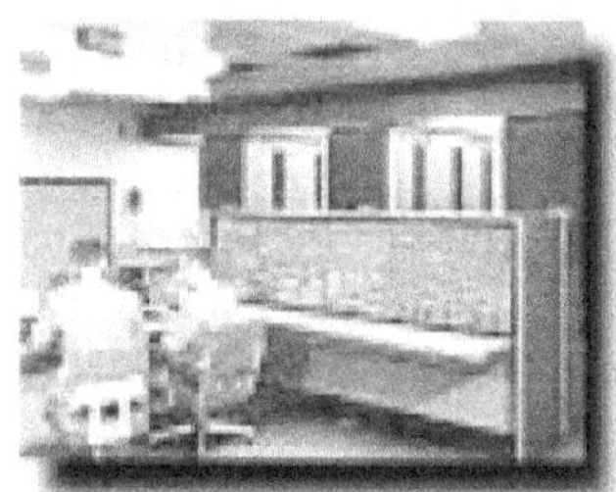

Mainframe Computers

The Important features of mainframe are :

- They are big computer systems, sensitive to temperature, humidity, dust etc.
- Qualified trained operators are required to operate them.
- They have a wide range of peripherals attached.
- They have a wide storage capacity.
- They can use wide variety of software.
- They are not user-friendly.
- They can be used for more mathematical calculations.
- They are installed in large commercial places or government organization.

3.2.2 Mini Computers

The term mini computer originated in 1960 when it was realised that many computing task do not require an expensive contemporary computers but can be solved by a small, inexpensive computer. Initial mini computers were 8 bit and 12 bit machines but by 1970s almost all mini computers were 16 bit machines.

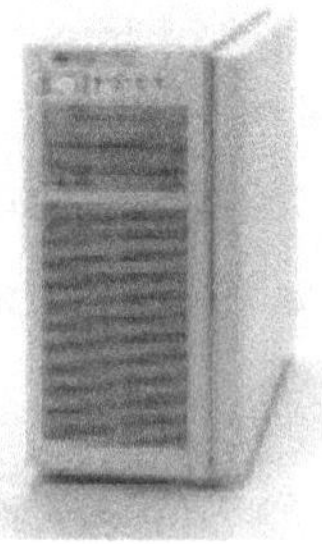

Mini computer

The 16-bit mini computers have the advantage of large instruction set and address field, and efficient storage to handling of text in comparison to lower bit machines. Thus, 16-bit mini computer was more powerful machine, which could be used in a variety of applications and could support business applications, along with the scientific application.

With the advancement in technology the speed, memory size and other characteristics developed and the minicomputer was then used for various stand alone or dedicated applications. The mini computer was also used as a multi-user system, which can be used by various users at the same time. Gradually the architectural requirement of mini computers grew and a 32-bit mini computer, which was called super mini, was introduced. The super mini had more peripheral devices, larger memory and could support more users working simultaneously on the computer in comparison to previous mini computers. A mini computer has a multiprocessing system capable of supporting 4 to about 200 users simultaneously.

Traditionally, mini computers have been used to cater to the needs of medium sized companies or departments within large companies, open for accounting or design and manufacturing (CAD / CAM). Mini computers are also becoming more important as 'servers'. A server is a computer on a network that manages network resources.

The entire network is called client server network.

Characteristics of mini computer are
- They have less memory and storage capacity.
- They offer limited range of peripherals.
- They can use limited range of software.
- End users can directly use it.
- They are not very sensitive to the external environment and hence are more generalized.
- They are used for data processing.

3.2.3 Micro Computers

A micro computer's CPU has a microprocessor. The micro computer originated in late 1970s. The first micro computers were built around 8-bit microprocessor chips. 8-bit chip means that the chip can retrieves instruction/data from storage, manipulate, and process an 8-bit data at a time or we can say that the chip has a built in 8-bit data transfer path.

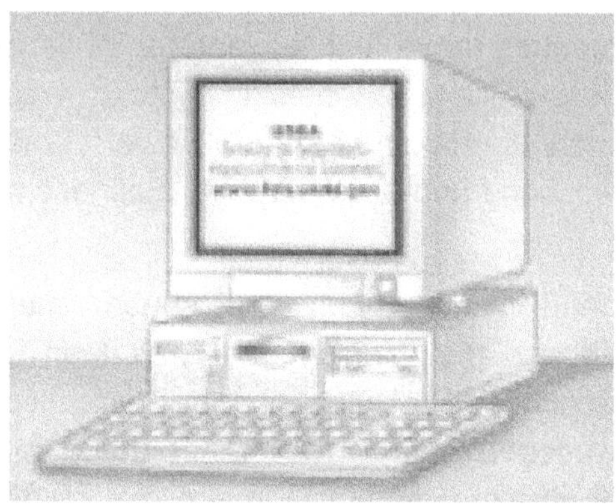

Micro Computer

An improvement on 8-bit chip technology was seen in early 1980s when a series of 16 bit chips, namely 8086 and 8088, were introduced by Intel corporation, each one with an advancement over the other.

8088 is an 8116-bit chip, i.e. an 8 primary storage, but processing is done within the chip using a 16-bit path at a time. 8086 is a 16116-bit chip, i.e. the internal and external paths both are 16 bits wide and these chips can support a primary storage capacity of up to 1 mega byte. Intel 80286 is 16/32-bit chip and it can support up to 16 MB of primary storage.

Similar to Intel chip series, exists another popular chip series of Motorola. The first 16-bit microprocessor of this series is MC 68000. It is a 16/32 bit chip and can support up to 16 MB of primary storage. An advancement over 16/32 bit chips are the 32/32 chips. Some of the popular 32 bit chips are Intel's 80386 and MC 68020 chip.

A small, relatively inexpensive computer is designed to cost a few thousand rupees to over fifty thousand rupees. Personal computers first appeared in the late 1970. One of the most popular and first personal computers was the Apple II, introduced in 1977 by Apple computer during the late 1970s and early 1980s. New models and competing operating systems seem to appear daily. Then, in 1981, IBM entered the fray with its first processor computer, known as the IBM PC. The IBM PC quickly became the personal computer of choice. In general, micro computers are considered to be of two types:

(a)   Personal computer   (b)   Workstation.

(a)   Personal Computer (PC)

The first personal computer produced by IBM was called IBMPC, and increasingly the term PC come to mean IBM or IBM – compatible personal computer, to the exclusion of other types of personal computers, such as Macintoshes. Micro computers or PC comes in various sizes.

Desktop models

A computer designed to fit comfortably on top of a desk, typically with the monitor sitting on top of the computer. Desktop model computers are broad and flat, whereas tower models computers are norms and tall. Based on their shape, desktop model computers are generally limited to three internal mass storage devices. Desktop model designed to be very small are sometimes referred to as slim line models.

Portable or luggable

Portable means small and lightweight. A portable computer is a computer small enough to carry. Portable computers include notebook and sub notebook computers, hand-held computers, palmtops and PDAS.

Laptop computers

A small, portable computer, small enough that can be sit on your lap. Now-a-days, laptop computers are more frequently called notebook computers. It is extremely lightweight personal computer. Notebook computers typically weight less then 6 pounds and are small enough to fit easily in a briefcase. Aside from size, the principal difference between a notebook computer and a personal computer is the display screen. Notebook computers use a variety of techniques, known as flat panel technologies, to produce a lightweight and non-bulky display screen. Notebook computers come with battery packs that enable you to run them without plugging them in electric socket. However, the batteries need to be recharged every few hours. The most common substances used in computer battery packs are nickel cadmiums (Nickel), Nickel metal hydride (NiMH) and Lithium gun.

Pocket or hand-held computer

A portable computer is small enough to be held in one's hand. Although extremely convenient to carry, hand-held computers have not replaced notebook computers because of their small keyboards and screens. Some manufacturers are trying to solve the small keyboard problems by replacing the keyboard with an electronic pen. However, these pen-based devices rely on handwriting recognition technologies, which are still in their infancy.

Pocket computers may be classified into as three types :

1. Electronic Organizers

Electronic organizers or electronic diary are specialized pocket computers that mainly store appointments, addresses, and ' to-do' lists.

2. Palmtop

A small computer that literally fits in your palm is called palmtop. Compared to full-size computers, palmtops are severely limited, but they are practical for certain functions such as phone books and calendars. Palmtops that use a pen rather than a keyboard for input are often called hand-held computer or PDAs.

3. PDA

PDA stands for Personal Digital Assistant, a handheld device that combined computing, telephone, face and networking features. A typical PDA can function as cellular phone, fare sender and personal organizer. PDAs are pen based, using a stylus rather than a keyboard for input. Some PDAs can also react voice input by using voice recognition technologies.

(b)   Workstation

Workstation are those computers which are used for engineering application, desktop publishing, software development and other type of applications that require a moderate amount of computing power and relatively high quality graphics capabilities.

Workstations generally come with a large, high-resolution graphics screen, at least 64 MB of RAM, built-in network support, and a graphical user interface. Most workstations also have a mass storage device as a disk drive, but a special type of workstation, called a diskless workstation comes without a disk drive. The most common operating systems for workstation are UNIX, LINUX and Windows 2000, The leading manufacturers of workstations are SUN Micro systems, Hewlett-Packards, Silicon Graphics Incorporated and Compaq.

Summarized features of Micro Computers are :

- They brought revolution in the history of computers.
- They are also known as personal computers.
- They are cheap and user-friendly.
- This type of computer uses wide range of software.

3.2.4 Super Computer

The fastest type of computer is called super computer. Super computers are very expensive and are employed for specialized applications that require immense amounts of mathematical calculations.

Weather forecasting requires a super computer; other uses of super computer include Space Technology, Animated Graphics, Fluid Dynamic Calculations, Nuclear Energy, Nano-Technology research, Petroleum Exploration, Image Processing, Biomedical applications, etc.

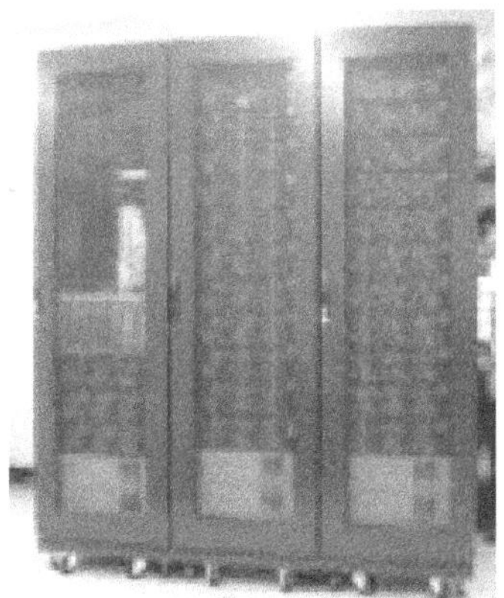

Super Computer

The chief difference between a super computer and a mainframe is that a Super computer channels all its power in to execute a few programs as fast as possible, where as a mainframe uses its power to execute many programs concurrently.

Super Computers are designed in two ways

Vector Processor

The traditional design of super computers, now 50 years old, is vector processing. In vector processing, a relatively few large, highly specialized processor runs calculations by a single large processor creating potential bottlenecks. In addition, the processors are costly to build, and they run so hot that they need elaborate cooling systems.

Parallel processors

The newer design is based on parallel processors, which spread calculations over hundreds or even thousand of standard, inexpensive microprocessors used in PCs. Tasks are parceled out to a great many processor, which work simultaneously.

Summarized features of super computer are :

- They are huge computers installed in Space Centres, Nuclear Power stations etc.
- They perform complete mathematical calculations.
- Only scientists and mathematicians can operate them.
- They have huge memories and tremendous processing speed.
- They are used for weather forecasting, image processing, Remote Sensing, animation graphics etc.

CHAPTER 4

Number System

A number system of base (also called radix r) is a system, which has r distinct symbols for r digits. A number is represented by a string of these symbolic digits. To determine the quantity that the number represents, we multiply the number by as integer power of r depending on the place it is located and then find the sum of weighted digits.

4.1 Decimal Numbers

Decimal number system has ten digits represented by 0, 1, 2, 3, 4, 5, 6, 7, 8 and 9. Any decimal number can be represented as a string of these digits and since there are ten decimal digits, therefore, the base or radix of this system is 10.

Thus a string of number 102.5 can be represented as:

$$1 \times 10^2 + 0 \times 10^1 + 2 \times 10^0 + 5 \times 10^{-1}$$

4.2 Binary Number

In binary numbers, we have two digits 0 and 1 and they can also be represented as a string of these two digits. The radix of this system is 2.

4.2.1 Conversion of Binary to Decimal

For converting the value of binary to decimal equivalent we have to find its quantity, which is obtained by multiplying a digit by its place value. For example, binary number 100101 is equivalent to

$$1 \times 2^5 + 0 \times 2^4 + 0 \times 2^3 + 1 \times 2^2 + 0 \times 2^1 + 1 \times 2^0$$

$$= 32 + 0 + 0 + 4 + 0 + 1$$

$$= 37$$

4.2.2 Conversion of Decimal to Binary

For converting the value of decimal to binary equivalent we have to successively divide the decimal number by 2, till the quotient reduces to 0. The remainders at each stage taken from the last stage upwards give the required notation. For example take 65 and let us see how to convert it into binary number.

2	65	
2	32	1 – Least significant bit
2	16	0
2	8	0
2	4	0
2	2	0
2	1	0
	0	1 –Most significant bit

Thus the binary equivalent of the number 65 is "1000001"

4.3 Octal Number

The octal number system is one where numbers are represented using 8 digits that is 0,1, 2, 3, 4, 5, 6, 7. This system has radix 8. A subscript 8 is used with a number to indicate that it is written in the octal number system e.g. $(4624)_8$ indicates that this number is written in the octal number system. The method for finding decimal equivalent of octal number is similar that of finding the decimal equivalent of binary number, the only difference being the value of weight 8 in place of 2

$$(4624)_8 = 4 \times 8^3 + 6 \times 8^2 + 2 \times 8^1 + 4 \times 8^0$$

$$= 4 \times 512 + 6 \times 64 + 2 \times 8 + 4 \times 1$$

$$= 2048 + 384 + 16 + 4$$

$$= 2452$$

Converting a decimal into octal number is equally simple. Divide the decimal number successively by 8, till we get the quotient as 0. Write the remainders in backward direction to obtain the octal equivalent of the number. Let us convert the decimal number 2452 in its octal equivalent.

8	2452	
8	306	4 – Least significant
8	38	2
8	4	6
	0	4 – Most significant

So the octal equivalent is $(4624)_8$

4.3.1 Octal to Binary conversion

Each digit in the number systems can be represented by a combination of 3-bit binary number. The binary equivalent of each octal number is follows :

Octal	Binary
0	0
1	001
2	010
3	011
4	100
5	101
6	110
7	111

To convert an octal to its binary equivalent, convert each octal digit to its binary equivalent and place them in the same order.

For example – $(463)_8$ convert equivalent binary number

Octal digits	-	4	6	3
Binary equivalent	-	100	110	011
$(463)_8$	-	$(100110\ 011)_2$		

4.3.2 Binary to Octal Number

The conversion of binary number to its octal equivalent is equally easy. The binary digits should be grouped from right hand side into a group of 3 bits each and the remaining bit/s is/are one or two, then 0 should be added at left to make the group of three bits. For each group of three bits the octal equivalent will be found and will be written in the same order to find the octal equivalent.

Let us convert the binary number $(100\ 110\ 011)_2$ to its

Octal equivalent $\dfrac{100\ 110\ 010}{4\quad 6\quad 3}$

Equivalent octal

$$\therefore\ (100\ 110\ 011)_2 = (463)_8$$

4.4   Hexadecimal System

The hexadecimal system has a base of sixteen as it uses the following sixteen symbols such as computer process binary data in groups that are in multiples of 4 bits, making the hexadecimal system very convenient. This is because each hexadecimal member represents a 4-bit binary as shown below:

Octal	Binary	Hexadecimal
0	0	0
1	0001	1
2	0010	2
3	0011	3
4	0100	4
5	0101	5
6	0110	6
7	0111	7
8	1000	8
9	1001	9
10	1010	A
11	1011	B
12	1100	C
13	1101	D
14	1110	E
15	1111	F

The base of hexadecimal number system (16) is used as subscript to indicate that the number is hexadecimal number system e.g. $(57A2)_{16}$.

4.4.1   Binary to Hexadecimal conversion

To obtain the hexadecimal equivalent of a number, arrange the bits in groups of 4 bits from right. Each remaining bit/bits should be made into group by adding required number of 0s at the left side of the remaining bit/bits. Each group of 4 bits is then assigned with the equivalent hexadecimal digit. Thus to convert binary 1100 1100 1001 into hexadecimal equivalent group, arrange the above bits into 3 groups 4 bits each as follows :-

$$110011001001 = \qquad 1100 \quad 1100 \quad 1001$$

Hexadecimal equivalent   C   C   9

The hexadecimal equivalent of $(110011001001)_2$ is $(C\ C\ 9)_{16}$

4.4.2 Hexadecimal to Binary conversion

Binary equivalent for each hexadecimal, which will be in the group of four bits, should be first found and placed below the respective hexadecimal. The hexadecimal (CC9) has C means 12 and its binary equivalent is 1100, binary equivalent 9 are 1001.

Thus the binary equivalent of $(CC6)_{16}$ is $(1100\ 1100\ 1001)_2$.

4.4.3 Decimal to hexadecimal conversion

The conversion of a number in decimal system into its hexadecimal equivalent is similar to the one used for converting number to the octal or binary system i.e. by successive division of the number by 16, till we get a gradient of zero and then assemble the remainders.

For e.g. 921 to be converted into the hexadecimal.

16	921	
16	57	9
16	3	9
	0	3

Thus, the hexadecimal equivalent of 921 is $(399)_{16}$

4.4.4 Hexadecimal to decimal conversion

The conversion of hexadecimal number to its decimal equivalent is similar to that of the previously discussed number system i.e., multiply each digit in the number by its equivalent weight and then add them up. Thus, if the number is $(399)_{16}$, its equivalent decimal number is

$$3 \times 16^2 + 9 \times 16^1 + 9 \times 16^0$$
$$= 3 \times 256 + 9 \times 16 + 9 \times 1$$
$$= 768 + 144 + 9$$
$$= 921$$

CHAPTER 5

The System Concept

5.1   Introduction

You might have observed by now that we have been referring to computer as a system (computer system). To know the answer let us first consider the definition of a system.

A system is group of integrated parts that have common purpose of achieving some objective(s). So, the following three characteristics are key to a system.

1. A system has more than one element.
2. All the elements of a system are logically related.
3. All the elements of a system are controlled in such a way that the system goal is achieved.

Since a computer is made up of integrated components (input and output devices, storage, CPU) that work together to process the data when the program is executed, it is a system. The input or output units cannot function until they receive signals from the CPU. Similarly, the storage unit or the CPU alone is of no use. So the usefulness of each unit depends on other units and can be realized only when all units are put together (integrated) to form a system.

A computer system can also be said to be consisting of:

1. Hardware   2. Software

5.2   Hardware

Hardware is a general term used to represent the physical components of the computer itself, i.e. those components, which can be seen and touched. In computer system the hardware includes devices like keyboards, monitor, printer and the central processing unit:

1. Input devices   2. Output devices   3. Central processing unit

4. Memory devices   5. Communication devices

The electronic circuits consist of resistors, capacitors, ICs, etc. in side a computer's cabinet are all examples of computer hardware. All input and output devices connected to computer are collectively known as peripherals. We can define peripheral as "any piece of hardware that is connected to a computer." Examples are the keyboards, mouse, monitor and disk drives.

5.3 Software

Software is defined as sets of instructions stored as programs that govern the operation of a computer system and make the hardware run. "Software or computer programs are the step-by-step instructions that tell the computer what to do". In general, software can be classified as "System Software" and "Application Software".

5.3.1 System Software

The user of a computer has at his disposal a large amount of software provided by the manufacturer. Most of this software contributes to the control and manage its internal resources and give optimum performance from the system.

A more detailed sub-division of such software is as follows:

Operating systems and control programs

Translators

Utilities and service programs.

5.3.2 Application Software

Application software is defined as software that can be used to perform a general-purpose or specific task. Word processing software is used to create a text document. Database software is used to create a database for a specific purpose. DTP software is used to create a document for electronic publishing. Application software may be either customized or packaged.

Customized software is that software which is designed for a particular customer and for particular use. Packaged software is the kind of program developed for sale for general-purpose applications. These softwares are more commonly used in organisation & business applications.

We will discuss software in great detail later. In this chapter we concentrate on hardware.

5.4 Input Devices

Data and instructions are entered into a computer through input devices. An input device converts input data and instructions into a suitable binary form accepted by the computer. The most commonly used input device is a keyboard. A number of other input device have also been developed which do not require typing for inputting information, for example: mouse, light pen, graphic tablet, joystick, track ball, touch\ screen etc. Each of these devices permits the user to select something on CRT screen by pointing to it. Therefore, these devices are called pointing devices. Voice input systems have also been developed. A microphone is used as a voice input device.

Input devices are categorised as keyboard entry and direct entry devices: In keyboard entry we use keyboard to enter the information into the computer readable form. Direct entry refers to many forms of data entry devices that do not use keyboard. Such devices create machine-readable data. These include pointing devices, scanning devices, smart and optical cards, voice recognition devices, etc.

Often keyboard and direct entry devices are combined in a single computer system. A Desk Top Publishing (DTP) system, for example, uses a keyboard, a mouse and an image scanner.

5.4.1 Keyboard

Programs and data are entered into a computer through a keyboard, which is attached to a micro computer of the terminal of a mini or large computer. A keyboard is similar to the keyboard of a typewriter. It contains alphabets, digits, special characters and some control keys. When a key is pressed, an electronic signal is produced which is detected by an electronic circuit called keyboard encoder. A keyboard encoder may be a special IC or a single-chip micro computer used as encoder. The function of an encoder is to detect which key has been pressed and send a binary code (corresponding to the pressed key) to the computer. The binary code may be an ASCII, EBCDIC or HEX code.

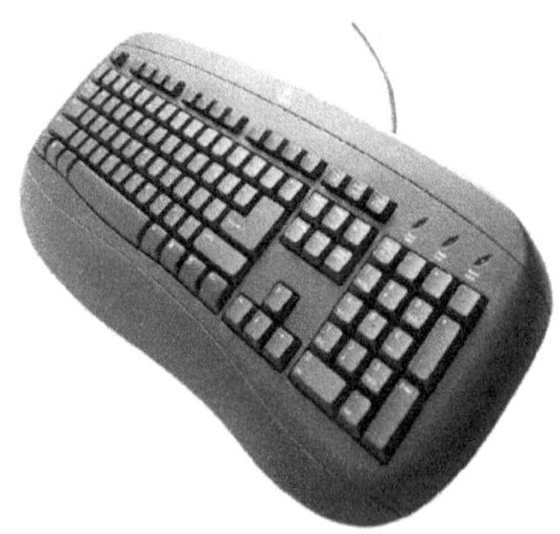

Conventional computer keyboards have all the keys that typewriter keyboards have plus others keys unique to computers. Actually, computer keyboards are easier to use than most typewriter keyboards because you can easily rectify your typing mistakes.

Standard typewriter keys : Typewriter keys are the same familiar QWERTY arrangement of letter, number, and punctuation keys found on any typewriter. QWERTY refers to the order of alphabet keys in the top left row on a standard typewriter keyboard.

The Space Bar, Shift, Tab, and Caps Lock Keys do the same things on the computer that they do on a typewriter. (When you press the Caps Lock Key, a light on your keyboards shows you are typing ALL CAPITAL LETTERS until you press the Caps Lock key again.)

An exception is the Enter (bent left arrow) key, which occupies the place where a carriage-return key would be on a typewriter. The Enter key, sometimes called the Return key, is used to enter commands into the computer.

Cursor-movement keys : The cursor is the symbol on the display screen that shows where data may be entered next. The cursor-movement keys, or arrow keys, are used to move the cursor around the text on the screen. These keys move the cursor left, right, up or down.

The keys labeled PgUp stands for page up and the key labeled PgDn stands for page down. These keys move the cursor one page or one screen at a time up (backward) or down (forward). Some software lets you use the Home key to move the cursor to the top of the document and the End key to move to the bottom of the document.

Numeric Keys : A separate set of keys, 0 - 9, known as the numeric keypad, is laid out like the keys on a calculator. The numeric keypad has two purposes.

Whenever the Num Lock key is off, the numeric keys may be used as arrow keys for cursor movement.

When the Num Lock key is on, the keys may be used for typing numbers, as on a calculator. A light is illuminated on the keyboard when the Num Lock key is pressed once and goes off when the Num Lock key is pressed again.

For space reasons, portable computers often lack a separate numeric keypad or the numeric keys may be superimposed on the typewriter letter keys and are activated by the Num Lock key.

Function Keys *:* Function keys are the keys labeled with a F and a number, such as F1 and F2 that are used for tasks that occur frequently. Desktop microcomputers usually have 12 function keys.

The software you are using defines the purpose of each function key. For example, pressing F2 may print your document in one program but save your work to disk in another. Special-purpose keys include Backspace, Del, Ins, Esc, Ctrl, and Alt. The uses of these special purpose keys are as follows:

Backspace (indicated by a left pointing arrow) erases as you move left over the preceding text you have typed.

Del (Delete) erases text to the right (on Macintoshes, to the left).

Ins (insert) allows you to type over (or push right) existing text, inserting new next.

Esc (Escape) may be used to cancel whatever task you are currently performing.

The purposes of Ctrl (Control) and Alt (Alternate) are defined by the software you are using. Some computers may have other special-purpose keys.

Light Pen *:* A light pen is a pointing device used to select a displayed menu option on the CRT. It is a photosensitive pen-like device. It is capable of sensing a position on the CRT screen when its tip touches the screen. When its tip is moved over the screen surface, its photocell-sensing element detects the light coming from the screen and the corresponding signals are sent to the processor. The menu is a set of programmed choices offered to the user. The user indicates his choice by touching light pen against a desired description of the menu. The signals sent by the light pen to the processor identify the menu option.

5.4.2 Mouse

A device that controls the movement of the cursor or pointer on a display screen. A mouse is a small object you can roll along a hard, flat surface. Its name is derived from its shape, which looks a bit like a mouse. Its connecting wire that one can imagine to be the mouse's tail, is in fact that one must make it scroll along a surface. As you move the mouse, the pointer on the display screen moves in the same direction. Mouse contains at least one button and sometimes as many as three, which have different functions depending on what program is running. Some new mouse also include a scroll wheel for scrolling through long documents.

Invented by Douglas Engel Bart of Stanford Research Center in 1963, and pioneered by Xerox in the 1970s, the mouse is one of the greatest breakthroughs in computer ergonomics because it frees the user to a large extent from using the keyboard. In particular, the mouse is important for graphical user interfaces because you can simply point to options and objects, and click a mouse button. Such applications are often called point-and-click programs. The mouse is also useful for graphics programs that allow you to draw pictures by using the mouse like a pen, pencil, or paintbrush.

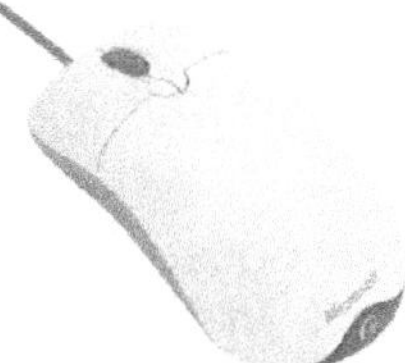

There are three basic types of mouse:

Mechanical : Has a rubber or metal ball on its underside that can roll in all directions. Mechanical sensors within the mouse detect that the direction, ball is rolling and move the screen pointer accordingly.

Opt mechanical : Same as a mechanical mouse, but uses optical sensors to detect motion of the ball.

Optical : Uses a laser to detect the mouse movement. You must move the mouse along a special mat with a grid so that the optical mechanism has a frame or reference. Optical mouse has no mechanical moving parts. They respond more quickly and precisely than mechanical and opt mechanical mouse but they are more expensive.

5.4.3 Joystick

A joystick is also a pointing device. It is just like a lever that moves in all directions and controls the movement of a pointer or some other display symbol. A joystick is similar to a mouse, except that with a mouse the cursor stops moving as soon as you stop moving the mouse. With a joystick, the pointer continues moving in the direction the joystick is pointing. To stop the pointer, you must return the joystick to its upright position. Most joysticks include two buttons called triggers.

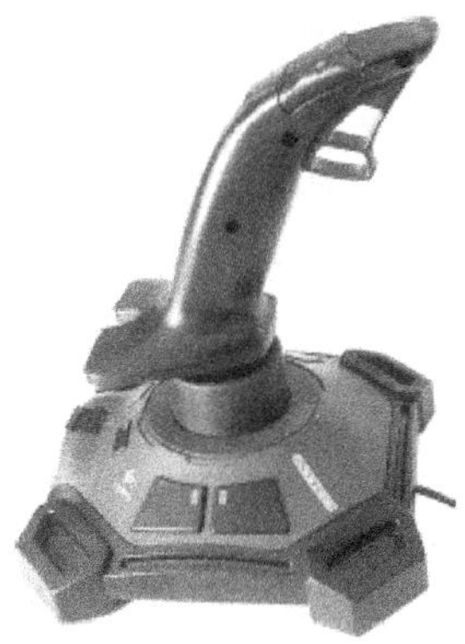

Joysticks are used mostly for computer games, but they are also used occasionally for CAD / CAM systems and other applications.

5.4.4 Trackballs

Trackball is also a pointing device. Essentially, a trackball is a mouse lying on its back. To move the pointer, you rotate the ball with your thumb, your fingers, or the palm of your hand. There are usually one to three buttons next to the ball, which you use just like mouse buttons.

The advantage of trackballs over mouse is that the trackball is stationary so it does not require much space to use it. In addition, you can place a trackball on any type of surface, including your lap. For both these reasons, trackballs are popular pointing devices for portable computers.

5.4.5 Scanners

Scanning device translates images of text, drawings, photos into digital form. Scanners are a kind of input devices. They are capable of entering information directly into the computer. The main advantage of direct entry of information is that users do not have to key the information. This provides faster and moves accurate data entry. Important types of scanners are optical scanners and magnetic-ink character readers.

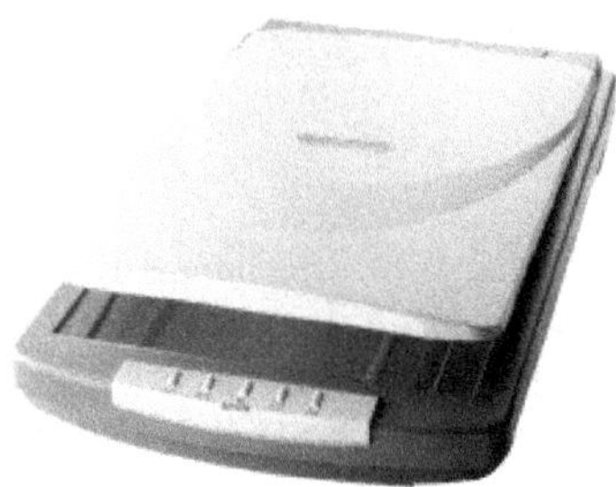

Optical Scanners: The optical scanners are capable of reading information recorded on paper, employ light source and light sensors. The information to be scanned is typewritten information. Information is coded as ink or pencil marks or bars.

5.4.6 Optical Character Reader (OCR)

An optical character reader detects alphanumeric character printed or typewritten on paper. The text which is be scanned is illuminated by a low frequency source. The light is absorbed by the dark areas and reflected from the lighted areas. The reflected light is received by photocells or charged coupled devices (CCDs), which provide binary data corresponding to dark and lighted areas. An OCR can scan several thousands of printed or typewritten characters per second. Optical character technology finds use in areas like office automation and electronic documentation.

5.4.7 Optical Mark Readers (OMR)

Special marks such as squares or bubbles are prepared on examination answer sheets or questionnaires. The users fill in these squares with soft pencil or ink to indicate their choice. An optical mark reader detects these marks and the corresponding signals are sent to the processor. If a mark is present, it reduces the amount of reflected light. If a mark is not present, the amount of reflected light is not reduced. This change in the amount of reflected light is used to detect the presence of a mark. This method is used for analysis of objective type questions, for example, market survey, population survey, etc. where choice is restricted to one out of a few choices available.

5.4.8 Optical Bar Code Readers

This method uses a number of bars (lines) of varying thickness and spacing between them indicates the desired information. Bar codes are used on most manufactured retail products. An optical bar reader can read such bars and convert them into electrical pulses to be processed by a computer. The most commonly used bar code is Universal Product Code (UPC). The UPC code uses a series of vertical bars of varying widths. These bars are detected as ten digits. The first five digits identify the supplier or manufacturer of the item. The second five digits identify the product. The code also contains a check digit to ensure that the information read is correct.

5.4.9 Magnetic Ink Character Readers (MICR)

MICR is widely used by banks in advanced countries to process large volumes of cheques and deposit forms written by customers every day. Special ink called magnetic ink (i.e. an ink which contains iron oxide particles) is used to write characters on cheques and deposit forms, which are to be processed by an MICR. MICR is capable of reading characters written with magnetic ink on paper. The magnetic ink is magnetized during the input process. The MICR reads the magnetic patterns of the written characters. To identify the characters these patterns are compared with special patterns stored in the memory. When a cheque is entered into an MICR, it passes through a magnetic field. The iron oxide particles are magnetized under the magnetic field. The read head reads the characters written with magnetic ink on cheque. It interprets the character and sends the corresponding data directly to the computer for processing. An MICR processes up to 2,600 cheques per minute.

5.4.10 CCD Camera

In many applications it is desired that a computer should be able to see its environment. For example, a robot must be able to see to perform its job; a computer-controlled security system must be able to see its environment etc. To provide vision to computers, sensors like video cameras, CCD cameras, OPTICRAM cameras, etc. are employed. These cameras act as sensors to provide signals proportional to the intensity of light falling on various spots of the image of an object. The computer can process these signals and recognize, and display the image of the object.

5.4.11 Sensors

A sensor is a type of input device that collects specific kinds of data directly from the environments and transmits it to a computer. Although you are unlikely to see such input devices connected to a PC in an office, they exist all around us, often in invisible form. Sensors can be used for detecting all kinds of things: speed, movement, weight, pressure, temperature, humidity, wind current, fog, gas, smoke, light, shapes, images, and so on.

For example, in metro highways there are sensors that detect the speed and volume of traffic. These sensors send data to computers that can adjust traffic lights to keep cars and trucks away from grid locked areas. In aviation, sensors are used to detect ice buildup on airplane wings or to alert pilots to sudden changes in wind direction. Government regulators also use sensors to monitor whether companies are complying with air-pollution standards.

5.5   Output Devices

5.5.1 Softcopy vs. Hardcopy

Output devices translate information processed by the computer into a form that humans can understand. The two principal kinds of output are hardcopy, which is printed, and softcopy, such as material shown on a display screen. Output devices include display screens, printers, plotters, and multi function devices; audio-output devices; video-output devices; and virtual reality.

Output devices translate information processed by the computer into a form that humans can understand. The principal outputs are hardcopy and softcopy.

Hardcopy *:* Hardcopy refers to printed output, whether text or graphics which are printed from printers. Film is also considered as hardcopy output.

Softcopy *:* Softcopy refers to data that is shown on a display screen or is in audio or voice form. This kind of output is not tangible; it cannot be touched.

There are several types of output devices. We will discuss the following ones.

- Display screens
- Printers, plotters, and multifunction devices
- Audio-output devices
- Video-output devices
- Virtual-reality devices.

5.5.2 Display Screen or Monitor

The term monitor usually refers to the display screen. There are many ways to classify monitors. The most basic is in terms of colour capabilities, which separate monitors into three classes:

Monochrome: Monochrome monitors actually display two colours, one for the background and one for the foreground. The colour can be black and white, green and black, or amber and black.

Gray-Scale: A gray scale monitor is a special type of monochrome monitor capable of displaying different shades of gray. The use of many shades of gray to represent an image is called gray-scalling. Continuous-tone images, such as black and white photographs, use an almost unlimited number of shades of gray.

Conventional computer hardware and software, however, can only represent a limited number of shades of gray (typically 16 or 256). Gray-scaling is the process of converting a continuous-tone image to an image that a computer can manipulate.

Colour: Colour monitors can display anywhere from 16 to over 1 million different colours. Colour monitors are sometimes called RGB monitors because they accept three separate signals – red, green, and blue.

After this classification, the most important aspect of a monitor is its screen size. Like televisions, screen sizes are measured diagonally in inches, the distance from one corner to the opposite corner diagonally. A typical size for small VGA monitors is inches. Monitors that are 16 or more inches diagonally are often called full-page monitors. In addition to their size, monitors can be either portrait (height greater than width) or landscape (width greater than height). Larger landscape monitors can display two full pages, side by side. The screen size is sometimes misleading because there is always an area around the edge of the screen that can't be used.

Therefore, monitor manufactures must now also state the viewable area i.e. the area of screen that is actually used.

The resolution of a monitor indicates how densely packed the pixels are. In general, the more pixels (often expressed in dots per inch), the sharper is the image. Most modern monitors can display 1024 by 768 pixels, the SVGA standard. Some high-end models can display 1280 by 1024, or even 1600 by 1200.

Another common way of classifying monitors is in terms of the type of signal they accept: analog or digital. Nearly all-modern monitors accept analog signals, which is required by the VGA, SVGA, 8514/A, and other high-resolution colour standards.

A few monitors have fixed frequency, which means that they accept input at only one frequency. Most monitors, however, are multi-scanning, which means that they automatically adjust themselves to the frequency of the signals being sent to it. This means that they can display images at different resolutions, depending on the data being sent to them by the video adapters.

Other factors that determine a monitor's quality include the following :

Bandwidth: Bandwidth is the range of signal frequencies the monitor can handle. This determines how much data it can process and therefore how fast it can refresh at higher resolution.

Refresh Rate: Refresh rate is, how many times per second the screen is refreshed (redrawn). To avoid flickering, the refresh rate should be at least 72 Hz.

Interlaced or no interlaced: Interlacing is a technique that enables a monitor to have more resolution, but it reduces the monitor's reaction speed.

Dot pitch: It refers to the amount of space between each pixel. The smaller the dot pitch, the sharper is the image.

5.5.3 Video Display Unit (VDU)

Video Display Unit also called monitors, or CRTs, are output devices showing programming instructions and data as they are input and after they are processed. Sometimes a monitor is also referred to as a VDT (Vide display terminal), although technically a VDT includes both screen and keyboard.

Display screens are of two types: cathode-ray-tubes and flat-panel display.

Cathode Ray Tubes (CRTs) : The most common form of display screen is the CRT. A cathode ray tube is a vacuum tube used as a display screen in a computer or video display terminal. This same kind of technology is found not only in the screen of desktop computers but also in television sets. Images are represented on the screen (whether CRT or flat-panel display) by individual dots or "picture elements" called pixels. A pixel is the smallest unit on the screen that can be turned on and off. A stream of bits defining the image is sent from the computer (from the CPU) to the CRT's electron gun, where the bits are converted to electrons. The inside of the front of the CRT screen is coated with phosphor. When a beam of electrons from the electron gun (deflected through a yoke) hits the phosphor, it lights up selected pixels to generate an image on the screen.

Flat-panel Displays : Flat panel display is much thinner, less weight and consumes less power and thus they are more useful as portable computers. There are three types of technology used in flat panel display – liquid-crystal display, electro luminescent display and gas plasma display.

Clarity of Picture on a screen : Whether for CRT or flat-panel, screen clarity depends on three qualities: resolution, dot pitch, and refresh rate.

Resolution : It refers to the sharpness and clarity of an image. The term is most often used to describe monitors, printers, and bit-mapped graphic images. For graphics monitors, the screen resolution signifies the number of dots (pixels) on the entire screen. For example, a 640-by-480-pixel screen is capable of displaying 640 distinct dots on each of 480 lines, or about 300,000 pixels. This translates it into different dpi measurements depending on the size of the screen. For example, a 15-inch VGA monitor (640 x 480) displays about 50 dots per inch.

Monitors, scanners, and other I/O devices are often classified as high resolution, medium resolution, or low resolution. The actual resolution ranges for each of these grades is constantly shifting as the technology improves. In the case of dot matrix and laser printers, the resolution indicates the number of dots per inch. For example, a 300-dpi (dots per inch) printer is one that is capable of printing 300 distinct dots in a line 1 inch long. This means it can print 90,000 dots per square inch.

Dot Pitch : Dot pitch is the amount of space between pixels; the closer the dots, the crisper the image. This is a measurement that indicates the diagonal distance between like-coloured phosphor dots on a display screen. Measured in millimeters, the dot pitch is one of the principal characteristics that determine the quality of display monitors. The dot pitch of colour monitors for personal computers ranges from about 0.15 mm to 0.30 mm. Another term for dot pitch is phosphor pitch.

Refresh Rate : Refresh rate is the number of times per second the pixels are recharged so that their glow remains bright. The refresh rate for a monitor is measured in hertz (Hz) and is also called the vertical frequency, vertical scan rate, frame rate or vertical refresh rate. The old standard for monitor refresh rates was 60 Hz, but a new standard developed by VESA sets the refresh rate at 75 Hz for monitors displaying resolutions of 640 x 480 or greater. This means that the monitor redraws the display 75 times per second. The faster the refresh rate, the sharper the image.

Monochrome Vs Colour Screens : Display screens can be either monochrome or colour.

Monochrome : Monochrome display screens display only two colours – usually black and white, amber and black, or gray and black.

Colour : Colour display screens can display between 16 and 16.7 million colours, depending on their type. Most software today is developed for colour, except for some pocket PCs.

Text Vs Graphics : *Character-Mapped Vs Bitmapped Display* : Another distinction in display screens relates to their capacity to display graphics. A screen lacking this capacity is referred to as character-mapped. A bitmapped screen can display graphics.

Character-Mapped : Character-mapped display screens display only text-letters, numbers, and special characters. They cannot display graphics unless a video adapter card is installed. Text is displayed in rows and columns, with rows measuring the height of the screen and columns measuring the width. Most computer screens display 25 rows and 80 columns, which means that a row or line can have up to 80 characters of text.

Bitmapped : A representation, consisting of rows and columns of dots, of a graphics image in computer memory. The value of each dot (whether it is filled in or not) is stored in one or more bits of data. For simple monochrome images, one bit is sufficient to represent each dot, but for colours and shades of gray, each dot requires more than one bit of data. The more bits used to represent a dot, the more colours and shades of gray can be represented.

The density of the dots, known as the resolution, determines how sharply the image is represented. This is often expressed in dots per inch (dpi) or simply by the number of rows and columns, such as 640 by 480.

To display a bit-mapped image on a monitor or to print it on a printer, the computer translates the bit map into pixels (for display screens) or ink dots (for printers). Optical scanners and fax machines work by transforming text or pictures on paper into bit maps.

Video Display Adapters

To display graphics, a display screen must have a video display adapter. A video display adapter, also called a graphics adapter card, is a circuit board that determines the resolution, number of colours, and how fast images appear on the display screen. Video display adapters come with their own memory chips, which determine how fast the card processes images and how many colours it can display. A video display adapter with 256 kilobytes of memory will provide 16 colours; one with 1 megabyte will support 16.7 million colours.

The video display adapter is often built on the motherboard, although it may also be an expansion card that plugs into an expansion slot. Video display adapters embody certain standards. New computer displays tend to favor VGA, SVGA or XGA standards.

VGA *:* Abbreviation of video graphics adapter, a graphics display system for PCs developed by IBM. VGA has become one of the *de facto* standards for PCs. In text mode, VGA systems provide a resolution of 720 by 400 pixels. In graphics mode, the resolution is either 640 by 480 (with 16 colours) or 320 by 200 (with 256 colours). The total palette of colours is 262, 144.

Unlike earlier graphics standards for PCs MDA, CGA and EGA, VGA uses analog signals rather than digital signals. Consequently, a monitor designed for one of the older standards will not be able to use VGA.

Since its introduction in 1987, several other standards have been developed that offer grater resolution and more colours, but VGA remains the lowest common denominator. All PCs made today support VGA, and possibly some more advanced standard.

SVGA *:* Short for Super VGA, a set of graphics standards designed to offer greater resolution than VGA. There are several varieties of SVGA, each providing a different resolution:
- 800 by 600 pixels
- 1024 by 768 pixels
- 1280 to 1024 pixels
- 1600 by 1200 pixels

All SVGA standards support a palette of 16 million colours, but the number of colours that can be displayed simultaneously is limited by the amount of video memory installed in a system. One SVGA system might display only 256 simultaneous colours while another displays the entire palette of 16 million colours. Monitor and graphics manufacturers called VESA develop the SVGA standards.

XGA : Short for extended graphics array, a high-resolution graphics standard introduced by IBM in 1990. XGA was designed to replace the older 8514/A video standard. It provides the same resolutions (640 by 480 or 1024 by 768 pixels), but supports more monitors to be non-interlaced.

For any of these displays to work, video display adapters and monitors must be compatible. Your computer's software and the display adapter must also be compatible. Thus, if you are changing your monitor or your video display adapter, be sure the new one will still work with the old.

5.5.4 Paper Output Devices: Printers, Plotters & Multifunction Devices

Printers, plotters and multifunction devices produce printed text or images on paper. Printers may be desktop or portable, impact or non-impact. Impact printers include daisywheel and dot matrix printers. Non-impact printers include laser, ink-jet, and thermal printers. Plotters are pen, electrostatic, and thermal. Multifunction devices combine capabilities, such as printing, scanning, copying, and faxing.

Printers are most popular output devices. They provide information in a permanent readable form. They produce printed outputs of results, programs and data. Printers used with computers can be classified as follows:

    (a)   Character printers   (b)   Line printers and   (c)   Page printers

A character printer prints one character of the text at a time. A line printer prints one line of the text at a time. A page printer prints one page of the text at a time.

The above classification of printers is based on as to how they print. There is one more classification based on the technology used in their manufacture.

Impact printers : An electro-mechanical that causes hammers or pins to strike against a ribbon and paper to print the text. Non-impact printers do not use any electro-mechanical printing head to strike against ribbon and paper. They use thermal, chemical, electrostatic, laser beam or inkjet technology for printing the text. Usually a non-impact type printer is faster than an impact type. The disadvantage of non-impact type printers is that they produce only a single copy of the text whereas impact printers produce multiple copies of the text.

Character Printers : Character printers print one characters at a time. They are low speed printers. Their printing speed lies in the range of 60-600 characters per second. Two types of impact character printers are available: dot-matrix printers and letter quality printers.

Dot Matrix Impact Type Character Printers : A character is printed by printing the selected number of dots from a matrix of dots. The print head contains a vertical array of 9, 18 or 24 pins. A character is printed in a number of steps. One dot-column of the dot matrix is taken up at a time. The selected dots of a column (i.e. the column of dot-matrix) are printed by the print head at a time as it moves across a line.

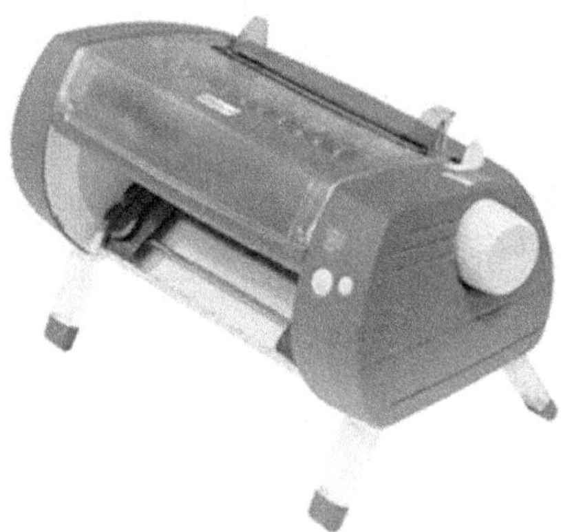

A dot-matrix printer is faster than a letter quality printer. Its printing speed lies in the range of 80-600 cps (character per second). Such printers operate at two or three speeds. The lower the speed, the better the printing quality. Higher speed is for draft printing and the lower speed is for near-letter quality (NLQ) printing, i.e. printing is as good as that of a letter quality printer. Many dot-matrix printers are bi-directional. A bi-directional printer, prints one line a text from left to right and then it prints the next line from right to left.

Dot-matrix printers are very flexible. They do not have fixed character fonts. The term font is used to refer to a character set of a printer. As fonts are not fixed, a dot-matrix printer can print any shape of a character by software. This permits printing special characters such as @, Ω, $\sqrt{}$, Θ, Φ, β, ∞, $\subseteq$, $\Leftrightarrow$, Ψ etc: various sizes of print, bold or expanded characters, italics characters of any languages and ability to print graphics.

Letter Quality Impact Character Printer (Daisy Wheel Printers) : An impact type letter quality printer is used where good quality of printing is needed. Such printers also called Daisy Wheel Printers. It is much slower compared to a dot-matrix printer. Its speed is in the range of 20-75 cps. It is costlier than dot-matrix printer. Its font is of fixed type. It cannot print graphics; Two-to-three types of fonts are available with Daisy Wheel. One can select a font having the desired style of characters.

A daisy wheel printer has a removable print wheel, the flower-like daisywheel consisting of spokes. Each spoke ends with a raised character, which is turned to align the desired letter, and then strike with a hammer.

Non-impact Character Printers

This type of printers uses thermal, electrostatic, chemical and inkjet technologies. They are briefly described below.

Thermal Character Printers : This type of printers use special heat-sensitive paper. Such papers have a special heat-sensitive coating. When a spot on the special paper is heated, it becomes dark. A character is printed with a matrix of dots. A print head consists of 5 x 7 or 7 x 9 matrix of tiny heating elements. Electric current heats the heating element. To print a character the printing head is moved first to the correct character position. Then the heating elements for the desired character are turned 'ON'. After a short time they are turned 'OFF'. Therefore the print head is moved to the next character position. Such printers have a speed of about 200 characters per second (cps).

For people who want the highest quality colour printing available with desktop printers, thermal prints are the answer. However, they are expensive and they require expensive paper. Thus they are not generally used for jobs requiring a high volume of output.

Ink-jet Character Printers : It uses dot-matrix approach to print text and graphics. Earlier ink-jet printers used one or more nozzles in print head that emit a steady stream of tiny ink drops. Each droplet is charged when it passes through a valve. Then it passes through horizontal and vertical deflecting plates. These plates deflect ink drops to direct them to the desired spots on the paper to form the impression of a character. In this type of printers the continuous stream of ink-jet approach is used. The speed of inkjet printers lies in the range of 40-300 cps. The average life of an ink-jet print head is about 10 billion characters, which is 5 times more than that of the print head of an impact type dot-matrix printer.

Inkjet printers use ink cartridges containing a column of tiny heaters. The print quality of such printers is very near letter-quality. Speed of such printers is in the same range as that of slow dot-matrix printers. Most colour printing is done on ink-jet because the nozzles can hold four different colours.

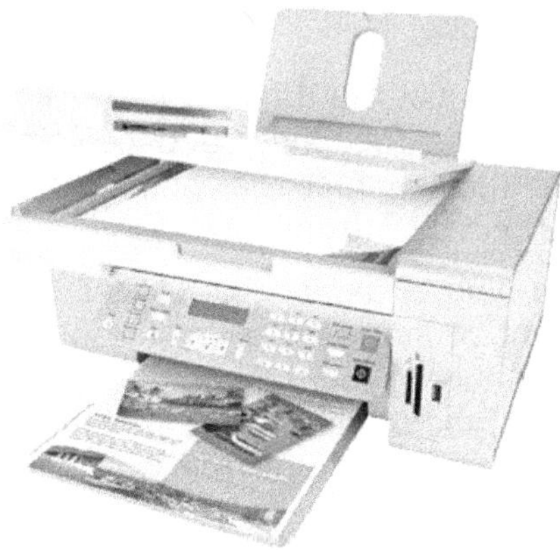

Line Printers :

The line printer prints one line of the text at a time. Its printing speed lies in the range of 300-3000 lines per minutes. It is used for large-volume printing jobs. It may be used with mini and mainframe computers.

   (a) Drum Printer   (b) Chain Printer   (c) Band Printer

Drum Printer : A drum printer uses a rapidly rotating drum (cylinder) which contains a complete set of raised characters in each band around the cylinder. Each character position along the text line contains a band of raised character set. There is a magnetically driven hammer in each character position of the line. The printer receives all characters to be printed in one line of the text from the processor. The hammers hit the ribbon and paper against the desired character on the drum when it comes in the printing position. Its noise level is high. Its speed varies from 200 to 2000 lines/ minute.

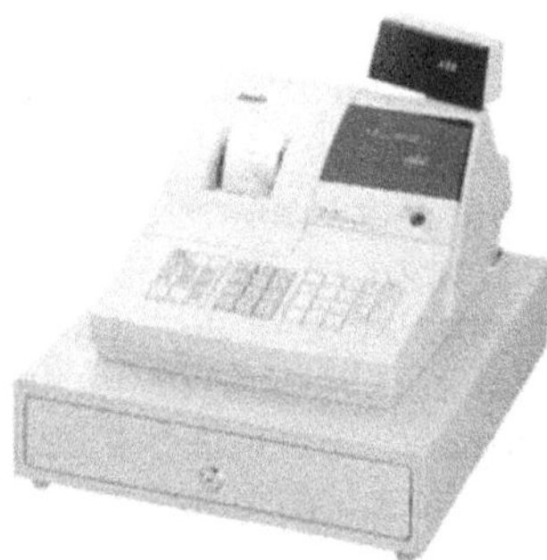

Chain Printer : Chain printer uses a rapidly rotating chain, which is called print chain. The print contains characters. Each link of the chain is character font. Magnetically driven hammers are located in each print position. The printer receives all the characters to be printed in one line from the processor. The printer prints one line at a time. A chain may contain more than one character set. When the desired character comes in the print position the hammer strikes the ribbon and paper against the character. The noise level of the printer is high. Its speed lies in the range of 400-2400 lines/m.

Band Printer : Band printer is just like a chain printer. It contains fast rotating steel print bands in place of chains. The print band contains a raised character set. Hammers strike the ribbon and the paper against the character to print the character. Some printers can print up to 3000 lines/m.

Laser Printers : This is a type of printer that utilizes a laser beam to produce an image on a drum. The light of the laser alters the electrical charge on the drum wherever it hits. The drum is then rolled through a reservoir of toner, which is picked up by the charged portions of the drum. Finally, the toner is transferred to the paper through a combination of heat and pressure. This is also used as a copy machine.

Because an entire page is transmitted to a drum before the toner is applied, laser printers are sometimes called page printers. There are two other types of page printers that fall under the category of laser printers even though they do not use lasers at all. One uses an array of LEDs to expose the drum, and the other uses LCDs. Once the drum is charged, however, they both operate like a real laser printer.

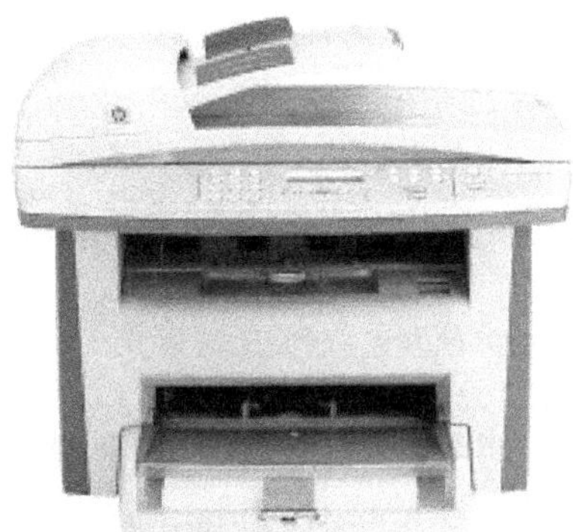

One of the chief characteristics of laser printers is their resolution i.e. how many dots per inch (dpi) they lay down. The available resolution range is from 300 dpi at the low end to 1,200 dpi at the high end. By comparison, offset printing usually prints at 1,200 or 2,400 dpi. Some laser printers achieve higher resolutions with special techniques known generally as resolution enhancement.

5.6   Units of Measurement or Storage

We will discuses the meanings of kilobytes, megabytes, gigabytes, and terabytes as unit of data storage. The same terms are also used to measure the data capacity of storage devices.

Bit : Short for binary digit, the smallest unit of information on a machine. A single bit can hold only on of two values: 0 or 1. More meaningful information is obtained by combining consecutive bit's larger units. For example, a byte is composed of 8 consecutive bits.

Byte : To represent letters, numbers, or special characters (such as $ or *), bits are combined into groups. A group of eight bits is called a byte and a byte represents one character, digit, or any other value. (For example, in binary scheme, 01001000 represents the letter P.) The capacity of a computer's memory of a floppy disk is expressed in terms numbers of bytes.

Kilo Byte : In decimal systems, kilo stands for 1,000, but in binary systems, a kilo is 1,024 (2 to the 10th power). Technically, therefore, a kilobyte is 1,024 bytes, but it is often used loosely as a synonym for 1,000 bytes. For example, a computer that has 256 KB main memory can store approximately 256,000 bytes (or characters) in memory at one time.

Mega Byte *:* Megabyte is frequently abbreviated as MB. This is equal to 1,048,576 (2 to the 20th power) bytes or 1024 kilo bytes.

Gigabyte *:* Gigabyte is often abbreviated as GB. One gigabyte is equal to 1,024 megabytes, or 2 to the 30th power (1,073,741,824) bytes.

Terabyte *:* This is approximately 1 million bytes. 2 to the 40th power (1,099,511,627,776) bytes. A terabyte is equal to 1024 Gigabytes.

Petabyte *:* 2 to the 50th power (1,125,899,906,842,624) bytes. A petabyte is equal to 1.024 terabytes.

Exabyte *:* 2 to the 60the power (1,152,921,504,606,846,976) bytes. An exabyte is equal to 1,024 petabytes.

Zettabyte *:* 2 to the 70th power bytes, which is approximately 10 to the 21st power bytes. A zettabyte is equal to 1,024 exabytes. The name zeta was chosen because it's the last letter of the Latin alphabet and also sounds like the Greek letter *Zeta.*

Yottabyte *:* 2 to the 80th power bytes, which is approximately 10 to the 24th power bytes. A yottabyte is equal to 1,024 zettabytes. The name yotta was chosen because it's the second-to-last letter of the Latin alphabet and also sounds like the Greek letter *iota.*

5.7 Primary Storage

Storage is categorized as primary or secondary. Primary storage is main memory working storage or temporary storage. Secondary storage is permanent storage. Examples are floppy disk, hard disk, optical disks, flash memory cards, and magtietic tape.

5.7.1 Primary Storage

Primary storage refers to physical memory that is internal to the computer. The word primary, internal or main is used to distinguish it from external mass storage devices such as disk drives. Another term for main memory is RAM.

The computer can manipulate only data that is in main memory. Therefore, every program you execute and every file you access must be copied from a storage device into main memory. The amount of main memory on a computer is crucial because it determines how many programs can be executed at one time and how much data can be readily available to the program.

Because computers often have too little main memory to hold all the data, they need a technique called swapping, in which portions of data are copied into main memory when they are needed. Swapping occurs when there is no room in memory for the existing data. When one portion of data is copied into memory, its equal-sized portion is copied (swapped) out to make that memory block vacant.

Primary storage is the computer's small storage capacity, determining the total size of the programs and data files it can work with at any given moment. Primary storage, which is contained on RAM chips, is temporary. Once the power to the computer is turned off, all the data and programs within memory simply vanish. For this reason, primary storage is said to be volatile. Volatile memory is temporary memory; the contents are lost when the power is turned off. If you accidentally kick out the power cord underneath your desk, or a storm knocks down a power line to your house, whatever you are currently working on will immediately washout.

RAM

A RAM is an acronym for Random Access Memory, a type of computer memory that can be accessed randomly; that is, any byte of memory can be accessed without touching the preceding bytes. RAM is the most common type of memory found in computers and other devices.

There are two basic types of RAM :

- Dynamic RAM (DRAM)
- Static RAM (SRAM)

Dynamic RAM *:* A type of physical memory used in most personal computers. The term dynamic indicates that the memory must be constantly refreshed or else it will lose its contents.

Static RAM *:* Static RAM pronounced ess-RAM. SRAM is faster and less volatile than dynamic RAM, but it requires more power and is more expensive.

ROM

ROM is acronym for Read Only Memory. Once data has been written onto a ROM chip, it cannot be removed and can only be read. Unlike main memory, ROM retains its contents even when the computer is turned off. ROM is referred to as being non-volatile, whereas RAM is volatile. ROM stores critical programs such as the program that boots the computer.

Types of ROM

PROM *:* Pronounced prom, is acronym for Programmable Read Only Memory. A prom is a memory chip on which data can be written only once. Once a program has been written onto a PROM, it remains there forever. The difference between RAM and PROM is that a ROM is programmed during the manufacturing process, whereas a PROM is manufactured as blank memory.

EPROM *:* Erasable Programmable Read Only Memory is a special type of memory that retains its contents until it is not exposed to ultraviolet light. The ultraviolet light clears its contents, making it possible to program. The memory write and erase an EPROM, you need a special device called a EPROM burner.

EEPROM *:* Electrically Erasable Programmable Read Only Memory is a special type of PROM that can be erased by exposing it to an electrical charges.

Cache

Cache pronounced cash is a special high-speed storage mechanism. It can be either a reserved section of main memory or an independent high-speed storage device. Two types of caching are commonly used in personal computers – memory caching and disk caching.

5.7.2   Secondary Memory or Secondary Storage

Refers to various techniques and devices used for storing large amounts of data. The earliest storage devices were punched paper cards, which were used as early as 1804 to control silk-weaving looms. Modern mass storage devices include all types of disk drives and tape drives. Mass storage is distinct from memory, which refers to temporary storage areas within the computer. Secondary storage is non-volatile i.e. data and programs are permanent, or remain intact, when the power is turned off. The main types of secondary storages are:

Floppy Disks

Floppy disk is round pieces of flat plastic that store data and programs as magnetized spots. The two principal sizes are 3½ inch and 5¼ inch. A disk drive copies or reads data from the disk and writes, or records data to the disk. Components of a floppy disk include tracks and sectors. Disks come in various densities. All have write protect features. Care must be taken to avoid data corruption on disks and users are advised to backup, or duplicate, the data on their disks.

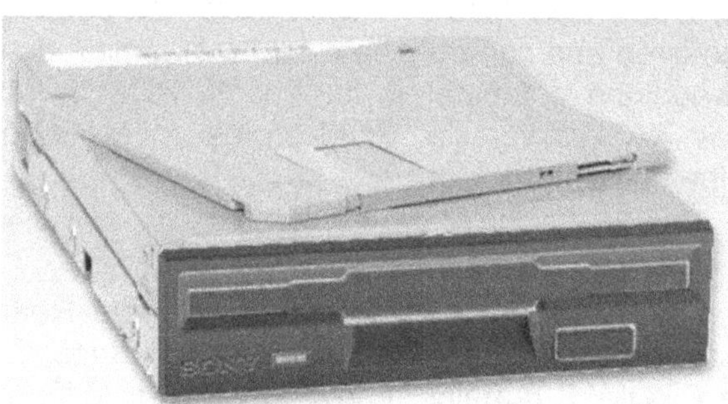

A floppy disk is a soft magnetic disk. It is called floppy because it flops if you wave it (at least, the 5¼ inch variety does). Unlike most hard disks, floppy disk (often called floppies or diskettes) is portable, because you can remove them from a disk drive. Disk drives for floppy disks are called floppy drives. Floppy disks are slower to access than hard disks and have less storage capacity, but they are cheaper and portable.

Floppies come in two basic sizes

5¼ inch : It is common size for PCs made before 1987. This type of floppy is generally capable of storing between 100 K and 1.2 MB (megabytes) of data. The most common sizes are 360 K and 1.2 MB.

3½ inch : Despite their small size, microfloppies have a larger storage capacity than their cousins (from 400 K to 1.4 MB of data). The most common sizes for PCs are 720 K (double-density) and 1.44 MB (high-density). Macintoshes support disks of 400 K, 800 K, and 1.2 MB.

Floppy disk drive

To use floppy disk we use a machine that reads data from and writes data onto a disk called Floppy Disk Drive. A disk drive rotates the disk very fast and has one or more heads that read and write data. Disk drives can be either internal (housed within the computer) or external (housed in a separate box that connects to the computer). The process of READ and WRITE means the following:

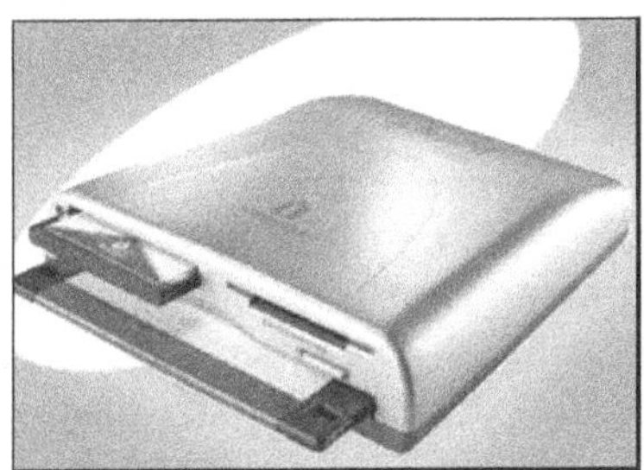

READ : To copy data to a place where it can be used by a program. The term is commonly used to describe copying data from a storage medium, such as a disk to main memory for the purpose of using the data for processing.

WRITE : To copy data from main memory to a storage device, such as a disk, i.e. the data recorded on to the disk from the main memory for later use.

Characteristics of Floppy Disks : Both 5 ¼ inch and 3 ½ inch disks work in similar ways, although there is some difference. The characteristics of floppy disks are as follows:

Tracks and sectors : Once a floppy disk data is recorded in rings it is called tracks. These tracks are not visible. A typical floppy disk has 80 (double density) or 160 (high density) tracks. Each track is further divided into a number of sectors. Sector is the smallest unit that can be accessed on a disk. The tracks are concentric circles around the disk and sectors are segments within each circle. For example, a floppy disk might have 40 tracks, with each track divided into 10 sectors. The operating system and disk drive keep tabs on where information is stored. They are measured in terms of tracks per inch (TPI). For example, double-density 5.25 inch floppies have a TPI of 48, while high density floppies record 96 TPI. High density 3.5 inch diskettes are formatted with 135 TPI.

Formatting *:* formatting means to prepare a storage medium, usually a disk, for reading and writing. When you format a disk, the operating system erases all book keeping information on the disk, tests the disk to make sure all sectors are reliable, makes bad sectors (that is, those that are scratched), and creates internal address tables that it later used to locate information. You must format a disk before you can use it.

Note that reformatting a disk does not erase the data of the disk, it only erases the address tables. Do not panic, therefore, if you accidentally reformat a disk that has useful data. A computer specialist should be able to recover most, if not all, of the information on the disk. You can also buy programs that enable you to recover a disk yourself.

The previous discussion, however, applies only to high-level formats, the type of formats that most users execute. In addition, hard disks have a low-level format, which sets certain properties of the disk such as the interleave sector. The low-level format also determines what type of disk controller can access the disk (e.g. RLL or MFM).

Data capacity – sides and density *:* Density means how tightly information is packed together on a storage medium (tape or disk). A higher density means that data are closer together, so the medium can hold more information. Floppy disks can be single-density, double-density, high-density, or extra-high-density. To use a double-density, high-density, or extra-high-density disk, you have a disk drive that supports the density level. Density, therefore, can refer both to the media and the device.

Write protect feature *:* 'Write-Protect' means to marks a file or disk so that its contents cannot be modified or deleted. When you want to make sure that neither you nor user can destroy data, you can write - protect it. Many operating systems include a command to write protect files. You can also write - protect 5¼ inch floppy disks by covering the write protect files. 3½ inch floppy diskettes have a small switch that you can set to turn on write protection. Write protected files and media can only be read; you cannot write to them, edit them, append data to them, or delete them.

Backup of important data *:* Backup means to copy files to a second medium (a disk or tape) as a precaution in case the first medium fails. One of the cardinal rules in using computer is:

'Back up your files regularly'.

Even the most reliable computer is apt to break down eventually. Many professionals recommend that you make two, or even three, backups of all your files. To be especially safe, you should keep one backup in a different location from the others. You can back up files using operating system commands, or you can buy a special-purpose backup utility. Backup programs often compress the data so that backups require fewer disks.

Hard Disk : Hard disk is a magnetic disk on which you can store computer data. The term hard is used to distinguish it from a soft, or floppy disk. Hard disks hold more data and are faster than floppy disks. A hard disk, can store data from MB to TB whereas most floppies have a maximum storage capacity of 1.4 MB.

A single hard disk usually consists of several platters. Platter is a round magnetic plate that constitutes part of a hard disk. Each platter requires two read/write heads, one for each side. All the read/write heads are attached to a single access arm so that they cannot move independently. Each platter has the same number of tracks, and a track location that cuts across all platters and is called a cylinder.

Removable Hard Disk

A type of disk drive system in which hard disks are enclosed in plastic or metal cartridges so that they can be removed like floppy disks. Removable disk drives combine the best aspects of hard and floppy disks. They are nearly as capacious and fast as hard disks and have the portability of floppy disks. Their biggest drawback is that they're relatively expensive.

Some Important terms related to Hard / Floppy Disk

Cylinder : A single-track location on all the platters makes up a hard disk. For example, if a hard disk has four platters, each with 600 tracks, then there will be 600 cylinders, and each cylinder will consist of 8 tracks (assuming that each platter has tracks on both sides).

Track : A ring on a disk where data can be written. A typical floppy disk has 80 (double-density) or 160 (high-density) tracks. For hard disks, each platter is divided into tracks, and a single-track location that cuts through all platters (and both sides of each platter) is called a cylinder. Each track is further divided into a number of sectors. The operating system and disk drive remembers where information is stored by noting its track and sector numbers.

The density of tracks (how close together they are) is measured in terms of tracks per inch (TPI).

CD-ROM

CD-ROM's abbreviation is Compact Disc-Read Only Memory. This is a type of optical disk capable of storing large amounts of data – up to 1GB, although the most common size is 650 MB (megabytes). A single CD-ROM has the storage capacity of 700 floppy disks, enough memory to store about 300,000 text pages.

The vendor stamps CD-ROMs, and once stamped, they cannot be erased and filled with new data. To read a CD, you need a CD-ROM player. All CD-ROMs conform to a standard size and format, so you can load any type of CD-ROM into any

CD-ROM player. In addition, CD-ROM players are capable of playing audio CDs, which share the same technology.

CD-ROMs are particularly well-suited to information that requires large storage capacity. This includes software applications, graphics, sound, and especially video.

CD-ROM Player

Also called a CD-ROM drive, a device that can read information from a CD-ROM. CD-ROM players can be either internal or external, which generally connect to the computer's SCSI interface or parallel port. Parallel CD-ROM players are easier to install, but they have several disadvantages: They're somewhat more expensive than internal players. They use up the parallel port which means that you can't use that part for another device such as a printer, and the parallel port itself may not be fast enough to handle all the data pouring through it.

There are a number of features that distinguish CD-ROM players, the most important of which is probably their speed. CD-ROM players are generally classified as single speed or some multiples of single-speed. For example, a 4X player access data at four times the speed of a single-speed player.

Constant Linear Velocity, or CLV is a method used by older CD-ROM player to access data. With CLV, the rotation speed of the disk changes based on how close to the center of the disk the data is. For tracks near the center, the disk rotates faster and for data outside the disk it rotates slower. The purpose of CLV is to ensure a constant data rate, regardless of where on the disk the data is being accessed. Because less data can fit on the inside tracks, the disk needs to rotate faster for these areas. An alternative technology, which is becoming increasingly popular, is Constant Angular Velocity (CAV).

Constant Angular Velocity, is a technique for accessing data of rotating disks, with constant speed regardless of what area of the disk is being accessed. This differs from constant linear velocity (CLV), which rotates the disk faster for inner tracks. Disk drives use CAV, whereas CD-ROMs generally use CLV, though some new drives use a combination of CAV and CLV. The advantage of CAV is that it is much simpler to design and produce because the motor doesn't need to change speed. In addition, CLV runs into problems for very high-speed CD-ROMs because there's a brief latency whenever the drive needs to change the rotational speed.

CD-R drive : Short for Compact Disk-Recordable Drive, a type of disk drive that can create CD-ROMs and audio CDs. This allows users to "master" a CD-ROM or audio CD for publishing. Until recently, CD-R drives were quite expensive, but prices have dropped dramatically.

A feature of many CD-R drives, called multi session recording, enables you to keep adding data to a CD-ROM over time. This is extremely important if you want to use the CD-R drive to create backup CD-ROMs.

To create CD-ROMs on audio CDs, you'll need not only a CD-R drive, but also a CDR software package. Often, it is the software package, not drive itself that determines how easy or difficult it is to create CD-ROMs.

CD-R drives can also read CD-ROMs and play audio CDs.

CD-RW DISK *:* Short for CD-Re-Writable disk, a type of CD disk that enables you to write onto it in multiple sessions. One of the problems with CD-R disks is that you can only write to them once. With CD-RW drives and disks, you treating the optical disk just like a floppy or hard disk, writing data onto it multiple times.

WORM *:* Short for Write Once Read Many, an optical disk technology that allows you to write data onto a disk just once. After that, the data is permanent and can be read any number of times. WORM is also called CD-R.

Erasable optical disk *:* A type of optical disk that can be erased and loaded with new data. In contrast, most optical disks, called CD-ROMs are read-only.

Digital Video Disk (DVD) *:* Short for Digital Versatile Disc or Digital Video Disc, a new type of CD-ROM that holds a minimum of 4.7 GB (gigabytes), enough for a full-length movie CD-ROMs, as well as VHS videocassettes and laser discs.

The DVD specification supports disks with capacities of from 4.7 GB to 17 GB and access rates of 600 KBps to 1.3 MBps. One of the best features of DVD drives is that they are backward compatible with CD-ROMs. This means that DVD players can play old CD-ROMs, CD-I disks, and video CDs, as well as new DVD-ROMs. Newer DVD players can also read CD-R disks. DVD uses MPEG-2 to compress video data.

DVD-RAM *:* A new type of re-writable compact disc that provides much grater data storage than today's CD-RW systems. The DVD Consortium is still hammering out the specification for DVD-RAMs. Meanwhile, a competing group of manufacturers led by Hewlett-Packard, Philips and Sony, have come up with a competing standard called DVD+RW. Whereas the DVD-RAM standard supports 2.6 GB per disk side, DVD+RW supports 3 GB per side.

DVD-ROM *:* A new type of read-only compact disc that holds a minimum of 4.7 GB (gigabytes), enough for a full-length movie. Many experts believe that DVD-ROMs will eventually replace CD-ROMs, as well as VHS video cassettes and laser discs. Currently, however, DVD-ROMs are more promise than reality. There are only a few DVD-ROM devices that can play old CD-ROMs, CD-I disks, and video CDs, as well as new DVD-ROMs. Newer DVD players can also read CD-R disks.

DVD-ROMs use MPEG-2 to compress video data.

Magnetic Tape

It is a magnetically coated strip of plastic on which data can be encoded. Tapes for computers are similar to tapes used to store music. This is the oldest storage media used till today.

Storing data on tapes is considerably cheaper than storing data on disks. Tapes also have large storage capacities, ranging from a few hundred kilobytes to several gigabytes. Accessing data on tapes is slower than accessing data on disks. Tapes are sequential-access media, which means that to get to a particular point on the tapes, the tape must go through all the preceding points. In contrast, disks are random-access media because a disk drive can access any point at random without passing through intervening points.

Pen Drive

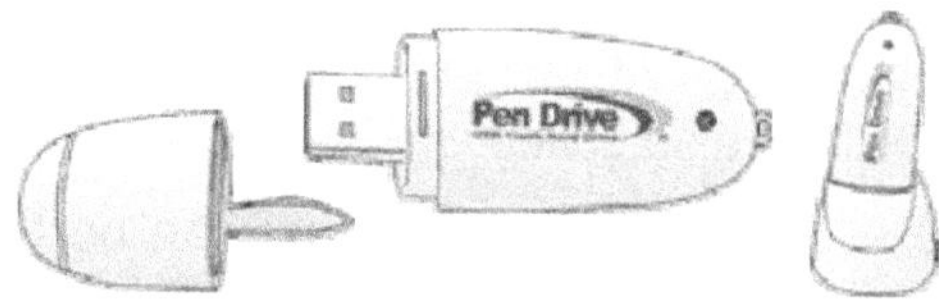

USB Pen Drive is a small key ring-sized device that can be used to easily transfer files between USB-compatible systems. Available in a range of capacities (and in some cases, with an MP3 player built-in), this handy little device can save all those data-transfer hassles.

Simple. Plug it into the USB port* of your PC (or Mac!) and watch the system automatically detects the new device. Take at look at your system drives... a new drive has been created! The operating system can now access your USB Pen Drive just like any ordinary Hard Disk Drive.

Copy across all the files you want to the 'new' drive, wait for the Read/Write LED on the USB Pen Drive to stop flashing then disconnect it. That's it. Your files are now safely stored on your USB Pen Drive. If you want to copy those files to another PC/Mac, just plug it in the new machine, wait for it to be detected and copy them off again.

* If you don't want to reach round to the back of your PC every time to plug it in, you can use the handy Docking Bay to give you USB Pen Drive access right from your desktop.

USB

USB – Universal Serial Bus, is a 'standard' developed by the computer industry to allow a vast number of different devices to be easily attached to one machine with the minimum requirement for extra drivers and software and still operate at an efficient speed.

Put simply, this means: We can plug a USB device in without switching the PC off. It will be automatically detected by the Operating System and will be ready for use in a few seconds. The USB Pen Drive is one of those devices.

CHAPTER 6

Fundamentals of Operating System

6.1 Definition and Need of Operating System

The operating system is the link between the hardware and software. An operating system (usually known as the OS) is an organised set or collection of software programs that control the overall operation of the computer system. It controls and directs the flow of data and instruction from one part of the computer to another.

A computer itself is nothing but a collection of various hardware devices such as the keyboard, the visual display unit, Central Processing Unit (CPU). It is the operating system that makes these independent hardware devices, although interconnected by cables, a single entity which is both easy to use and manage. Operating system acts as an interface between the user and the computer system. It is only due to presence of the operating system that the user doesn't have to bother about the technical details and functional aspects of each of the hardware components of the system. All that the user needs to do is to present the problem to the operating system in a language that can be understood by the operating system and get the results. The computer hardware provides the raw processing power or ability. It is the job of the operating system to make this ability conveniently available to the users.

6.2 Function of Operating System

An operating system (OS) is an integrated set of programs that is used to manage the various resources and overall operations of a computer system. It is designed to support the activities of computer Installation. Its prime objective is to improve the performance and efficiency of a computer system and increase facility with which a system can be used. Thus, like a manager of a company, an operating system makes the computer system user friendly. That is, it becomes easier for people to interact with and make use of the computer.

Operating system is known by many different names, depending on the manufacture of the computer. Other terms used to describe the operating system are, executive, supervisor, controller and master control programs. Operating System performs the following functions.

1. **Process Management** – That is assignment of processors to different tasks being performed by the computer system.
2. **Memory Management** – That is, allocation of main memory storage to the system programs.
3. **Input/Output management** – That is coordination and assignment of the different input and output devices while one or more programs are being executed.
4. **File management** – The storage of files on various storage devices and the transfer of these from one storage device to another. It also allows all files to be easily changed and modified through the use of text editors or some other file manipulation routines.
5. **Setting Priority** – It determines and maintains the order in which jobs are to be executed in the computer system.
6. Automatic transition from job to job, directed by special control statements.
7. Interpretation of commands and instructions.
8. Coordination and assignment of compilers, assemblers, utility programs, software.
9. Production of dumps, traces, and error message and other debugging and error detection aids.
10. Facilitates easy communication between the system and the computer operator.

6.3 Useful Terms of Operating System

6.3.1 Multi-Programming

Overlapped or interleaved execution of two or more processes is terms as multiprogramming. In other words, multiprogramming implies that two or more processes are active at the same time and are available for execution. The operating system may select one of these active programs for allocation to CPU or processor on the basis of some selection technique. The next process in the queue is allocated to the CPU, when either of the following takes place.

(i)   The executing process issues an I/O request,
(ii)   The executing process completes execution, or
(iii) The time allocated to the executing process is over.

In this way, the CPU or the processor can be kept busy by the operating system, which switches from one process to a waiting process, whenever the first process either terminates or requests an I/O activity or its allocated time is over, while the I/O is outputting the data. All active processes that are not executing are kept on the secondary storage and when one of these is to be executed, it is loaded from there along with the intermediate results that it had computed when the CPU was allocated to it last time. Note that at any time one and only one process is executing.

6.3.2 Multi-Processing

Multiprocessing is a term used with the processing on a system which contains more than one CPUs. In a system with more than one CPU, more than one instruction can be executed by the system at the same time. Thus more than one process can be simultaneously executed in such systems.

A multiprocessing operating system is an operating system that has been designed for a multiprocessor system, that is, a system having more than one CPUs output from system. It is the job of the multiprocessing operating system to schedule and balance the input, output and the processing capabilities of a system to schedule processors. Since scheduling and coordinating the activities of multiple CPUs is a very complex task, a multiprocessing operating system is a very complex and sophisticated operating system.

6.3.3 Real Time

A real-time operating system is one in which the input data is to be processed and the result produced within a stipulated time period. That is, the processing of data should take very small amount of time. Real-time operating systems are generally used in industry as monitors. Such systems are very useful in places where a close watch is kept on the surroundings of the system and some corrective action is to be taken in case one particular thing happens. For examples consider a heat furnace whose temperature is to be kept constant for 30 hours at 300° Centigrade and that the maximum allowable temperature variation is $+ 1^\circ$ centigrade. In such a situation, manual monitoring is virtually impossible. Here a real-time system can be used very conveniently. Such a system (that is the one that can be used in such a situation) will have heat sensors, which will provide the input – the temperature of the furnace – to the system. The system will process this input and accordingly try to adjust the temperature of the furnace.

6.3.4 Time Sharing Technique

In the manner in which processors working with higher speed were developed, the technique of batch processing proved to be unproductive in view of the use of processing capacity. On the one hand, input and output applications work with a very slow speed and the time taken to read any information from the memory forces the processor to remain free. On the other hand, as all programs are not of one size, the main memory is not utilized and the capacity of the main memory also cannot be fully utilized. After doing other work and after sometime, it again starts doing the first job from where it had left earlier. In this way the time of the processor can be fully utilized. The activities are assessed by the operating system.

If 16 terminals are attached with one system and if work is going on all terminals, then for sometime the computer does the work of one user and then serial wise of other users. It works with such high speed that every one feels that the computer is working method in which you don't have to wait. It is called Online Processing technique. The method in which computer does the work of many users together and distributes it in time slices is known as time-sharing technique.

6.4   Various Types of Operating System

Types of operating system :

On the basis of the number of users working on the system, O. S. can be classified into the following types.

6.4.1   Single-User O.S

The O.S. on which one user can work at a time is known as single operating system. DOS belongs to this category.

6.4.2   Multi-User O.S

When two or more users can work on the same O.S. simultaneously it is known as multi-user O.S. Unix is a multi-user O.S., as two or more persons can work at a time in this type of O.S.

On the basis of the mode of working, the O.S. are again classified into following types.

6.4.3   Character User Interface (CUI)

When the user operates the system by means of characters it is known as CUI. Ex: DOS. Here the USER gives command to the system by means of characters i.e., in order to copy a file we have to give exact syntax of copy command ex: in DOS : Copy A: FILE1 B: FILE1

6.4.4   Graphical User Interface (GUI)

When the user operates the system by means of pictorial or graphical representations it is known as GUI. Windows is an operating environment, which provides the feature of GUI, i.e. in order to copy a file in windows we have to select the option of copy and it will be copied.

6.5   Disk Operating System (DOS)

DOS can support a wide range of disks. At the lower end of the range are the disks with storage capacity of a few hundred bytes and at the higher end are the disks having enormous storage capacity of the order of tens of mega bytes.

DOS organizes these disks depending on their storage capacities. Each disk surface is divided into tracks. The number of tracks on the disk's surface depends upon the type of the disk. These circular tracks are further subdivided into sectors. A sector is the basic unit of storage for disks. Even the number of sectors contained in a track is dependent on the type of disks.

Most floppy disks have 40/80 tracks per surface. Floppy disks with 40 tracks are called the double disks and those with 80 tracks are known as the quad-density disks. On a double density disk, track is divided into 9 sectors. On a quad density disk too, a track contains 9 sectors. Each sector can store up to 512 bytes of information on any type of disk. Even in a hard disk the number of bytes a sector can have the same, that is, 512 bytes.

MS-DOS

MS-DOS stand for Microsoft Disk Operating System developed by the Microsoft Ltd.

Most of the DOS programs are stored in two files, namely IO.SYS and MSDOS.SYS. Another file, which contains DOS routines, is the COMMAND.COM. The IO.SYS and MSDOS.SYS are hidden files and are not visible to ordinary user. These are all present in the boot sector of the system.

The IO.SYS file contains the extensions to the ROM-BIOS. These may be additions to the exiting set of elementary routines stored in ROM and can be changed in already existing routines stored in ROM.

The MSDOS.SYS file contains the MS-DOS service routines. These routines provide better control over various peripheral devices. But these routines are not as flexible as the ROM-BIOS routines.

The COMMAND.COM files are the third part of the DOS. It contains the command interpreter of the DOS. This command interpreter first accepts any command that we give to the system. If what we have entered is correct and it exists as a command by the name then COMMAND.COM invokes the specified command. In case of an error, COMMAND.COM gives an appropriate error message. So any interaction that a user may have with the system or DOS can only be through COMMAND.COM.

6.6 Explanation of DOS Terminology

File

File is a collection of data, instruction or programs. Every set of program and data is given specific name to identify it. There are various types of files such as;

Date file : Collection of characters, letters etc.

Program file : Collection of instructions.

File naming rules in DOS

In DOS, a file name consists of two parts:

(i) *First Name or Primary file Name :*

It can be 1 to 8 characters long. There should not be any space in between the characters of first name. The characters in primary file name can be A to Z, 0 to 9 and any special characters like &, # % etc.

(ii)*Second name or extension name :*

This is optional and can be 0 to 3 characters long. It can also include any alphabet, digit or special character. The primary and extension name of the file is always separated by a dot (.).

Ex. PAYROLE.EXE

IES.COM

Ram.TXT

DIRECTORY : A directory is an index of the files stored on the disk. This includes a file name that primary name, extension name, memory occupied, date of creation and date of last updating. For ex: 2 directories are created in DOS for storing the 2 different types of files. USER directory stores all files of various users. Another directory is meant for storing system files.

(a) Subdirectory

Subdirectory is a directory within a directory. It is just like a child directory of parent directory made for maximum use of disk and maintains the records and files properly. With the help of subdirectory we can recognize our files in such a way that the files related to one person are in one place and those related to the second are at other place. Thus using subdirectories we can organize the disk in a better way. For ex. :- User1, User2 and User3. 3 subdirectories are created under the directory user, to organize the files for each user specifically in his own directory.

(b) Default Directory

This directory in which working presently is the default directory. For example, after loading DOS the default directory is C:/ (In Hard Disk) or A:/ (In floppy disk).

(c) Root Directory

The main directory or the topmost directory is called the root directory. All other directories are branches of the directory, like the roots of a tree. Root directory can include files, programs, other directories or subdirectories. It is designation by a backslash (\).

(d) Parent Directory

The directory one level above the current working directory is known as parent directory. For ex: The user directory is parent directory for the 3 subdirectories user1, user2 and user3.

Wild card characters

When you want to work with a group of files, you can use wild cards. There are two types of wild cards: asterix (*) and a questions mark (?). That is abc. * means a file has any extension whose name is abc, (?) used only for one word while * used for many words.

(a) FAT

FAT stands for File Allocation Table. It is a table, which contains mappings of physical locations of all the clusters or files on the disk storage.

(b) Special files

There are certain files, which have special meaning for DOS.

When you first start DOS, it looks for a file called AUTOEXEC.BAT. This file is nothing but a series of DOS commands which you have to execute every time you start your computer. This file must be stored in the root directory. When DOS starts, it finds the file, and executes it. This file may include commands that control different settings. For example, you might include a command that controls different programs.

6.6.1 File Arrangement in DOS

In DOS, files are arranged in hierarchical manner, i.e. an inverted tree structure. For example, If there are 4 users working on a system such as, USER1, USER2, USER3 and USER4 and they have 16 files as follows :

		ROOT	
USER1	**USER2**	**USER3**	**USER4**
FILES1	FILES2	FILES10	FILES3
FILES12	FILES5	FILES11	FILES4
FILES13	FILES6	FILES14	FILES8
FILES16	FILES9	FILES7	FILES15

6.7 Booting Process

The process of starting your computer is called booting. Typically, you will start your computer at the beginning of the day and leave it on until you're done at the end of the day. At that time, you'll exit any programs you're running, return to the DOS command prompt, and turn off the power.

If we reboot our system, we have two options: a warm boot or a cold boot.

6.7.1 Warm Booting

A warm boot is "gentler" and often quicker because the computer stays powered on during the procedure. To perform a warm boot, press the key combination CTRL+ALT+DEL. To use this key combination, hold down the Ctrl Key, then hold down the Alt key, then hold down the Del key. Release all three keys after the screen clears and the computer restarts.

6.7.2 Cold Booting

If a warm boot doesn't seem to clear up the problem completely, you can perform a cold boot. To do so, turn off the power, preferably using the switch on your computer's surge protector. Wait until the computer's hard disk has stopped rotating (counting to 30 slowly should do it!), then turn the power on again.

6.8 DOS Commands

Types of DOS Commands

DOS commands are basically of following two types.

6.8.1 Internal DOS commands

Internal DOS commands are stored in the COMMAND.COM file, which is loaded into the memory, when you start your system. They include the simpler; you need on a regular basis. Because internal commands are part of COMMAND.COM, you never get to see their names in a directory listing. These commands remain resident in memory and are available to you at all times.

6.8.2 External DOS Commands

External DOS Commands exist as separate files on your disk. When you use the dir command to view the files on your MS-DOS system disk, you see the external command in the list of filenames and directory names. The filename of an external command is COM, EXE or BAT extension. External commands need special DOS files for execution.

6.8.3 Switches Available in the Commands

A switch is a forward slash (/) usually followed by a single letter or number you use. Switches are used to modify the way a command performs a task. For example, suppose you want to use the dir command to view a listing of a directory, that contains a large number of files. When you type the dir command by itself, the /p switch, you can view the list of files on screen at a time.

MS-DOS commands do not have any switches, whereas others have several. If a command has more than one switch, you type them one after the other. You can separate switches with a space but the space is optional.

Internal Commands

To create a file

COPY CON

COPY CON < file name >. txt >

This command creates a file in the specified directory. Pressing ENTER would take the cursor to the next line. Now we can type the data we want to feed into the file.

Once this is done. Press Ctrl+Z. The following message appears.

1. File (s) copied

Directory : There might be times when you want to keep some related files together and at the same time separate it from other files. To help this situation, directories can be made to hold these files.

A directory is a collection of files or in other words, it is a folder that contains related files.

To create a directory

Make Directory

MD < Name > Enter

Or

MKDIR <Name>

We can make another directory within this directory, but to do that we have to be in the directory we had just created.

C:\IES

To change a directory

CD <name>

The prompt would look like

C: \<IES>

Here we can create another directory using the MD MKDIR command. This directory is called as the sub directory within a directory. For e.g.

C:\IES > MD ONE

C:\IES > CD ONE

C:\IES\ONE>

Here ONE is a sub directory of IES.

And IES itself is a sub directory of the root directory, denoted by backslash (\). A subdirectory is also called as the child directory and the directory within which it is present is called as its parent directory.

To change from a subdirectory to its parent directory

CD...

To change from a directory to the root directory

CD\

Note: - To change from one directory to another write the whole path name.

To remove a directory

RD < >

Note: - To remove a directory, it is necessary that the directory to be removed must be empty, i.e. there should be no files or sub directories in that directory. To remove sub directories we have to come to its parent directory and then do the following.

C: \IES\RD ONE

To Delete a File

DEL <filename>

Del [Drive] [path] [filename [\p]

\p – Prompts for confirmation before deleting each file.

ERASE (Drive;] [Path] Filename [\p]

VIEWING the contents of a file

TYPE <filename>

VIEWING the contents of a directory.

Online Help with Commands

MS-DOS version 5.0 includes online help for MS-DOS commands. To get Help with the syntax, parameters, and switches of any MS-DOS command, type the command name followed by / ? on the command line or type Help followed by the command name, for example, for help information about the copy command.

Getting Help

Online Help provides a quick way to get information about MS-DOS shell basics, and using menus, Commands dialog boxes, dialog boxes, dialog box option, and procedures. You can get Help in three ways : by pressing F1, by selecting the Help button that appears in most dialog boxes or by using the Help menu.

To request Help on a menu:

1. Press ALT.
2. Select the menu you want Help by using the LEFT ARROW or RIGHT ARROW key.
3. Press F1

Help window containing information about the selected menu appears.

To request help on a command:

Mouse

1. Click the menu that contains the command we want help on.
2. Select the command we want help on by using the UP ARROW or DOWN ARROW key.
   #. Press F1.

A help window containing information about the selected command appears.

Keyboard

1. Press ALT to select the menu bar.
2. Select the menu that contains the command you want help by using the LEFT ARROW and RIGTH ARROW keys.
3. Select the command you want help on by using the UP ARROW and DOWN ARROW keys.

To request Help on a dialog box option:

1. Open the dialog box you want Help on.
2. Select a command button or option by clicking it, or by using TAB or the arrow keys.
3. Press F1.

If you have selected the Search For box in the Search File dialog box you press F1. MS-DOS shell displays the following help window.

Getting Help on a Related Procedure

Often Help refers to a related procedure. For example, the following Help on the Colour Scheme dialog box contains a reference to the procedure for changing colours.

In Help, related procedures are displayed in colour in reverse video, depending on the color scheme we have selected.

Mouse

Double-click the related procedure.

Help window containing information about the related procedure appears.

Keyboard

1. Press TAB until the related procedure is selected.

2. Press ENTER.

Help window containing information about the related procedure appears.

Using the Help Menu

We can use the commands on the Help menu to view an index of Help topics ; information on the keys we can use with MS-DOS shell : basic skills for working with MS-DOS Shell commands and procedures and information about using the Help system.

To use the Help menu:

Mouse

 From the Help menu, choose the Help category you want.

Either information about the subject or a list of topics related to the subject appears.

Keyboard

1. Press ALT, H.

2. Press the highlighted letter for the help category we want.

Or press the UP ARROW or DOWN ARROW key to select the Help category you want, and then press ENTER.

Either information about the subject or a list of topics related to the subject appears.

The following items are on the Help menu:

Index provides a list of all MS-DOS shell help topics.

MS-DOS shell provides an introduction of using MS-DOS Basics shell.

Keyboard Lists and key combinations we can use with MS-Dos shell.

Commands Explains all MS-DOS shell commands. This information is organized according to the menu in which the command appears. (We can get the same information by selecting a command and then pressing F1.)

Procedures : Provides step-by-step instructions for performing tasks in MS-DOS shell.

Using Help : Provides an introduction to using MS-DOS shell help.

About Shell : Displays copyright and version information of MS-DOS shell.

6.9 Explanation of the DOS Commands

ATTRIB

Displays or charges file attributes. This command displays, sets or removes the read only, archive, system and hidden attribute assigned to files for an introduction to attrib command.

> SYNTAX: ATTRIB [+R-R][+A-A][+S-S][+H-H]
>
> [DRIVE:] [PATH] [FILENAME] [/S]

To display all attributes of all files in the current directory use the following syntax. attrib [drive:] [path] filename

PARAMETERS

Specify the location and name of the file or set files we want to process.

SWITCHES   +R   SETS the read only files attributes.

-R   CLEARS the read only file attributes.

+A   SETS the archive file attributes.

-A   Clears the archive file attributes.

+S   Sets the files as a system file.

-S   Clears the system file attributes.

+H   Sets the files as hidden file.

-H   clears the hidden file attributes.

/S   Possess files in the current directory and all of subdirectories.

CHKDSK

Creates and displays a status report for a disk.

The status report shows logical errors found in the file allocation table (FAT) and file system. If errors exist on the disk, CHKDSK alerts us with a message. You should use CHKDSK occasionally on each disk to check for errors.

The CHKDSK command, available on all versions of DOS, checks the status of selected disk. It is an external DOS command, and displays several important items of information. These include: resident program.

The general form of the CHKDSK command is CHKDSK [drive:]

Syntax

CHKDSK [drive:] [path] [filename [/f] [/v]

To display the status of the disk in the current drive, use the following syntax : chkdsk

Drive : Specifies the drive that contains the disk that we want chkdsk to check [path]. Filename: Specifies the location and name of the file or set of files that we want chkdsk to check, for Fragmentation can use wild cards (*, ?) to specify multiple files.

Switch

/f Fixes errors on the disk

/v Displays the name of each file in every directory as the disk is checked.

CLS

Starts a new instance of instance of the MS-DOS Command interpreter, COMMAND.COM.

DELTREE

Delete a directory and all of its files and subdirectories, including hidden files. Be careful with DELTREE, as it can be very destructive and we not be able to undo our deletions.

Syntax: -

DELTREE [/y] [drive:] path

/y deletes the directory and its files without prompting for confirmation.

Notes

For safety, do not use the Y option.

You can use wildcards in the path, but be extremely careful because wildcards can match filenames as well as multiple directory names.

DEVICE

DEVICE, used only in CONFIG.SYS, installs for optional devices, such as a mouse, RAM disk extended memory.

Loads into memory devices driver we specify.

Syntax: -device high [drive:][path]filename[parameters].

Option: -[drive:][path]filename, drive, directory location, and filename of device driver parameters.

Command line information required by the device driver.

DISKCOMP

The DISKCOMP command is an external command that compares the contents of two floppy disks to ensure they are identical. DISKCOMP is available on all versions of DOS.

The general form of the DISKCOMP Command is :

DISKCOMP A:B:

DISKCOPY

The DISKCOPY command is an external command that is available with all version of DOS. It makes a copy of one removable disk (the source disk) on another (the target disk). The involved diskettes must be of the same size and format for DISKCOPY to operate property. Never specify a fixed disk with the DISKCOPY command. If the target disk is unformatted, DISKCOPY formats it for you during the copy operation.

The form of the DISKCOPY command is,

DISKCOPY A: B:

Where A: is the source disk (the disk being copied) and B: is the target disk (the disk to which the copy is transferred).

With the introduction command makes as exact replica of the source disk. If it is single sided or contains data errors, then the resulting copy is also single sided or contains data errors, also. If we want to copy the first side of a disk, we can use the /1 parameter in the form:

DOSKEY

Start the Doskey program, which recalls MS-DOS commands. edits command lines and creates macros.

The Doskey program is a terminate-and-stay-resident program. Doskey occupies about 3 kilobytes of resident memory.

Syntax :

Doskey [/reinstall] [/bufsize=size] [/macros] [/history] [/insert/overstrike].

FDISK

The FDISK command is an external DOS command that prepares a fixed (or hard) disk to organize our disk into partitions, which allocates disk space to separate usable areas.

Each partition is assigned a logical drive letter, like C, D, and E when more than one partition is used on a single disk device. Because the maximum amount of disk space addressed by DOS versions released prior to 4.014 was 32 megabytes, it was necessary to be familiar with partitioning strategies offered by the FDISK command in order to organize disk drives having storage capacities in excess of the 32 megabyte barriers. Smaller disks are normally given a single DOS partition.

The FDISK command is used after our fixed disk has received a low-level format. The low-level format process is described briefly in Module 37. You may have to perform a low-level format yourself if you purchase a new fixed disk and controller card directly from the manufacturer or distributor. If you purchase a new fixed disk and controller card directly from the manufacturer, distributor or you purchase your computer from a reputable dealer, the fixed disk should be partitioned and formatted for you.

FIND

Beginning with DOS version 2.00, several external commands, called filters, were introduced. These filter commands are used to intercept rearrange, and output selected data. Three filter commands are : SORT, FIND, and MORE.

The find filter is used to search a file for one or more designated characters depending upon the form of the FIND command. Each line having the text string is sent to an output device, such as display on the screen, a file or the printer. The test string is always typed within quotes. There are three parameters available with the FIND command.

/V Display lines not having the designated text string.

/C Counts and displays the number of lines containing the text string.

/N Display the relative line number in front of each line containing the text string.

/i ignore uppercase or lowercase during the search.

A few examples of how the FIND filter is used are shown below. Like SORT, piping commands are also available for use with the FIND command.

ECHO

Turns the command-echoing feature on or off, or displays a message.

When we run a batch program, MS-DOS typically display (echoes) the batch program's commands on the screen. We can turn this feature on or off by using the echo command.

SYNTAX ECHO [ON/OFF]

To use the echo command to display a message, use the following syntax:

ECHO [MESSAGE]

Parameters on/off

Specifies whether to turn the command – echoing feature is on or off. To display the current echo setting, use it without parameter.

FORMAT

When you purchase new floppies, they have to be formatted before they can be used. The FORMAT command is executed by FORMAT followed by a space and then the drive you want to format. Don't forget to put: (colon) after the drive letter.

You can format your floppy with the following command:

FORMAT [drive:] format command creates tracks in the new floppy used.

PATH

The path command is an internal DOS command. The PATH command is used to tell DOS, which directories it should search and where it has to look for a program given in the PATH command.

c:\> path=c:\DBASE <-

MS-BACKUP

The MSBACKUP command available in DOS Ver.6 and later replaced the backup command. The new command combines improved backup capability with easier use. The first time you run the MSBACKUP it configures your system.

For performing proper backup after the command, work automatically through a menu driven interpreter.

To start backup type:

C:\MSBACKUP <-

Now follow the steps given below:

1. At the main screen press Alt-B to backup. The next screen is the backup configuration screen.

(In DOS 6.2 we have the facility to save our setting in the MS backup program in a setup files. If you want to save your own custom setup files then before step 5, press Alt-F, A and then give our setup filename.)

Then the next time we are MSBACKUP press Alt F, o and select setup file from disk or you can start MSBACKUP with the name of a setup file.

Ex=c:>MSBACKUP MSSETUP

MSSETUP is the name of setup file.

TIME

This command is used to set time in current system.

Let's we view or change the system time.

Syntax- Time (hh:mm:ss) (a/b)

hh-hour

mm-minutes

ss-seconds

a/b -A.M./P.M

TREE

Shows graphical display of the names of all directories on a disk. It is an external command.

Tree will also show the names of all files on each directory and subdirectory.

Syntax-TREE (drive:)(path)(/F)(/A).

?F = displays each dir files.

/a = displays the dir with text character rather than GRAPHICS.

TYPE

Provides a quick and easy way to look at the contents of a file.

Syntax – Type (drive:)(path) filename.

To interrupt the TYPE command press Ctrl + Break (or Ctrl+c).

UNDELETE

Allows you to restore files that were erased with the DEL or ERASE command. UNDELETE provides their labels of protection against deletion.

UNFORMAT

You can recover files from an accidental disk format, with the help of this command.

Syntax

UNFORMAT drive: / switches

Switch

/L Lists all files and subdirectories found on the formatted drive.

/P Echoes program messages to the standard printing device.

/TEST Processes, but does not write any changes to the formatted disk.

VER

The VER command was introduced in DOS version 2.00. It is an internal DOS command that displays the version of DOS we are using. To run the VER program, type VER and press Return.

Because several different version of DOS are available, we may wish to determine which version we are using.

VOL

The volume command is internal DOS command that display volume label (or name) of the specified disk. The VOL command is used to check the name of volume.

Syntax

VOL [drive:] (press return)

XCOPY

The XCOPY command is an external command introduced with DOS version 3.20. It is used to selectively copy files from one disk to another, or those files that have been created or modified since the last backup. With the introduction of DSO 6.2, XCOPY prompt you before overwriting an existing file having the same name. The general form of the XCOPY command is,

> XCOPY A: C:\PATH\FILENAME.

This form of the command operates like the copy command. There are a number of options that are added after the target filename to control file selection. The option letter, represented by /X in the following command line example, is quite useful.

> XCOPY A: C: \PATH\FILENAME/X

The value of/X controls the way XCOPY operates. Each of the available value are described in the following list.

/A   Copies files that the archive bit, which is set with the BACKUP and ATTRIB commands, set or a value of one.

/D copies all files that are the same or later than a specified data. The data is added to the command as shown:

> XCOPY A:C: /D:06-21-88

The data is entered in the format mm-dd-yy, or yy-mm-dd

/E   subdirectories are created on the target disk even if the new subdirectory empty. This happens when the command option used prevents the transfer of files within the directories because they do not meet selection criteria.

/M   Copies files having an archive bit value of one. When copied, the archive bit is reset to zero on the source file. This lets you use XCOPY IN BACKUP operations. An archive bit value of one indicate that the file was created or modified since the last BACKUP or XCOPY /M operation.

/P   Displays a (Y/N)? Prompt before copying a file to allow selection.

/S   files Copies from the source disk that are within and subdirectory to the active (or logged) directory path, as XCOPY searches through the directory tree.

This option does not create new directory path on the target disk unless the /E option is also used. If/S is omitted, XCOPY works only within the named directory.

/V   This options verify that data is written properly. As in the COPY command, the /V option slows the copy process.

/W   Displays the prompt "press any key to being copying files(s)". This option is used to let you insert a diskette.

6.10   Special DOS File

6.10.1 The AUTOEXEC.BAT

The AUTOEXEC.BAT file is the most important batch file located in the root directory. This file is read automatically when you boot your PC. This file is useful because it executes a sequence of commands, like setting the path and prompt, etc., as soon as the computer is switched on.

Creating AUTOEXEC.BAT is similar to the creation of any other batch file.

For example, if we want to include the commands for changing the prompt on our screen, setting the path and then clearing the screen, type the following commands:

C:\> COPY CON AUTOEXE.BAT ↵

The cursor will appear on the next line.

TYPE

PROMPT PG ↵

PATH = C:\DOS;C: \LOTUS;C: \DBASE;C: \WE ↵

CLS

After you have finished entering the command, press

^Z ↵

Now each time you switch on your computer, your prompt (C>) will be changed so that it displays the current directory. The PATH command tells DOS to look in the DOS, LOTUS, Dbase and WS directories for program files. At the end, your screen will be cleared by the CLS command.

Note : The name of this file must be spelt correctly; otherwise this batch file will not be executed automatically. Also, this file must be present in the root directory.

6.10.2   The CONFIG.SYS

When we start our computer, DOS carries out certain commands and this batch file will not get your hardware and reserve space in memory for information processing. The file, which contains the command, is called CONFIG.SYS. This file helps enhancing your PC's performance. The commands in your CONFIG.SYS determine how your hardware should work.

Now create the CONFIG.SYS file, go to the root directory and type the following commands:

C:\COPY CON CONFIG.SYS

FILES = 50

BUFFERS =30

^Z

First line creates a file named CONFIG.SYS

In the second line, we specify the maximum number of files that can be opend at a time. Here, we specified 50. This number can be increased or decreased, but this is most option setting. The third line specifies how much memory DOS reserves for transferring information from and to the disks.

^Z is pressed to end the file creation.

To execute CONFIG.SYS, reboot the computer.

Various Important Commands Used in these Files

AUTOEXEC.BAT FILE

"A batch file executed automatically whenever the computer is booted up."

AUTOEXEC.BAT is a batch program that's executed automatically when you start your computer.

Simply type C:\autoexec at the command prompt.

A SIMPLE AUTOEXEC.BAT FILE

```
@ ECHO OFF
C:\DOS\SMARTDRV.EXE
SET DIRCMD=/ON/P
PROMPT$p$g
PATH C:\DOS;C: \WINDOWS,C: \C: \WP51
C: \DOS\CHKDSK C:
C: \DOS/CHKDSK D:
Set Temp=C: \WINDOWS\TEMP
Set Winpmt=Type 'exit'to return to windows $p$g
Mode con rate=32 delay=1
C:\DOS/DOSKEY
undelete/load
```

The command @ECHO OFF prevents DOS from displaying each command as it is executed in the batch program. Most people place '@echo off' Command at the beginning of every batch program.

The Command C:\DOS\MARTDRV.EXE executes the SMART Drive disk caching program.

The Set DIRCMD=/on/p sets the DIRCMD environment variable to specify two automatically switches for the DIR command.

The command PROMPT pg defines the message displayed by the command prompt. This example shows the most widely used prompt command, which displays the current drive and path name followed by the greater than symbol (>). Thus, when we are in the windows directory of drive C the command prompt will display C:\WINDOW> as it awaits our next instruction. We can use any text (Hello, for example) as well as verity of special character combination in the message following the prompt command. The PATH command tells DOS which drives and directories to search and the order in which to search, if a command or program can't be found in memory of the current directory. To enter several paths on the same line separate them with semicolons (;). Do not include any spaces in the line.

The two CHKDSK command check drives C and D for logical errors.

The command SET TEMP = C:\WINDOWS/TEMP

Associates the directory named C:\WINDOWS/TEMP with the TEMP environment variable. DOS uses the TEMP variable.

TABLE: Character Combinations for the prompt command.

TO DISPLAY THIS.....   USE THIS CHARACTER.

$ (DOLLER SIGN) $$

< (LESS THEN SIGN) $L

= (EQUAL SIGN) $Q

> (GRATER THEN SIGN) $G

| (PIPE) $B

ASCII ESCAPE (COAD 27) $E

BACKSPACE (for deleting a $H character written to the command file)

CURRENT TIME $T

CURRENT DATE $D

CURRENT DRIVE AND PATH $P

ENTER LINE FEED (for starting text on the next line) $_

VERSION OF DOS $V

CONFIG.SYS COMMAND

As you known the CONFIG.SYS file is read whenever you start up your computer and contains special commands used to configure your computer's hardware components. A CONFIG.SYS can include any of the commands listed in Table below.

Table 6.1 CONFIG.SYS file command.

FUNCTION	CON.SYS. COMMAND
To specify where DOS should look for keyboard interrupts.	BREAK
To specify the number of buffers and caches	BUFFERS
To designate the time, data decimal separators and other conventions used in a particular country	COUNTRY
To tell DOS which drives to load	DEVICE
To load drives into upper memory	DIVICEHCH
To specify where to load DOS	DOS
To define block device parameters	DRIVPAKM
To specify how many file control blocks (FCBs) can be open at the same time.	FCBS
To include the contents of a configuration block for a specific menu block	INCLIDE
To load memory resident programs	INSTALL
To specify the number of drives	LAST DRIVE
To set the startup menu colours	MENUCOLOUR
To specify the default item in the startup menu	MENUDEFAULT
To set the number key	ON/FF NUMLOCK
To include comments or remarks	REM
To display set or remove environment variable	SET
To specify name and location.	SHELL
To use data stacks for hardware interrupts	STACKS
To define a set of menu item under a Startup menu item.	SUBMEN
To provides special device options	SWITCHES
To verify accuracy of a file written to a disk	VERIFY

6.11   Unix Operating System

6.11.1 What is UNIX?

UNIX is an operating system which was first developed in the 1960s, and has been under constant development ever since. By operating system, we mean the suite of programs, which make the computer work. It is a stable multi-user, multi-tasking system for servers, desktops and laptops.

UNIX systems also have a graphical user interface (GUI) similar to Microsoft Windows, which provides an easy to use environment. However, knowledge of UNIX is required for operations, which aren't covered by a graphical program, or for when there are no windows interface available, for example, in a telnet session.

They are many different versions of Unix, although they share common similarities. The most popular varieties of Unix are Sun Solaris, GNU/Linux and Marcos X.

The UNIX operating system

The UNIX operating system is made up of three parts; the kernel, the shell and the programs.

The Kernel

The kernel is the hub of the operating system: it allocates time and memory to programs and handles the file storage and communication in response to system calls.

As an illustration of the way that the shell and the kernel work together, suppose a user types **rm myfile** (which has the effect of removing the file **my file**). The shell searches the file store for the file containing the program **rm**, and then requests the kernel, through system calls, to execute the program **rm** on **myfile**. When the process **rm myfile** has finished running, the shell then returns the UNIX prompt % to the user, indicating that it is waiting for further Commands.

The Shell

The shell acts as an interface between the user and kernel, when a user logs in, the login program checks the username and password, and then starts another program called the shell. The shell is a command line interpreter (CLI). It interprets the commands the user types in and arranges for them to be carried out. The commands are themselves programs: when they terminate, the shell gives the user another prompt.

The adept user can customize own shell, and users can use different shell on the same machine. Staff and students in the school have the trash shell by default. The trash shell has certain features to help the user inputting commands Filename Completion – by typing part of the name of a command, filename or directory and pressing the [**Tab**] key, the tics shell will complete the rest of the name automatically. If the shell finds more than one name beginning with those letters you have typed, it will beep, prompting you to type a few more letters before pressing the tab key again. History the shell keeps a list of the commands you have typed in. If you need to repeat a command, use the cursor keys to scroll up and down the list or type history for a list of previous commands.

Files and process

Everything in Unix is either a file or a process. A process is an execution program identified by a unique PID.

A file is a collection of data. Users using text editors, running compilers etc, create them.

Examples of files:

- A document (report, essay etc.).
- The text of a program written in some high-level programming language.
- Instruction comprehensible directly to the machine and incomprehensible to a casual user, for example, a collection of binary digits (an executable or binary file).
- A directory, containing information about its contents, which may be a mixture of other directories and ordinary files.

The Directory Structure

All the files are grouped together in directory structure. The file system is arranged in a hierarchical structure, like an inverted tree. The top of the hierarchy is traditionally called **root.**

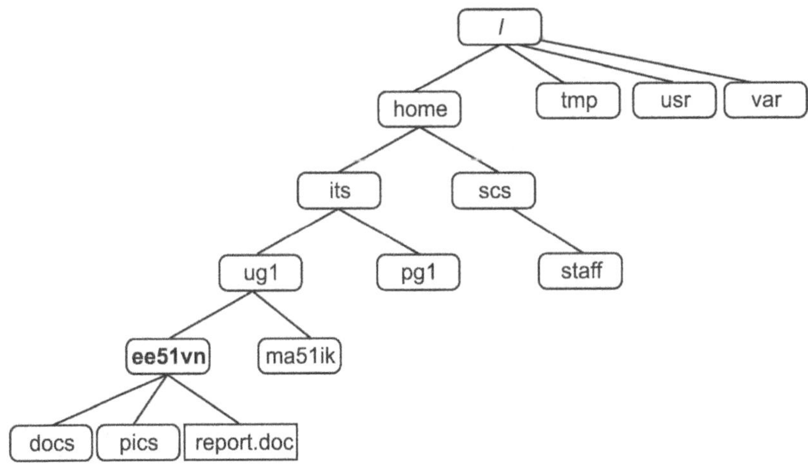

The Directory Structure

CHAPTER 7

Computer Languages

7.1 Introduction

A language is a system of communication. With a natural language such as Hindi, we can communicate with one another our ideas and emotions. Similarly, a computer language is a means of communication. With the help of a computer language, a programmer tells a computer what he wants it to do. A Computer Programming Language is a set of rules that tells the computer what operations to perform. All natural languages (Hindi, French, German etc.) use a standard set of symbols for the purpose of communication. Everyone using those languages understands these symbols. We normally call this set of symbols the vocabulary of that particular language. All computer languages have a vocabulary of their own. Each symbol of the vocabulary has a definite, unambiguous meaning, which can be looked up in the manual of that language. Hence, each symbol of a computer language is used to tell the computer to do a particular job. The main difference between a natural language and a computer language is that computer language uses a very limited or restricted vocabulary. This is mainly because a programming language by its very nature and purpose does not need to say too much. Each and every problem to be solved by a computer has to be broken down into discrete (simple and separate), logical steps which basically comprise four fundamental operations – input and output operations, arithmetic operations, movement of information within the CPU, and logical or comparison operations.

The symbols of a particular computer language must also be used as per prescribed rules, which are known as the syntax rules of the language. Computers, being machines, are receptive only to exact vocabulary used correctly as per syntax rules of the language. Thus, in case of a computer language, we must stick by the exact rules of the language if we want to be understood by the computer. As yet, no computer is capable of correcting and deducing meaning from incorrect instructions. Computer languages are smaller and simpler than natural languages but they have to be used with great precision. Unless a programmer adheres exactly to the syntax rules of a programming language, even down to the correct punctuation marks, the computer will not understand his commands.

7.2   Characteristics of Programming Language

A programming language should possess the following characteristics to be considered as a good high-level language:

(a)   The language should be relatively independent of a given computer system. That is, instead of being machine based, it should be oriented more towards the problem to be solved.

(b)   Each statement of the language should be a macroinstruction that gets translated into many machine language instructions.

(c)   The language should enable the programmers to write instructions using familiar words and mathematical symbols. It should be natural and should use abbreviations and words used in everyday communication.

(d)   The language should be independent of machine language instructions and other pieces of system software except for the compiler or the interpreter.

(e)   The language should not be experimental in nature and should exist on more than one computer system.

7.3   Types of Programming Languages

Programming languages have improved just as computer hardware improved. They have progressed from machine-oriented languages that use strings of binary 1's and 0's to problem-oriented languages that use common mathematical and/or English terms. However, all computer languages can be classified into the following five broad categories:

Machine languages (First Generation Languages – 1945)

Assembly languages (Second Generation Languages – mid 1950s)

High-level languages (Third Generation Languages – early 1960s)

Fourth Generation languages (Very High Level Languages or SQL – early 1970s)

Fifth Generation languages (Natural Languages – early 1980s).

7.3.1   Machine Languages

The set of instruction codes, whether in binary or decimal, which can be directly understood by the CPU of a computer without the help of a translating program, is called a machine code or machine language. This is the basic language of the computer, representing data as 1s and 0s. Machine language programs vary from computer to computer. i.e. they are Machine Dependent.

Advantages and Limitations of Machine Languages

Machine Language is the fundamental language of a computer and is normally written as strings of binary 1's and 0's. The circuitry of a computer is wired in such a way that it immediately recognizes the machine language and converts it into electrical signals needed to run the computer. An instruction prepared in any machine language has two-parts. The first part is the command or operation, and it tells the computer what function to perform. The second part of the instruction is the operand, and it tells the computer where to find or store that data or other instructions that are to be manipulated. Thus, the data field that is involved in the operation. Typical operations involve reading, adding, subtracting, writing, and so on.

As all computers use binary digit (0's and 1's) for performing internal operations, most computers' machine language consists of strings of binary numbers and this is the only number system the CPU directly understands. When stored inside the computer, the symbols, which comprise the machine language program, are made up of 1's and 0's. For example, a typical program instruction to print out a number on the printer might be look like,

    101100111111010001100011000

The program to add two numbers in memory and print the result might look something like the following :

    001100111110001110011001

    110001000011110000110011

    000110000100000010000100000

    100001000001000001000100

This is obviously not a very easy language to learn, because it is difficult to read and understand and it is written in a number system with which we are not familiar.

Programs written in machine language can be executed very fast by the computer. This is mainly because machine instructions are directly understood by the CPU and no translation of the program is required. However, writing a program in machine language has several disadvantages, which are discussed below.

Machine Dependent : The internal design of every type of computer is different from every other type of computer and needs different electrical signals to operate; the machine language differs from computer to computer.

Difficult to Program : Although easily used by the computer, machine language is difficult to program. It is necessary for the programmer either to memorize the dozens of code numbers for the commands in the machine's instruction set or to constantly refer to a reference card.

Error Prone : For writing program in machine language, since a programmer has to remember the op-codes and he must also keep track of the storage location of data and instructions, it becomes very difficult for him to concentrate fully on the logic of the problem. This frequently results in program errors. Hence, there is a large likelihood to make errors while using machine code.

Difficult to Modify *:* It is difficult to correct or modify machine language programs. Checking machine instructions to locate errors is as tedious as writing them initially. Similarly, modifying a machine language program at a later data is so difficult that many programmers would prefer to code the new logic afresh instead of incorporating the necessary modifications in the old program.

7.3.2 Assembly Languages

Assembly languages are one step ahead of machine languages. Assembly language (also called Low Level Language) is a language that allows a programmer to use abbreviations or easily remembered words instead of binary numbers. Each assembly language statement is translated into one-machine instructions by the assembler program. To program in an assembly language, we have to be well-versed in the computer's architecture. Unless well-documented, assembly language programs can be extremely difficult to maintain.

Assembly languages are hardware dependent; there is a different assembly language for each CPU series, and their language statements are quite different. In the past, systems software (operating systems, database managers, etc.) was written in assembly language to maximize the machine's performance.

Advantages of Assembly Languages over Machine Languages

Assembly languages have the following advantages over machine languages:

Easier to Understand and Use *:* Assembly languages are easier to understand and use because mnemonics are used instead of numeric op-codes and suitable names are used for data. The use of mnemonics means that comments are usually not needed; the program itself is understandable. Symbolic programming also saves a lot of time and effort of the programmer because it is easier to write as compared to machine language programs.

Easy to Locate and Correct Errors *:* While writing programs in an assembly language, fewer errors are made, and those that are made are easier to find and correct because of the use of mnemonics and symbolic field names. Furthermore, assemblers are so designed that they automatically catch errors. If we use an invalid mnemonic or a name that has never been defined, the assembler will print out an error indication. For example, suppose one instruction in the symbolic program reads ADD SUM, and we forget to define what SUM is, the assembler will look through its table to find whether SUM is earlier defined or not. If not, it will indicate the error.

Easier to Modify *:* Assembly language programs are easier for people to modify than machine-language programs. This is mainly because they are easier to understand and hence it is easier to locate, correct, and modify instructions as and when desired. Moreover, insertion or removal of certain instructions from the program does not require change in the address part of the instructions following that part of the program. This is required in case of machine languages.

No Need to Track Addressee : One of the greatest advantages of assembly language is that it relieves us of worrying about addresses for instructions and data. This is more important than it seems at first glance. Suppose we have written a long machine language program involving many steps and many reference to itself within the program, such as looping, and address modifications, and so on. At the very end, we may suddenly discover that we have left out an instruction in the middle. If we insert that entire program to check any reference to other steps, it is a tedious job. But if we write the same program in symbolic language, we merely add the extra instruction at their right place, and the assembler will take care of step numbering automatically.

Easily Relocatable : Suppose that an assembly language program starts at address 2000 and we suddenly find that we have another program to be used with this program and this program also starts at location 2000. Obviously, one of the two programs will have to be rewritten or moved somewhere else. In machine language, this can be a complicated job. But in case of assembly language, we merely have to change the first statements. For example, instead of:

  START PROGRAM AT 2000 AND START DATA AT 3000,

  we merely change this first statement to :

  START PROGRAM AT 3000 AND START DATA AT 4000,

  and run the symbolic program once more through the assembler.

Efficiency : In addition to the above-mentioned advantages, an assembly language program also enjoys the efficiency of its corresponding machine code because there is one-to-one correspondence between the instructions of an assembly language program and its corresponding machine language program. There is one-to-one relationship between symbolic and machine codes.

Limitations of Assembly Languages

Machine Dependent : Because each instruction in the symbolic language is translated into exactly one machine language instruction, assembly languages of the processor being used.

Knowledge of Hardware required : Since assembly languages are machine dependent, so the programmer has to be aware of particular machines' characteristics and requirements as the program is written. An assembly language programmer must know how his machine works and should have a good knowledge of the logical structure of his computer in order to write a good assembly language program.

Machine Level Coding : In case of an assembly language, instructions are still written at the machine-code level, i.e. one assembler instruction is substituted for one machine-code instruction.

Machine and assembly languages being machine dependent, are referred to as low-level language. In general, assembly languages are termed one-for-one in nature, i.e. each assembly language instruction will result in one machine language instruction.

A language in which each statement is directly translated into a single machine code is known as a low-level language. Examples of low-level languages are assembly languages of various processors.

7.3.3 High-Level Languages

To overcome the difficulties associated with assembly languages, high-level or procedure-oriented languages have been developed. High-level languages permit programmers to describe tasks in a form, which is problem-oriented rather than computer-oriented. One can formulate problems more efficiently in a high-level language. The programmer does not need to have a precise knowledge of the architecture of the computer he is using.

The instructions written in high-level languages are called statements. The statements more clearly resemble English and mathematics as compared to mnemonics in assembly languages. Examples of high-level languages are BASIC, PASCAL, FORTRAN, COBOL, ALGOL, PL-II, PROLOG, LISP, ADA, SNOBOL, etc.

Advantages of High-Level Languages

High-level languages enjoy the following advantages over assembly and machine languages:

Machine Independence : High-Level languages are machine independent. This is a very valuable advantage. Thus a program written in a high-level language can be run on many different types of computers with very little or practically no modification.

Easy to Learn and Use : These languages are very similar to the languages normally used by us in our day-to-day life. Hence they are easy to learn and use. The programmer need not learn much about the computer he is using. The programmer does not have to necessarily know the machine instructions, the data format, and so on.

Few Errors : In case of high-level languages, since the programmer need not write the entire small steps carried out by the computer, he is much less likely to make errors. The computer takes care of all the little details, and will not introduce any error of its own unless something breaks down. Furthermore, compilers are so designed that they automatically catch and point out the errors made by the programmer. Hence, diagnostic errors, if any, can be easily located and corrected by the programmer.

Lower Preparation Cost *:* Writing programs in high-level language requires less time and effort, which ultimately leads to lower program preparation cost. Generally, the cost of all phases of program preparation (coding, debugging, testing, etc.) is lower with a high-level language than with an assembly language or with a machine language.

Better Documentation *:* A high-level language is designed in such a way that its instructions may be written more like the language of the problem. Thus a person familiar with the problem can easily understand the statements of a program written in a high-level language. For the documentation of such programs, very few or practically no separate comment statements are required.

Easier to Maintain *:* Programs written in high-level languages are easier to maintain than those in assembly languages or machine languages. This is mainly because high-level language programs are easier to understand and hence it is easier to locate, correct, and modify instructions as and when desired. Insertion or removal of certain instructions from a program is also possible without any complication. Thus, major changes can be incorporated with very little effort.

Limitations of High-Level Languages

Two disadvantages of high-level languages are:

Lower Efficiency *:* Generally, a program written in an assembly language or machine language is more efficient than the one written in a high-level language. That is, the programs written in high-level languages take more time to run and require more main memory.

Lack of Flexibility *:* Because the automatic features of high-level languages always occur and are not under the control of the programmer, they are less flexible than assembly languages. An assembly language provides programmers access to all the special features of the machine they are using. This lack of flexibility means that some tasks cannot be done in a high-level language, or can be done only with great difficulty.

In most cases, the advantages of high-level languages far outweigh the disadvantages. Most computer installations use a high-level language for most programs and use an assembly language for doing special tasks that cannot be easily done otherwise.

Difference between Assembly Languages and High-Level Language

One statement of a high-level language corresponds to many instructions of the assembly language program. Hence, a high-level program is much shorter compared to an assembly language program.

Many high-level languages have been developed; some are for general purpose and some for special purposes. For example, PASCAL, PL-II and ADA are general purpose languages. FORTRAN and APL are for scientists and engineers. They are designed to solve mathematical problems. COBOL is for business applications. BASIC is for newcomers to programming. PROLOG is based on logical reasoning and used for artificial intelligence (i.e. expert system). SNOBOL is suitable for text processing. APT is used in manufacturing applications to control machine tools.

Brief Description of some popular High-Level Languages

Ada : A high-level programming language was developed in the late 1970s and early 1980s for the United States Defense Department. Ada was designed to be a general-purpose language for everything from business applications to rocket guidance systems. One of its principal features is that it supports real-time applications. In addition, Ada incorporates modular techniques that make it easier to build and maintain large systems. Since 1986, Ada has been the mandatory development language for most U.S. military applications. In additions, Ada is often the language of choice for large systems that require real-time processing, such as banking and air traffic control systems. Ada is named after Augusta Ada Byron (1815-52), daughter of Lord Byron, and Countess of Lovelace. She helped Charles Babbage develop programs for the analytic engine, the first mechanical computer. She is considered by many to be the world's first programmer.

BASIC : It is an abbreviation for Beginners All-purpose Symbolic Instruction Code. It is a very simple and easy language. It is suitable for scientific computations. But it is not as powerful as FORTRAN. It was introduced in 1965 by Dartmouth College, UK. It is a widely-used language for simple computations and analysis. It is the most popular high-level language used in personal computers. To translate BASIC instructions into machine language codes, interpreters are frequently used in PC systems. But BASIC language compliers are also available for these systems.

FORTRAN : It is an abbreviation for *Formula Translation*. IBM introduced it in 1957. It is a very useful language for scientific and engineering computations as it contains many functions for complex mathematical operations. It is a compact programming language. Huge libraries of engineering and scientific programs written in FORTAN are available to users. It is not suitable for processing large business files i.e. COBOL. It has a number of versions. Earlier, FORTRAN IV was very popular. In 1977 the American National Standard Institute (ANSI) published a standard for FORTRAN called FORTRAN 77 so that all manufacturers could use the same form of the language. The latest version is known as FORTRAN 90.

APL : IBM has developed APL. It is a very powerful language. It permits users to define instructions. It contains a large library of pre-determined functions. It is used with personal computers and also with larger systems. It can perform complex arithmetic-logic operations with a single command. It is designed for mathematical work and provides more facilities than FORTRAN. It is very complex and has no commercial applications. Mathematician uses it. It requires special keyboards and terminals because its instructions entirely consist of geometric shapes and symbols.

C Language : A high-level program developed by Dennis Ritchie and Brian Kernighan at Bell Labs in the mid-1970s. Although originally designed as a systems programming language, C has proved to be a powerful and flexible language that can be used for a variety of applications, from business programs to engineering. It is a popular language for personal computer programmers because it is relatively small – it requires less memory than other languages.

The first major program written in C was the UNIX operating system, and for many years C was considered to be interlinked with UNIX. However, C is important independent language of UNIX.

Although it is a high-level language, C is much closer to assembly languages than other high-level languages. This closeness to the underlying machine language allows C programmers to write very efficient code. The low-level nature of C, however, can make the language difficult to use for some types of applications.

C++ : A high-level programming language developed by Bjarne Stroustrup at Bell Labs. C++ adds object-oriented features to its predecessor; C. C++ is one of the most popular programming languages for graphical applications, such as those that run in Windows and Macintosh environments.

PROLOG : It is suitable for developing programs involving complex logical operations. It is used primarily for artificial intelligence applications. It was developed in France. The Japanese have chosen this language as a standard language for their fifth generation computer project. It is quite suitable for handling large databases and for producing rules-based expert systems applications. PROLOG stands for *Pro*gramming in *Log*ic. It is based on mathematical logic. Most of high-level languages like BASIC, COBOL, FORTRAN or PASCAL are not based on the principles of mathematical logic. These languages were designed to provide efficient computation and data manipulation. They enable us to use computers for computations data manipulation purposes. But today computers are also being used to provide conclusions based on intelligent reasoning. For such a purpose programming languages based on the principle of mathematical logic are needed. PROLOG is based on the first order predicate calculus. PROLOG consists of a set of facts and rules that describe objects and relations between objects in a given domain. The statements that are unconditionally true are called facts, while rules provide properties and relations which are true depending on given conditions. Many expert systems have been developed. They perform operations based on logical reasoning and provide conclusions.

LISP : It stands for *LIS*T Processing. McCarthy developed this language in the early 1960s. It is suitable for non-numeric operations involving logical operations. It is used extensively in artificial intelligence and pattern recognition. It is also used in game playing, theorem proving etc. It is capable of searching, handling and sorting long string of lists of text. So it has often been used to implement computerized translators. It is used primarily on larger computers but LISP compilers are also available for PCs.

SNOBOL : It stands for String Oriented Symbolic Language. A group led by Griswold in the mid 1960s developed this language. It can manipulate strings of characters and hence it is used in text processing. It is capable of performing various types of operations on strings of characters such as combining strings, splitting strings, matching strings etc.

LOGO : Seymour Papert and his colleagues at MIT developed it in the late 1960s. It has also been popularized as a first educational language that children can use to achieve intellectual growth and problem-solving skills. LOGO has graphics capability. Children can easily use it to make drawings. They can draw colour and animate images. It runs of PCs. It is used to compose music, manipulate text, manage data, etc.

APT : It stands for Automatically Programmed Tooling. It is used in manufacturing applications to control machine tools.

MODULA-2 : Nicklaus Wirth, the creater of PASCAL, has developed it. Although it retains the merits of PASCAL, it is more powerful and easier to use. PASCAL programs can easily be translated into MODULO-2 codes. It is a strongly structural language. It is easier for the compiler to find programming errors than it is with other languages. Structured programming also results in well-planned program steps, which produce more efficient and trouble-free software.

JAVA : A high-level programming language developed by Sun Microsystems. Java was originally called OAK, and was designed for handheld devices and set-top boxes. OAK was unsuccessful. So in 1995 Sun changed the name to Java and modified the language to take advantage of the World Wide Web.

Java is an object-oriented language similar to C++, but simplified to eliminate language features that cause common programming errors. Java source code files (files with a java extension) are compiled into a format called byte code (files with a class extension), which can then be executed by a Java interpreter. Compiled Java code can run on most computers because Java interpreters and runtime environments, known as Java Virtual Machines (VMs), exist for most operating systems, including UNIX, the Macintosh OS, and Windows. Byte code can also be converted directly into machine language instructions by a just in time compiler (JIT). Java is a general purpose programming language with a number of features that make the language well suited for use on the World Wide Web. Small Java applications are called Java applets and can be downloaded from a Web server and run on your computer by a Java-compatible Web browser, such as Netscape Navigator or Microsoft Internet Explorer.

7.3.4 Fourth Generation Languages (4GLS)

A very high-level language is often a 4GL (4th generation language). 4GLs are much more user-oriented and allow programmers to develop programs with fewer commands compared with third-generation languages. 4GLs are called non-procedural because programmers cannot write the programs that need only tell the computer what they want done, not all the procedures for doing it. That is, they do not have to specify all the programming logic or otherwise tell the computer how the task should be carried out. This saves programmers a lot of time because they do not need to write as many lines of code as they do with procedural languages.

Fourth generation languages consist of report generations, query languages, application generators, and interactive database management system (DBMS) programs. Some 4GLs tools are applicable for end-users and some for programmers.

Difference between 4GLs and High-Level languages

   (i) The 4GLs are often easier to use than high-level languages.

  (ii) The 4GLs are not supported by the industry standards. They offer less control over output results than do high-level languages.

 (iii) 4GLs do not use hardware resources as efficiently as do the high-level languages. Therefore, most application programs are written in high level languages only.

4GLs will probably not replace third-generation language because they are usually focused on specific tasks, hence offer options, still, they improve productivity because programs are easy to write.

7.3.5 Fifth Generation: Natural Languages

Natural languages are of two types: The first are ordinary human languages : Hindi, English, German, French, Spanish, and so on. The second are programming languages that use human language to give people a more natural connection with computers. Some of the query languages mentioned above under 4GLs might seem pretty close to human communication, but natural languages – which are still in their infancy – try to be even closer.

Natural languages allow questions or commands to be framed in a more conversational way or in alternative forms. For example, with a natural language, you might be able to state:

"I want the sales of personal computers for Madhya Pradesh and Chhatisgarh broken down by city for January and February. Also, I need January and February sales list by cities for laser printers sales in Keral and Madhya Pradesh".

Natural languages are part of the field of study known as artificial intelligence. Artificial intelligence (AI) is a group of related technologies that attempt to develop machines to emulate human like qualities, such a learning, reasoning, communicating, seeing and hearing.

Query languages : A Query language is an easy-to-use language for retrieving data from a database management system. The query may be expressed in the from of a sentence or the query may be obtained from choices on a menu.

Examples of query languages are SQL (Structured Query Language), QBE (Query-By-Example), and Intellect. For example, with Intellect, which is used with IBM mainframes, you can pose an English language command such as 'Tell me the number of employees in the purchase department.'

CHAPTER 8

Concept of Programming

8.1 Introduction

Systems analyst, familiar with both management and data processing, would probably be assigned the responsibility for working out a detailed, technical solution that satisfies the user.

The first event leading to the preparation of a computer task is someone's decision that here is a need for information – perhaps management requests the preparation of a report, or operating personnel may request a new or improved record-keeping procedure to prove data for decision making, or it may be as subsystem in the master information system development. The starting point for the design of any computer program must be a proper specification of its intended behaviors. It is most usual to describe this behaviors pattern in terms of the necessary inputs and the required outputs. The programmer's problem is then transferred to design a process (or algorithm), which will, give the correct inputs, derive from them the required output.

In addition to the descriptions of these input and outputs, a program specification may include a description of any constraints, which must apply to the solution. These may include details of run time and/or space limitations, available equipment and utilities, as well as project deadlines.

Within a program specification, the definitions of the inputs and outputs must include a description of their meaning, so that the programmer can understand the relationship between them.

For instance, one may need a program to find the area of a triangle given the lengths of its three sides. Such statement of the problem is almost a complete specification the programmer needs to know only the properties of triangles in order to handle it. The problem as stated has meaning only because we understand the terms "triangle" "area" and "side", and their inter-relationships. If, on the other hand, the specification is "given X, Y and Z, compute A". It would be meaningless without a definition of A, X, Y and Z.

A program needs to be fully specified, because it is part of a larger system and its design must be consistent with the method used overall. In a commercial environment, the specification would come from a systems analyst, or systems manager, who studies user requirements and is responsible for the design and coordination of a software project. The analyst hands over the specifications to a team of programmers, each of who works on a set of programs.

To help a programmer understand a particular program's position, the entire system should be clear. Since an overall system's specification should be known before individual programs are specified, all the programmer needs to do is study the documentation. He or she should find, among other things, an overall system description in diagrammatic form. This may take the form of a system run chart, showing all files and programs involved or it may be a data flow diagram, in which specific files are not mentioned. In either case the role played by the particular program under consideration should be clear.

The program gains a name according to the naming in use; also, in addition to a description of the program, inputs and outputs in the form of details record formats, the programmer will probably receive a description of the function of the program in some form.

8.2 Task Analysis

Any program written in a business environment is part of a software system to carry out a certain processing task. An actual data processing package would consist of a large number of programs, each handling one activity. For example, in a software package used by a sales department, one program may enter daily sales into data files. Another program uses the records to these data files to produce a particular report.

Information is the basis for action both by personnel within an organization and by persons outside (e.g. customers, suppliers, government agencies). The analysis of need and development of specification should involve both a system's analyst and the people who will use the program. The participation of those who need the data is important because of their knowledge of the function being studied and because of the human relations problems, which develop, if a system is designed for their use without them handling it.

Participation by a system's analyst early in the definition stage is important because he or she has the background to perceive ways in which the full power of the computer may be used to assist the decision process. Frequently, a program is designed from the specifications furnished by the users without considering the decisions to be made and other uses for the output. The resulting programs have frequently been found to be inadequate because the definition was incomplete or did not consider the use of new computer based analytical and computation techniques.

Based on the rough specifications for the application, the programmer designs a program which best meets the need considering the limits imposed by the facilities and personnel which can be used and the costs which can be justified by the value of the results to be achieved. He or she must make decisions with respect to processing method, types of file media, frequency of processing, etc., to balance the cost and value or alternative approaches. In all matters affecting the users, he or she should consult with them so that these decisions will be understood and accepted.

Some of the questions, which need to be answered in the task analysis and design phase, are:

For Source Documents

- What source documents must be provided, how often, any by whom?
- How will information on the source document be transcribed to machine-readable forms?
- What is the layout of the source document and computer input form?

For Files

- Which computer files will be maintained?
- What type of file media and file organization will be used?
- What will be the size of the file and the growth rate?
- What is the layout of the computer record and the computer file?

For Processing

- What processing, computerized or mechanical is required?
- How frequently must processing be performed?
- What volume of transactions must be processed?
- What processing approach will be used?
- What off-line equipment will be necessary?

For Output

- What is format of the report?
- To whom will the report be distributed?

The result of this analysis of need is a set of specifications outlining the information needs. The specifications describe the problem, the data to be provided, the persons to receive the output, the frequency of output, and an estimate of the volume of transactions to be processed. Essentially, it is a statement of user needs.

8.3 Data Analysis and Input Design

Input design is the process of converting an external, user-oriented description of the inputs into a machine-oriented format. In most business systems, devices operated by humans generate inputs. In these cases, the input design must take into account the human element in order to ensure rapid and accurate data entry from a source document. This will prevent error and speed up data entry. Two important rules to follow in designing source documents for data entry are:

1. Lay out the data elements in sequence so that the data entry operator can follow easily. The normal sequence of data entry is from left to right and from top to bottom of the page.

2. Group the data elements to be entered separately from those that are not to be entered. This means that the data entry operator does not have to hesitate while skipping over fields that are not to be stored or processed.

It must be remembered that digital computers do not make any mistakes. This implies that computer errors can generally be traced to incorrect input data or unreliable programs – both caused by human failures and not due to computer fragilities.

8.4 Output Identification and Specifications

8.4.1 Printer and Page Layouts

The next step is the production of output. Printing on screens provide one option, but printed reports are more permanent. The stationery used can be continuums or consist of single sheet. Sometimes the system design will demand preprinted forms (documents containing fixed spaces which will be filled in with printed data from the computer).

The page length and width used on the printer are standardized as part of the specification. The number of characters per line would normally vary from 80 to 160 normal sized characters (with a larger range if the size is changed, this is only possible in case of dot matrix printers). The page contains heading lines, data lines and footer lines spaced by top, bottom, right, and left margins.

A line of column headings normally follows the main heading, such as the name of the company, and one or more subheadings, such as the name of the report. The main body of the report contains the detail-lines of figures filling the columns. At the end, footing lines contain such data as page totals and page numbers. Some of the headings would be repeated on every new page if the report goes to more than one page, while the footing line is generated as soon as the compute senses that a page is about to end. At the end of the report there may be special lines giving final totals and messages.

To prepare a print layout chart, people use special sheet, marketed like graph paper, with a square for every print position (character space) on the printed page. The print layout is indicated on this by specifying print positions, margins, and messages.

The length of the paper and the number of characters to appear on each line are usually fixed by the programmers; the number of lines is a maximum of six per inch ; for example, 11 inch paper will allow up to 66 lines on each page. Normally there are unused areas of between three and ten lines at the top of the page, and between five and ten lines at the bottom – the top and bottom margins. The rest of the page forms the print area. This is further divided into a heading area, a place for the body of the report, and a footing area. The header usually comprises a main heading line, one or more blank lines, and then a line of column headings. Between these and the details lines, there is usually a line of dashes, or other special characters.

8.4.2 Screen and Page Layouts

A display screen, on the other hand, normally allows up to 24 lines with 80 characters per lines. Within this area there can be heading, prompts, data lines, and error messages. Note that it may be necessary to overlay on the screen several times with new data within a program, without erasing the entire screen each time. A screen layout chart is similar to the print layout chart except that the number of lines is restricted to 24.

	Top Margin *	
	Header	
Left Margin	Data Lines (Details lines)	Right Margin
	Footer	
	Bottom Margin	

On a display screen the same area is used over and over again with screen formats of different types replacing each other, or being overlaid. When writing a program which uses the screen, take care to erase the remains of printed messages when they are not longer required.

A significant difference compared to producing a printed report is, in the "scrolling" which screens offer instead of a page by report, is in the "scrolling" which screen offer instead of a page report display.

It is often a temptation for a programmer to introduce special variations into the screen display, but do not forget that using a monitor is a strain on the eyes. It is therefore important to minimize the amount of reading that the user has to do, and to avoid extremes of intensity (brightness and colour) and unnecessary intensity variations.

Special effects at sing-on or between screens may be attractive to first- time users of an application, but if they are time-consuming, they can become irritating to someone who uses the package frequently. The main aim of having a computer is to speed up the work of the user – let your programs give the maximum assistance with the minimum of interference.

Having a standard design philosophy ensures that there is no major variation in the method of data entry from screen to screen within the application. The user quickly learns the conventions of the package and does not have to adjust to each new screen in different way.

The messages the program offers the user are of many types :

- Error reports produced by validation routines, and by procedures that write to files.
- Help messages explaining difficult or unusual procedures.
- Prompts (requests) for data entry.
- System message explaining long delays or system problems.

One standard practice is to allot special areas on the screen to different message types. This allows the user to adjust to each new screen more easily, and also given the programmer the freedom to display and erase messages of one type without affecting any of the others.

The same errors and special conditions can come up at any different point within a program – so it is a good idea to have a consistent approach when handling these. It is therefore better to have module dedicated to error and special conditions, and to re-use these at different points, as required.

Concurrently, most programs accept data on to backing storage work interactively via a screen. The usefulness of these programs depends on the programmer's ability to design screens which:

- Are easy to read and fill out as forms.
- Allow free cursor movement for easy correction and verification of the input data.
- Give message that are easy to interpret.

One of the most important facilities required by the user is the ability to abort an entry at the point. Thus do not make it necessary to fill out an entire form if one wishes to cancel the entry. This requires certain flexibility in the control, which terminates the entry of one screen of data.

Data entry programs allow the user to enter new or to edit (amend) existing data. A screen for editing previous data looks like a data entry screen, but, instead of having blank areas to be filled in, shows the existing record so the user can decide whether to make any changes or not. A good program will allow you to move to any data field easily, either retaining or amending the intermediate data items as you wish.

Any screen-oriented menu-driven program must ask users what they want done. This normally involves listing a number of options with a prompt saying how to choose. The choice lands to the next appropriate screen. This gives us a hierarchy ("tree") of screens through which the user can enter of leave any option.

As in all applications you must allow the user to quit or return to an earlier one (or quit the program altogether) whenever desired. Thus, if a wrong key entry is made, the situation can immediately be as one of the choices. Similarly, when a particular action has been concluded, it is better to present the next higher level menu again and allow the user to decide the next move, rather than asking "Do you wish to continue?" over and over again.

8.4.3 Designing

It is essential that the overall program strategy should be completely charted out before the detailed programming actually begins. The way the programmer can concentrate initially on the general program logic, without bothering for the syntactical details of the individual instructions. This overall planning process may then be repeated several times, with more programming detail added at each stage. Thus, the programmer can gradually shift his or her attention from the overall computation strategy to the details of the individual instructions. Such an approach is often referred to as "top-down" programming.

A problem specification is generally given in terms of a desired relation between inputs and outputs, which specifies what is to be computed. An algorithm or program for a given problem specifies how the given relation between inputs and outputs is to be achieved. It is the task of the programmer to convert "static" input/output specifications of what is to be computed into dynamic specifications that specify how the computation is to be performed.

A given input/output relation may be realized by a wide variety of different algorithms, and each algorithm may in turn be realized in a variety of different programming languages. Thus there is considerable freedom in developing a program for the solution of any given problem. This freedom of choice in developing programs lead to the notion that programming is an art rather than a science.

Although the set of all programs for realizing a given problem specification is in general infinite, there are a number of criteria other than correctness, which may be used to restrict the class of acceptable programs that realize a given problem specification.

A good program should economize both computation time and the storage space required to represent the program and data structures. A well-defined sub program should specify it. Modular design of a program is important because it makes the program easier to understand, facilitates debugging, and allows modifications to be made more easily. It is usually worth paying a price in computation time and memory space in order to achieve greater modularity. Modular construction is especially important in large programs. Since the human mind is severely limited in the complexity it can handle, and systematic modularity reduces the number of factors the human mind must handle at any given moment, thereby allowing the understanding of a large system than would otherwise be possible.

Programming is the process of converting broad system specifications into usable machine instructions that produce desired results. Programmers must answer the following questions during the program design.

1. Have the problem specifications been spelled out clearly and completely? Little significant progress can be made until the programmer can answer "yes" to this question.

2. Am I familiar with a solution method that will solve the problem?

   If the programmer knows a procedure that will solve the problem, the solution may then be coded in a selected language. If this is not the case, the next question must be considered.

3. Can I locate a solution method to solve the problem from other people or from books or journals? If a method can be located, the solution may be coded. Otherwise, the next question must be answered.

4. How can I develop a procedure that will solve this problem?

This question often challenges programmers, and a modular design approach (considered below) is often used at this time to reduce a large (and seemingly unmanageable) problem into smaller tasks that are easier to solve.

Several programming analysis tools are available to help people develop problem solutions. One such tool is the program flow chart. It is a detailed chart to represent steps to be carried out within the machine to produce the needed output.

A commercial program is designed to meet the needs of the customer who will be its ultimate user. The outputs and reports, the screen messages and questions, and the inputs required – the user must understand all these and find them similar to those already in use. The users should therefore have as close connection as possible with specifying the requirements. When they are satisfied, they will generally have to issue a formal "acceptance" of the specifications, by signing relevant documents. Because the programmer may not get a chance to interact with the users themselves, they must be able to understand the specifications and follow them rigidly. Any improvements, which they would like to suggest, should be raised at the appropriate meetings.

Moreover, because he or she is part of a team, the programmer must document his or her programs in a predetermined way, so that the rest of the team can easily understand them. This sometimes means that programmers who are new to a team have the additional burden of adapting to the standards for specifications and documentation that are already in use by the team as a whole.

Following steps are involved in designing the solution :

1. Planning the program

2. Coding of instructions

3. Translation (compilation)

4. Debugging

5. Documentation.

8.4.4 Decision Tables

Decision tables are graphic method for describing the logic of decisions. In a tabular format, the decision table lists a set of conditions plus a set of actions and identifies different combinations of decisions, which lead to different combination of actions. These different combinations are termed rules.

A decision table is simply a table showing the various actions to be taken for different combination of conditions. Since it specifies only the logic rules involved, and says nothing about the procedure used, a decision table is more problem oriented than a flowchart (which is solution oriented). The tables are more useful than flowcharts as an aid to program design.

The four basic elements of a decision table are:

- Condition stub

- Condition entry

- Action stub

- Action entry.

The condition stub and condition entries describe the conditions to be tested, while the action stub and action entries concern the actions to be taken. In a decision table these four elements form quadrants, as shown below :

Condition stub	Condition entries
Action stub	Action entries

Fig. 8.1 Layout of Decision tables.

The table lists all the conditions relating to a procedure, one below the other, in the condition stub; the action stub lists all possible actions. The condition entries and actions entries together constitute one or more "rules", which run vertically through the two right-hand quadrants. Each rule indicates the actions needed when a particular set of conditions applies.

There are two types of decision tables:

1. Limited Entry Table:

- It gives the simple conditions as Yes/No, so the actions related are: "execute" or "do not execute".

2. Extended Entry Table

- It has conditions more than two possible states Yes/No. So there are many options of actions related.

Conditions and actions are connected by "if...then..." relationship. If the specified condition exists then perform the indicated action.

If condition is met   (Yes)

If condition is not met   (No)

If conditions is in between   (-) (neither Yes nor No)

Another form of decision table is Mixed table in which all values like (Y), (N) & (-) are entered.

Since an extended entry table is an extension of limited entry table the explanation will concentrate first on the latter, and some comments about the former will follow. The action stub lists all actions, which can follow from the stated conditions. The action entries identify with X whose actions are to be taken for a rule. A black means the action is not to be taken for that rule

Heading	Rule numbers
Condition Stub	Condition entries
Action Stub	Action entries

Fig. 8.2 Basic configuration of decision table.

One of the powerful analytical features of a limited entry decision tables is that for a given set of conditions and actions, one can analyze whether or not all the rules have been stated. There are theoretically two rules for separate conditions. This follows from the number of combinations of the two conditions Y and N. In other words, four conditions would result in 24 or 16 rules. A set of eight conditions would require 256 rules, which give a large table. However, in practice the table need not be so large, because many of the rules are redundant. It is also possible to eliminate conditions, decision table should be eliminate of unnecessary conditions, testing for completeness, and elimination of redundant (unnecessary) rules.

A decision table may be used in conjunction with flowchart. For example, the flowchart may have a section that is more clearly represented by a decision table. As shown in the margin, a predefined process box in the flowchart represents this section ion, which reference the decision table.

The decision table may be used both for manual procedures and for computer program logic. It is very useful when collecting data from users on the logic they wish to have applied to a problem to organize it into a decision table. It helps to bring out any undefined rules (conditions without specified actions) and is more understandable to the users than a flowchart.

One of the useful applications of decision tables is in the analysis of rules, regulations, and procedures, For example, using decision tables to analyze government regulations, French officials discovered 44 classes of persons, the regulations excluded from entering France who where supposed to be admissible.

1. List conditions and actions.
2. Combine conditions that describe both possibilities.
3. Make yes or no responses (Y or N).
4. Mark actions to be taken for each rule with X.
5. Check for completeness.
6. Combine redundant rules to simplify table.
7. Record table for most understandable order of rules.

The explanation will emphasize a systematic procedure for developing a decision table. As an analyst or programmer develops some skill, he/she may be able to arrive more directly at the final table. The beginner should proceed carefully and systematically.

Example

A university has the following criteria for deciding to admit students to its graduate schools.

Admit a student who has undergraduate grades of A or better, has test scores on the admission test of over 500, and has a grade average of A or better for the past two years. Also, admit if the overall grade average is less than A but the last two-year's average is A or better and the test score is over 600. Admit on probation if the overall and 2-year grade averages are A or better but test score is 600 or less. Admit on probation if overall grade is A or better and test score is above 600 but last 2 years are below A. Also, admit on probation if overall grades are less than A average and test score is 600 or less, but grades for past two years are A or better. Refuse to admit all others.

Solution

Step first: to write down all of the conditions and actions.

Conditions

1. Undergraduate grades of A or better.
2. Test scores of over 600.
3. Grade average of A or better in past 2 years.
4. Test score of 600 or less.
5. Grades less than A last 2 years.
6. Overall grade average less than A.

Action

1. Admit.
2. Admit on probation.
3. Do not admit.

In second step we will combine conditions, which describe the only two possibilities of a single condition. In this case, "Test scores over 600" and "test scores of 600 or less" can be combined. A single condition "test scores over 600" can represent both because a "No" answer means test score 600 or below. The same reasoning allows the combination of 1 and 6 and also 3 and 5. There are thus only three conditions.

1. Undergraduate of A or better.
2. Test scores of over 600
3. Grade average of a better past 2 years.

Step three is to prepare the yes and no responses using Y and N all possible combinations and conditions. Then for each set of conditions mark the action(s) to be taken with an X. The number of rules to be handled in the step is 2, where N is the number of conditions. In the example there are three conditions, so there will be 2, 3 or 8 rules. The Y's and N's can be inserted in any order, but a systematic method will reduce the effort of filling in the table and then alternating between N and Y. Writing two Y's and four N's fill in the row above this. This doubling of the sets of Y's and N's continues until the table is complete. Then analyze each rule and fill in the action entries. Fig 8.3 shows the completed table at this stage.

Graduate school admission	1	2	3	4	5	6	7	8
Undergraduate grades of A or better.	Y	Y	Y	Y	N	N	N	N
Test scores of over 600	Y	Y	N	N	Y	Y	N	N
Grade average of A or better in past 2 years	Y	N	Y	N	Y	N	Y	N
Admit to graduate school	X				X			
Admit on probation		X	X				X	
Do not Admit				X		X		X

Fig. 8.3 Condition table.

The next action is to combine rules that are redundant. Two rules can be combined into a single rule if all of the conditions except one have the same Y and N (or -) condition entries and the actions are the same for both. Combine the two rules into one and replace the condition entry of Y and N with a dash (-), which means the condition does not affect the actions to be taken. Using these procedure rules 1 and 5 can be combined, as shown in the margin. In other words, if grades are A or better in the past two years, the student is admitted without regard to overall average.

The completed table with only five rules must represent the eight possible rules. To check for completeness of the rules, analyze as follows:

1. Count number of dashes in the condition entries for each rule. The number of rules "represented" by each rule is 2^m where m is the number of dashes. Where there are no dashes, the number represented is 20, or 1. A single dash means two rules have been combined (21-2), etc.

2. Sum the number of rules represented by the different rules as computed above.

3. Compare the number of rules represented by the table with the number to be accounted for, which are 20 (n-number of conditions). If they are equal (and all other features are correct), the table is complete.

In the example, rules 1, 3 and 4 have one dash (21 for each, or 6), and rules 2 and 5 have two dashes (20 for each, or 2). The sum of 6 plus 2 is equal to 23, or 8, rules required by the three conditions.

Example: A CAR SERVICING

Let us take a simple example of servicing a car. We might ask is oil low? Is Petrol consumption high? there two conditions lead to four possible combinations.

- Both petrol consumption high and oil low;
- Only petrol consumption high;
- Only oil low;
- Neither oil low nor petrol consumption high.

Each of the above will result in a different activity;

- Get oil and Servicing;
- Servicing only;
- Get oil only;
- No action required.

	Condition	Rules			
		1	2	3	4
1	Is consumption high petrol	Y	Y	N	N
2	Is Oil is low	Y	N	Y	N
ACTION					
1	Servicing required	X	X		
2	Get Oil	X		X	
3	No action				X

Fig. 8.4 Car Conditioning Decision Table.

Example : MAIL ORDERING

Let us now take another example, suppose that we have a mail ordering firm sending out literature to various groups of people. These groups are:

G1-   females between 18 and 60

G2-   females under 18

G3-   males under 60

G4-   males and females 60 and over

If our firm computerized its mailing system, then a program will exist which will check data on sex and age of a given individual and place him/her in one of the groups and print his or her address in the list of that group. Forgetting about decision tables for the moment let us attempt to construct that part of the program plan which will identify the group and an individual will be classed in. We will show the flowchart, as well as the "tree-chart". Various charts could be drawn, the ones we have shown find G4 and G3 more quickly since they 'recognize' an individual in one of these groups more quickly than in G1 or G2.

Both the chart shows the similarity of the necessary programming logic (conditions, decisions) to arrive at any one of the four groups. This is all a decision table will show – just the logic – but in a more direct manner. Fig 8.5 shows the decision table and it is useful to point out that the order of the condition is not important. Any order could be used whereas with the flow and tree charts many different charts could be drawn each one arriving at a particular group first.

CONDITION		RULE NUMBER			
		1	2	3	4
1	Age les then 60	Y	-	Y	N
2	Age grader then 18	Y	N	-	-
3	Sex is male	N	N	Y	-
Action					
	CLASSIFY AS GROUP	G1	G2	G3	G4

Fig. 8.5 E-mail condition table.

The dashes (-) used in the columns under the rule heading indicate that the corresponding conditions are irrelevant. Note that the action is an extended entry since the complete action to be taken can only be fully stated by looking (extending one's search) into the action entry quadrant.

Had dashes not been used, how many rules would we have ended up with ? There is a simple way to find out if stands for the number of conditions, then 2 will be the number of rules. In our case n=2, r=3, thus, $n^r = 8$ is the correct number of rules. Fig shows all eight rules.

However, certain rules can be combined, e.g. rules 1 and 4 both lead to a G3 result, therefore one is redundant and both rules may be combined. It can be seen that the answer to condition 2 (age greater than 18) is irrelevant and can be replaced with a dash. The same technique can be applied to rules 5 and 7. Both lead to a G4 indicating that the answer to condition 3 is irrelevant and may be replaced with a dash and the two rules combined. It can also happen because of a impossible relationship between some conditions that an apparent ambiguity or impossible situation arises. If we look more closely at rules 6 and 8 it is not possible for either of these rules to occur because the answer to conditions 1 and 2 cannot both be NO at the same time. Therefore, by combining rules 1 and 4, 5 and 7 and removing rules 6 and 8, the number of rules can be reduced from eight to four as we had in Figure.

A little more study will reveal that only one answer is really necessary to arrive at a G4, viz, a negative reply to condition 1 (AGE less than 60). It is sheer redundancy to ask for an answer to condition 2. This also be seen for rule 2 of Figure, hence the redundancy of condition 1.

It is clear that decision tables do not describe the total program but only that part which involves the logic /decisions of a certain section of the program. Since this logic information is captured in tabular form, it is easier to read than an equivalent flowchart or tree chart which in addition to the logic must also show the sequence in which alternative to flowcharts or tree charts but as a supplement or complement.

They are useful to determine whether any combination of conditions have been omitted, this is less easy to achieve with a flowchart.

1. Advantages of Decision Tables

The decision table has a number of advantages as a tool for analysis and communication.

1. The table provides a framework for a complete and accurate statement of processing or decision logic.
2. The table is compact and easily understood, making it very effective for communication between analysts or programmers and others.
3. The table allows mechanization of some programming tasks.
4. Decision tables can serve as a compact means of describing or specifying operations. How compact they are depends on the number of conditions included, and on the number of different actions to be taken. In general the compactness of decision table decreases in proportion to the sum of the number of variables included and the number of possible actions.
5. Because of its compactness, the decision table provides a convenient way of tersely stating logically complex problems. Larger decision tables can be split and linked together. The procedures for creating decision tables provide rules for checking for four types of possible errors: completeness, size, redundancy, and inconsistency.

   These offer valuable aids in systems design and programming, but people must go through the elaboration process of doing most of the checking work.

6. Decision tables can be used to summarize much information in documentation, but in this case they are sometimes regarded as being too concise. In programming, their precision and conciseness are major advantages, when supported with additional documentation.

2. Disadvantages

1. Decision tables have no theoretical size limit, but there are real practical limits imposed by people. Large decision tables become incomprehensible, and can be neither checked nor used well by people. Fortunately, the size usually is reduced by rule consolidation.

2. Decision tables do not reduce the human labor of thinking or discovery. Human beings still must do the work of defining, specifying, and following to its logical consequences, watch chain of conditions and actions. Decision tablet take away from people none of this arduous work, but they can be used to pinpoint where that work can be best concentrated.

3. Decision tables ignore the delicate interleaving of logic and action that seems so natural when people think about conditions and actions to be taken. Decision tables force the human user to consider conditions separately from actions.

The advantages of decision tables are drawing an increasing number of supporters, but their groups of users are fairly small. Typically, the experience of the first-time user is that he must increase the time and effort he puts in, in order to prepare the decision table. This additional investment may pay off in less debugging and in more efficient user or decision tables, but the additional investment by the user is difficult to justify.

8.5   Flowcharts

For writing algorithm to solving problems, we take the help of flowcharts. A flow-chart is a diagrammatic representation of the various steps involved in the solution of a problem. Flow-chart is a diagrammatic representation of the logic paths contained within a solution to the given problem. Flow-charts are drawn as a pictorial guide for assisting in writing of an algorithm.

The flow-chart indicates the direction of flow of a process, relevant operations and computations, points of decisions and other information which are a part of the solution. Once developed and properly checked, flow-chart provides an excellent guide for writing the program.

Flowcharts are of two types :

- System flowcharts
- Program flowcharts.

A system flowchart describes the data flow and operations for a data processing system. The flowchart shows how the data processing is to be accomplished.

A program flowchart describes the sequence of operations and decisions for a particular program. Program flowcharts are sometimes referred to as block or logic diagrams.

After the program has been defined and the processing system designed, the first step in the programming for the application is the preparation of a description of the computer procedures required performing the required processing. Program flowcharts are usually the most convenient methods of preparing this description. Program flowcharts are prepared in the same way as for lower-level language programs, except that less detail is required for describing higher-level program steps.

8.5.1 Flowchart Symbols

A flowchart is a drawing giving a suitable step-by-step solution of a problem, using suitable annotated geometric figures (having predefined meanings) connected by flow lines. The flowcharts are used for designing and documenting a process of a program. They represent the program logic and the sequence of steps to be performed for writing the program.

Each symbol in the flowchart has a well-defined shape meaning and expresses operation or flow of data. Sufficient annotation is incorporated within the symbols to make a flowchart self-explanatory. Templates are available for drawing the flowchart symbols. Flowcharts are helpful in devising algorithms for solving problems.

There is sufficient creativity and flexibility in the design of flowcharts, so much, so that no two people will draw them exactly alike. Flowcharts go by many other names like the diagram, system chart, run diagram, process chart, procedure chart, and logic chart. As a programming aid, flowcharts are often prepared by system analysts and designers to describe systems and to specify the work to be accomplished by programs. Programmers use flowcharts as a basis for writing programs and as a means of communication among each other, particularly when the programming is done as a team effort. Programmers as well as system analysts also use flowchart as a source of information for maintenance work on program and systems.

Flowchart is more widely used than decision tables, publication languages, or abstract notations. This popularity is due to their advantages. The flowchart provides an excellent means for depicting the flow of program logic. In this diagram different types of boxes represent the different steps. These boxes and other symbols used in flowchart are shown in Table along with their use/ meaning. In flow-charting, it is customary to label each box to show the action performed by it. For example, the figures indicate the start of a process or procedure and its end.

Symbol	Name	Meaning / Use
	Terminal Box	A flattened oval box. It denotes 'start' and 'stop' of a program. A flowchart starts from it and ends into it.
	Input / Output Box	A parallelogram shaped box, showing the location where data is required to be input into the program and the point where the results are output by the program.
	Processing Symbol	A rectangular box, used for indicating the types of process or action which result in singular outcome. They indicate arithmetic processes, assignment statements, macro instructions. It can also be a command for moving data from one place of storage to another.
	Decision Box	It is a diamond (rhombus) shaped box. It contains a logical question with a Yes or No (True of False). The branch followed by the program depends on the outcome of the questions.
	Connector	Long flow charts spanning more than a sheet of paper can be terminated at the bottom of the sheet and labeled with a number. The activity can begin at another connector with the same number on the next sheet. Exit connectors and entry connectors are depicted as shown.
	Flow lines and	Flow lines connect symbols to show the sequence of logical steps. An arrowhead indicates the direction of flow. Usually the direction of flow is indicated but in the absence of an arrow head flow is assumed from top to bottom and from left to right.
	Preparation Symbols	The symbol indicates the preparation for some procedure like initializing certain variables. Some programmers indicate a preparation by the process symbol (3) – a rectangular box.

In flowchart where the program branches into more than one direction – one along the "yes" path and the other along the "no" path. Decision is possible as the computer is able to tell whether the values stored in two fields of its main memory are equal or not. In case they are not equal it can also tell which one contains the higher value.

8.5.2 Rules for making a flowchart

1. Only those symbols should be used which are discussed above. Using conventional symbol the flowcharts are easy to understand.

2. The arrows in flow-chart represent the direction   of flow or data in the problem.

3. The logic of a program flowchart should flow from top to bottom and from left to right. This follows Standard English convention and imposes consistency upon the drawing.

4. Normally flow lines should not cross each other.

5. Horizontal arrow inside the box indicates that the terms on both sides of the arrow are synonyms. It can be taken as symbol for the words "Let the term on left hand side represent the expression on right hand side" or let the number be incremented by one".

6. Each symbol (except decision box) used in program flowchart should have one entry point and one exit point. A computer thinks linearly i.e., one step at a time in a sequential fashion. This rule forbids multiple exits from processing symbols or input / output symbols. The one exception to this rule is the decision symbol, which, by definition, is a branching symbol with more than one exit.

7. As far as possible, the instructions within the symbols of a program should be independent of any particular programming languages. Sometimes, it is not known what computer language will be used to write a particular program. At other times, a program will be written in one language and then, rewritten in another language. This rule keeps the flowchart at the logic level rather at the language-coding level that follows.

8. All decision branches should be labeled. Decisions usually ask questions that require labels like "Yes" and "No" or "True" or "False". Without labels, the different logic paths that data processing can take remain undefined.

8.5.3 Where to use Decision Tables and Flowcharts?

The decision table is best for presenting a problem with many conditions; it is not well suited to show the flow of processing where there are few decisions. Decision tables have been used much less frequently than flowchart. The reasons for this are partly the fact that many applications do not lend themselves to decision tables, but also the lack of training in their uses. On balance, than, the decision table is a very useful tool for some applications and should therefore be one of the methods that the analysts or programmers can use when appropriate.

8.5.4 Examples of Flowcharts

Example 1

Fig 8.6 is a flowchart for finding the sum S, the average A, and the product P of three numbers X, Y, and Z.

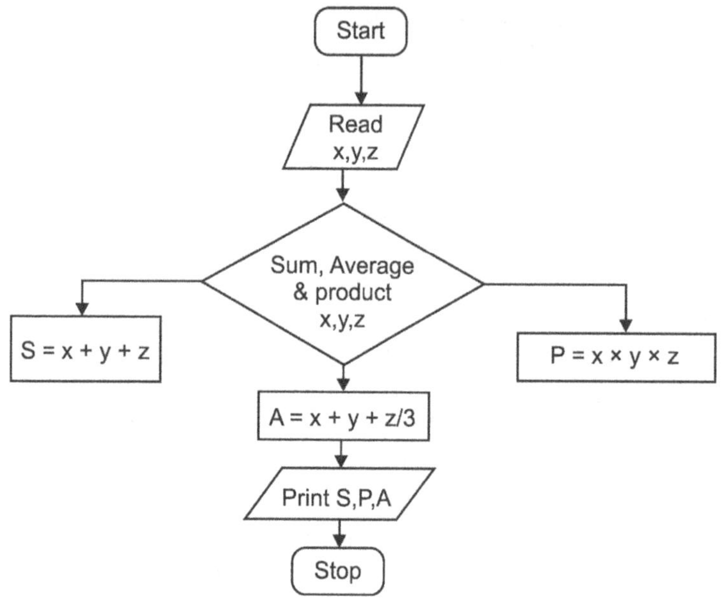

Fig. 8.6 Flowchart for sum, average and product.

Example 2

Fig. 8.7 shows a flowchart which reads two numbers, A and B and prints them in decreasing order, after assigning the larger number to BIG and the smaller number to SMALL. Observe the two arrows leaving the decision "Is A < B ?" One labeled "No" and the other labeled "YES".

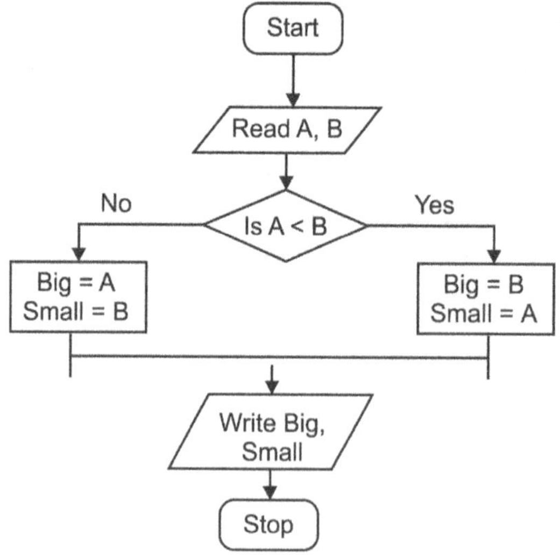

Fig. 8.7 Flowchart for finding Big and Small.

Example 3

(Solution of Quadratic Equation) : Recall that the solution of the quadratic equation

$$ax^2 + bx + c = 0$$

Where a # 0, are given by the formula $X = \left(-b \pm b^2 - 4ac / 2a\right)$

The quantity $D = Sqr(b^2 - 4ac)$ is called the discriminate of the equation. If D is negative, then there are no real solutions. If D = 0, then there is only one (double) real solution, x = b/2a. If D is positive, than we gate two distinct real solutions, Fig. 8.8, is a flowchart, which inputs the coefficients a, b, c of a quadratic equation, and outputs the real solutions, if any. Observe how the three alternate routes have been implemented with two decision symbols. It is not possible to do so in single decision as three outputs cannot be taken from a single decision diamond.

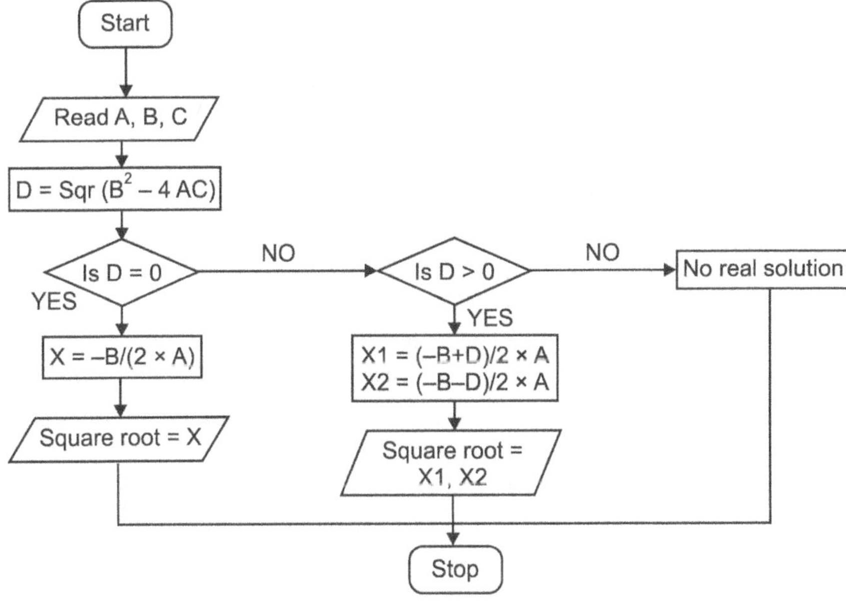

Fig. 8.8 Flowchart for Mathematical functions.

8.5.5 Advantages of Flowcharts

Flowcharts are used for a broad variety of applications in different types of work. For example, they are as convenient to use in administrative file handling as in scientific or engineering computation. This popularity, born out of wide applicability, generates further so much so that flow-charting is a lingua among persons of various disciplines working with computers.

- Flowcharts give a clear graphical/ pictorial representation of the various paths that must be followed to perform the acts to accomplish the goals of the program.

- Flowcharts are invaluable at the time when modifications must be made to the original program to perform additional services not planned originally. They help to locate the exact spots in the program where the changes should be made. A good flow chart enables the programmer to visualize whether or not such changes might upset program features.

- Flowcharts are languages independent. Knowledge of a programming language is not normally necessary to be able to use them or to create them. This is always true for the pictorial part of flowcharts, and ideally should be true for the wording inside the symbols in a flowchart.

- Flowcharts are constraining and precise in ways that they useful to programmers and analysts. These are a limited means of description that force the user to give attention to many significant matters while suppressing attention to a host to less important details.

- Flowcharts are a visual representation, and hence provide a convenient alternative to the usual narration description for a program or system. This enables a more rapid scan or search of a flowchart than is possible with a description when particular items of information are sought. The graphic format enables a user to comprehend a lot in a single glance.

- Flowcharts offer a controllable level of details. They are usable from the most summary systems level to the most detailed programming level. The wide range of detail options greatly enhances the communication value of the flowchart. It is generally concluded that the flowchart is more valuable to the summary than what is provided by the programming language (for flow diagrams) or in the English language narrative (for system charts). For this reason, arranged from very summary to quite detailed, so that the user may choose the level for detail most convenient for his particular purposes. In this regard it should be noted that the system chart variety of flowchart inherently provides a more summary view than does the flow diagram variety of flowchart.

8.5.6 Disadvantages of Flowcharts

- On the disadvantages side, some programmers and analysts complain that flowcharts are a waste of time, since people do not think in graphic terms. In their view, a flowchart is unnatural means of communication.

- Flowcharts are something new and strange to work with for beginners. They are reluctant to accept them.
- When modifications are made in the original program corresponding changes must be made in the flow charts of the program in the documentation. If the programmer is too busy, or other wise, forgets to up-data the flow charts each time.
- It is often difficult to draw the line as to the extent of details of the program to be incorporated in the flowchart. When too many details are included in the flowchart it may become obscure to other programmer.
- Flow charts may not reveal significant steps to be followed in actual coding. Also, they do not guide the programmer, how to code a step as given by the flow chart.
- Flowcharts are often cumbersome to use and costly to produce. Because of their graphic format, flowcharts may devote more than a page of space to present what may requires from a few lines to less than a half-page of equally detailed description in some other format. Manual preparation of flowcharts is slow, although detailed flow diagrams can be prepared by computer if the program to be flow-charted exists in source form.
- Flowcharts do not constitute programming languages. They are person-to-person means of communication, not person-to-computer. No translators exist for accepting program systems described in flowchart form.
- The flow diagram variety of flowchart does not fit well with all programming languages. Although flow diagrams go well with Cobol, Algol, PL/1, and Basic. They seem less compatible with SNOBOL, COMIT, Lisp, and IPL-V.
- Flowcharts may not highlight what is important. Each operation commonly receives as much attention in a flowchart as any other, given the level of detail at which the flowchart is prepared. Yet, individual people feel that some operations are more significant than others. The flowchart does not possess any convenient, automatic way to highlight these.
- Flowcharts are difficult to produce at a summary level. No consistent logical rules have yet been developed to aid the process of producing meaningful summary flowcharts.

8.5.7 Types of Flowcharts

Presently two major varieties of flowcharts are used in practice :

- System chart
- Program flow diagram.

The flow diagram in figure connects rates on part of what a system chart shows. The unit of data transformation for the two is thus very different. For a flow diagram, the unit of data translation is usually an operation or short sequence of operations that a computer can perform (such as an instruction or a series of instructions that comprise a subroutine). An example is testing for the presence of leading zeros in a number.

By contrast, in a system chart the unit of data transformation is usually the work done by an entire computer program. Example are : sorting a file of data, inverting a matrix, or producing a report. Flow diagrams commonly have an algorithmic orientation, stressing how data is transformed, whereas systems charts primarily identify inputs and outputs to algorithms, stressing what data is used or produced at various point in a sequence of operations.

8.5.8 Uses of Flowcharts

Flowcharts are the most widely used graphic method for describing computer operations. They are adaptable to wide from the early days of the computer programming.

The major use of flowcharts is in documentation and programming. As a documentation device, the flowchart is a way of communicating, from one person to another, the nature of the operation to be performed and of the data upon which it is to be performed, regardless of the programming language or computer used.

Since a flowchart is a graphic means of communication, this feature makes it a good choice for use the usual programming languages and English language. All the flow charts we have drawn, which give details of each step of a process or procedure. But these are more common in the flowcharts of large engineering project. Micro-level flowcharting is seldom used in computer programming.

8.6 Pseudo Code

Pseudo-code is a series of statements in unambiguous natural language that describes the actions to be taken by the program to produce that output required by the program. Pseudo implies that the program code is not written in any high-level language but in brief natural language phrases. At this stage programmers are not encumbered with the rule of the computer language but are free to write, in their nature language, statements, which will guide the flow of control in the program.

The objective of pseudo code is to set up a structure for the program so that the goals will be achieved in the most efficient manner possible. The first level of pseudo code gives the overall outline of the program. Additional levels of refinement may be developed to guide the details of the program.

Pseudo code has not been standardized; hence, a programmer is free to write the plan for the program in natural phrases. The thoughts, plans and ideas contained in the pseudo code phrases written by one programmer are equally understandable by other programmers.

Pseudo-code use phrases such as, it-then-else, repeat, until, while-do, read, print, copy etc. It also uses variable names and assignment symbol. Common logical and mathematical symbols are shown in the table.

Symbols used in pseudo code

Symbol	Example	Meaning
<	a< b	"a is less than b".
<=	a <= b	"a is either less or equal to b".
=	a = b	"a is equal to b".
>	a > b	" a is greater than b".
> =	a >= b	" a is greater or equal to b".
< >	a < > b	"a is not equal to b".
< -	a <- b	" a is assigned the value b, destroying the old value of a".

Some symbols, operators, key words and constructs enumerated below are used in writing pseudo-code;

(a)   The assignment symbols "<-" means "takes the value of";

C <- A+B

Means C takes the value of A plus B.

(b)   The sequencing operator (say ;) delimits each statement in a compound statement:

DO this; DO that; DO the other.

(c)   Key words allow data input to and output from the program:

Read: to input data from memory, e.g., READ next – Value of A

WRITE: to output data to memory, e.g., WRITE Result

ACCEPT: to input data from a keyboard, e.g. ACCEPT operator-response;

DISPLAY: to output data to a screen, e.g., DISPLAY Result

PIRNT: to output data to a printer, e.g. PRINT Data.

(d)   There are various looping constructs;
REPEAT a command sequence;
UNTIL condition;
WHILE condition
DO a command sequence;
ENDDO;
FORIFROM a to b (STEP x)
DO a command sequence;
ENDDO;

(e)   Conditional branching may use the IF-THEN-ELSE Construct;
IF Condition
THEN
Command sequence 1;
ELSE
Command sequence 2;
ENDIF;

(f)   We call procedures using the PERFORM or CALL key words;
PERFORM label; or
CALL label;

(g)   We obtain branching (or selection) with nested If;

IF conditions 1	Or we can use the CASE structure
(Which better);	
THEN	DO CASE OF index
Command sequence 1;	CASE index condition 1
Command sequence 2	
THEN	command sequence 1;
ELSE IF condition 2;	CASE index condition 2
THEN….	CASE index condition 3
:	:
ELSE	CASE index condition N
Default command sequence;	command sequence N;
ENDIF;	
	OTHERWISE
Default command sequence;	
	END CASE;

8.6.1 Logical Constructs in Pseudo code

A pseudo code program consists of a list of statements. Some of these statements are among those used in flowcharts, e.g. Read statements, Write statements, Assignment statements, Condition. However, instead of arrows of flow lines to indicate the logic an algorithm, the pseudo code program uses three types of organization.

- Sequential logic,
- Selective logic, and
- Iterative logic.

1. Sequential Logic

    Under this logic, and instructions in a pseudo code program are executed in order, from the top to the bottom. Although it is not necessary to have Start statement or Stop statement (since the program begins at the top and ends at the bottom), we frequently signal the completion of a pseudo code program by writing END at the bottom of the program.

    Read NAME, PRINCIPLE, RATE

    INTEREST = PRINCIPAL x RATE

    Write NAME, INTEREST

    END

    Sometimes we begin the program with a title, e.g. here "Calculating Interest".

2. Selective Logic

    This logic employs a number of structures, called IF-structures, each of which is essentially a selection of one out of several alternatives. Each such structure begins with a statement of the form.

    IF condition

    And ends with statement

    ENDIF

Single alternative: The appropriate structure is called an IF THEN structure ; its logic is illustrated in Fig. 8.7. That is, IF the condition holds, THEN procedure A, the coding of which may involve one or more statements, is executed; otherwise procedure A is skipped, and control transfers to the first, statement following the ENDIF statement.

The following pseudo code program, which calculates an employee's WAGES given his hourly RATE of pay and number of HOURS worked, used an IF THEN structure:

```
Read NAME, RATE, HOURS
WAGES = HOURS x RATE
IF HOURS > 40
WAGES = WAGES + (HOURS – 40) x 0.5 RATE
ENDIF
Write NAME, WAGES
END
```

In other words, WAGES equals HOURS times RATE, but if the employee has worked overtime (more than 40 hours), then there is an additional payment at half rate for those hours over 40. Observe that the IF-procedure is indented, a pseudo code convention that makes programs much easier to read.

Double Alternative: An IF THEN ELSE structure is used for decision involving two distinct alternatives. Observe that a THEN ELSE statement separates two procedures. As indicated by the flowchart, IF the condition holds, THEN procedure A (above the ELSE statement) is executed; ELSE procedure B (below the ELSE statement) is executed.

Example : Following is a pseudo code program for, whose flowchart appears in Fig. 8.7.

```
Read A, B
IF A < B
BIG = B
SMALL = A
ELSE
BIG = A
SMALL = B
ENDIF
Write BIG, SMALL
END
```

Again observe how the procedure blocks are indented for easier reading Multiple alternatives. Decisions that involve more than one alternative may be handled by means of nested. If structures, wherein one IF structure is contained in the procedure component of another IF structure. An example is the ELSE IF structure use one or more statements on the form.

ELSE IF Condition between the IF ELSE statements. Observe that only one of the procedures will be executed, the one the follows the first condition which holds. If none of the conditions holds, then the procedure following the ELSE statement is executed. If this procedure is empty, then the ELSE statement itself may be omitted.

Example: Following is a pseudo code program for Example 8.3 (flowcharted in Fig. 8.8)

Pseudo 1:	read a,b,c
Pseudo 2 :	$D = (b^2 - 4* a * c)$
Pseudo 3 :	IF D > 0
	$X1 = (-b + D) / (2 * a)$
	$X2 = (-b + D) / (2 * a)$
Pseudo 4 :	write X1 , X2
Pseudo 5 :	ELSE IF D = 0
	$X = -b / (2 \times a)$
Pseudo 6 :	write 'UNIQUE SOLUTION', X
Pseudo 7 :	ELSE
	write 'NO REAL SOLUTION'
Pseudo 8 :	ENDIF
	END

Again observe the indented procedure block.

Iteration Logic

This logic refers to structure involved loops, of which there are three types. One type, begin with a DO statement, which has the form.

DO K = 1 TO N or DO K = INIVAL = End value and INCR = Increment.

8.6.2 Advantages of Pseudo code

The pseudo code possesses the following major advantages:

1. The pseudo code instructions are midway between English and high level languages but free ambiguities of English language. That is why pseudo code is often called structured English. The pseudo code displays the programming logic beautifully and can be converted to complete programs very easily.

2. Pseudo code consisting of simple sentences in English and mathematical symbols and are easier to write and understand. On the other hand, charts are cumbersome to draw.

3. Pseudo code, being very closed to high level languages, can easily be translated to a computer program whereas flow charts cannot be coded directly into a computer program very easily.

8.7 Algorithm

In our daily life we encounter with a number of problems, which can be solved by two methods.

- Algorithm
- Heuristic

In algorithm, there is set procedure to solve the problem in such a manner that solution is definitely obtained. Heuristic is the method of obtaining optimum solution of the problem intuitively by experienced guess.

For solving a problem by computer, we have to be very clear in writing the instructions for the computer. The set of instructions is known as program. The solution is obtained by breaking the contents of the problem and given data in such a manner, that all instructions are given in sequence. This procedure is known as algorithm and has to be devised prior to the actual coding of the computer program.

Actual computer program is written in coded languages, known as programming language. Algorithm is thus a design or plan of obtaining a solution to the problem. It is logical process of analyzing a mathematical problem and data step by step so as to make it easier to understand and implement solution to the problem. Certain operations must be performed on data for producing the required results. In order that a computer can perform an operation, it must be converted into a form that the computer is able to execute. Moreover the operations must be carried out in a specific sequence. In our day-to-day work, the brain automatically performs the algorithms by experience but not in a systematic and error-free way. But for processing on computer, one has to be systematic and to the point, as computer does not know alternatives. For example we must read a record before using its content in calculations. Sometimes it is necessary to perform an operation only if the data satisfies a particular condition. For example, income tax must be deducted from the salary of an employee only if income exceeds a certain limit.

Writing algorithm for solution of a problem is a method of successive iterations. Algorithm is first roughly estimated and written. Then it is carefully gone through a number of times and refined each time. The final form of an algorithm emerges through a number of stepwise refinements carried out successively, till the detailed steps become precisely clear to the person or machine, which is going to execute the steps. In an algorithm, all items of instructions are listed in the order in which they are to be carried out. This is done with the help of flowcharts.

However complex the problems may be (numeric, or non-numeric), they can always be broken into a set of smaller sequence of steps and procedures. We can always think it to be solved with the help of a systematic step problem solving procedure, which if follows meticulously, will lead us to a definite solution. This step-by-step procedure is technically known as algorithm. In contrast to this, there are heuristic procedures, which most of the time may offer a person some optimum solution to correct solution or any solution at all will be achieved all the time. Algorithm may constitute of sequence, selections and repetitions. Therefore, it is necessary that all these terms be understood.

8.7.1 Efficient Algorithm

The following points must be born in mind before writing an efficient algorithm :

- Every procedure should carefully specify the input and output variable.
- The meaning of all variables should be defined.
- The flow of the program should generally be forward except for normal looping and unavoidable instances.
- Indentation rules should be established and followed, so that computation units of program text can more easily be identified.
- Documentation should be short, but meaningful. Avoid commands like "J is increased by one."
- Use subroutines, where appropriate.

Let us see method of evolving by writing the steps for solving certain day to day problems.

It is not sufficient that only the method of solving a problem is written and solution is obtained through computer. But we expect that computer also prints results in a systematic manner such that the user is able to identify the set of results. Suppose in a problem we want to calculate the value of three variables A, B and C and get the results printed. Now computer will print 3 values, but it may not be easy for user to identify which is the value of A out of these 3 results. So for this purpose remarks such as "Answer A=", or "Answer: Temp in Celsius is" are also printed.

Example

Develop an algorithm for converting given temperature in Celsius scale into Fahrenheit scale.

From our knowledge of physics, we know the relationship between temperature in the two given scales i.e. temperatures in Fahrenheit and Centigrade. This is,

$$C / 5 = (F-32) / 9$$

First, we have to write this formula in such a way so that values of temperature in degree Fahrenheit are equated to value in centigrade, namely,

$$F = 1.8 \times C + 32$$

Now we can write down steps for writing the algorithm for solving this in such a manner that any person with average intelligence can go on follow the procedure and come to definite solution. The algorithm shall be similar to following algorithm:

1. Read (obtain) the given values of C i.e. temperature in Celsius.
2. Multiply this value with 1.8 and equate it equal of F i.e. F-1.8 × C.
3. Now replace this value of F by F+32.
4. Write the Answer.
5. STOP.

Explanation

1. For deriving or obtaining any value from the given problem, we have written "Read" because in most of the computer programming languages, "Read" is a statement which causes the computer to read the given value of a data item. We have to feed this value in computer's memory and computer will read this value in the program automatically as and when necessary.
2. The value of F is in two parts which are 1.8 × C and + 32. In computer applications it is customary to calculate the value in part and equate them equal to the required parameter and store this part value in memory. This part value is further added with remaining part and replaced with original value.
3. It is customary to write stop at the end, otherwise sometimes due to mistake in designing the algorithm the computer may continue to work infinitely. Now we will define the algorithm by writing.

Refined Algorithm

1. Read value of C
2. F = 1.8*C
3. F = F + 32
4. Print "Answer: The value of F is = "; followed by the calculated value of F.
5. STOP

Explanation

1. In second step of the algorithm we have written F = 1.8 * C instead of F = 1.8 × C to indicate that computer is to replace value in storage location F by 1.8 × C which is its part value. In next step it replaces this part value of F i.e. F = F + 32 by any value of F which is equal to F = 1.8 C + 32 in the same location.

2. The calculated value i.e. result obtained, if printed simply numerically will not make any sense on the paper unless we write the words "The answer is equal to"; and fill in the blanks with the answered value. For making the computer to print these words' it is necessary that they are written under the quotes "…" because computer understands either the numeric values written without quotation marks or the strings of words written under quotation marks. This is one of the rules of BASIC Programming language.

3. Observe carefully that we have placed semi-colon, symbol immediately after quote marks. This is necessary according to rules of the programming languages like BASIC that allow the answered value to be printed immediately after the result after a space. Here the computer will not print the quote marks, or the semicolon. Actually these two symbols are a part of the instruction.

8.8 Data Validation

All data entry programs must also have routines that validate the data input. As one of the safeguards against incorrect entries, it is necessary to accumulate and display data-entry statistics giving the number of records entered and the errors found. The data entry operator can then check these incorrect records against the original source. Control totals (a sort of data entry check) should also be shown to ensure all data has been entered.

A good practice in a data entry program is to present some kind of key to the latest value entered – an operator often has to continue to work through interruptions which cause the last entry made to be forgotten.

Outputs also have to be validated, particularly those, which are little unusual, such as, the nil statement and the multi page Invoice. Testing is a vital but time-consuming activity. It is inevitable that errors will be found. These may be due to incorrect programming, misunderstanding of specifications or simply omissions in the original design. The programmer must code the amendments required, and the programs and system retested. This retesting is very important because the requested amendments may have caused unwanted side effects and so new errors and problems may appear. One of the most common sources of faults in programs is the fixing of others' faults!

Input Validation

At the point data is entered into the computer, it should be subjected to input validation procedures in which data is tested for errors to the extent possible or appropriate in the light of the consequences of input errors. A separate input validation run or input editing run is usually performed in systems where the data is vetted and transferred to run or during subsequent processing, the erroneous transaction or record was found to contain and error is shunted rather than stopping the computer on the console typewriter or printer explaining why item was rejected.

There will thus usually be a file of rejects and an error run should be carefully controlled to make sure they are corrected and reentered at a later run.

In the case of on-line processing of unmatched transactions, data items are tested in the same manner as the batch processing validation run. An error message to the input station describing the error is the basis for rejecting the transaction and requesting a resubmission of a correct input (or submission of a correction to one or more fields of the input record).

Before testing the data items themselves, the input validation run should test that the file being used is the correct one (correct data, correct records). Checking the internal file label does this. A file label is a record at the beginning and also possibly at the end of the file which contains identification or master file is used and that the entire file has been processed. At the beginning, is the header label, which identifies the file. Typical contents are:

- Name of file
- Creation data
- Purge date
- Identification number
- Reel number (for magnetic tape)

    Date 05-07-07

    Payroll edit run

    Operator no. 5

    Invalid records rejected

No.	246751DEPT NO.6 INVALID	23 REG 0 OT
No.	8673105HOURS EXCEED LIMIT	50 REG 29 OT
No.	7451123INVALID EMPLOYEE NO.	64 REG 37 OT

       CONTROL FIGURES

INPUT RECORD COUNT	177
RECORDS REJECTED	3
CALCULATED COUNT	174
OUTPUT RECORD COUNT	174
TOTAL HOURS HASH-DIFFERENCE	0
INPUT HASH TOTAL-TOT HOURS	3267
HOURS ON REJECTED RECORD	92

CALCULATED TOTAL HOURS   3351

OUTPUT COUNT – TOTAL HOURS   3351

TOTAL HOURS HASH-DIFFERENCE   0

END OF PAYROLL EDT RUN

The label also be used at the end of data input to check for completeness of the input. A trailer label is written as the last record and contains a record count, control totals, etc.

The input validation tests seek to establish that the data is within the limits established for valid data. Some examples of programmed checking which can be done are:

- *Valid Code*

  If there is only limited number of valid codes, say for coding expenses, the code being read may be checked to see if it is one of the valid codes.

- *Valid Character*

  If only certain characters are allowed in a data field, the computer can test the field to determine that no invalid characters are used.

- *Valid Field Size, sign, and composition*

  If a code number should be specified number of digits in length, the computer may be programmed to test the field size as is specified. If the sign of the field must always be positive or always negative, a test may be made to determine that the field does indeed contain a proper composition of characters.

- *Valid Transaction*

  There is typically a relatively small number of valid transactions which are processed with a particular file. There is a limited number, for example, of transaction codes, which can apply to accounts receivable file updating. As part of input error control, the transaction code can be tested for validity.

- *Valid Combinations of Field*

  In addition to each of the individual fields being tested, combinations may be tested for validity. For example, a salesman code, may be associated with only a few territory codes, this can be checked.

- *Missing Data Test*

  The program may check the data field to. make sure that all data field necessary to code a transaction have data field necessary to code a transaction have data in them.

- *Check Digit*

  Check digit are one or more digits carried within a unit item of numerical data to provide information about the other digits in the unit in such a manner that, if a transaction or transposition error occurs in subsequent data entry, the check tails, and an indication of error is given.

- *Sequence Test*

  In batch processing the data to be processed must be arranged in a sequence, which is the same as the sequence of the file. Both the master file and the transaction file may be tested to ensure that they are in a proper sequence, ascending or descending as the case may be. The sequence check can also be used to account for all documents, if these are numbered sequentially.

- *Limit of Reasonableness Test*

  This is a basic test for data processing accuracy. Input data should usually fall within certain limits. For example, hours worked should not be less than zero and should not be more than, say, 50. The upper limit may be established from the experience of the particular firm. Input data may be compared against this limit to ensure that no input error has occurred or at least no input error exceeding certain reestablished limits.

Examples : The total amount of a customer order may be compared with his average order amount. If this order exceeds, say, three times the amount of his average order, then an exception notice may be printed. A material receipt, which exceeds two times the economic order quantity established for particular item, might be subject to question. A receiving report amount may be compared with the amount requested on the purchase order. If there is more than a small percentage variance, then there is an assumption of error in the input data. In a utility billing, consumption is checked against prior periods to detect possible errors or trouble in the customer's installation.

8.9 Coding

Writing the program involves translating the algorithm or flowchart into a programming language. This processing is known as coding. The language chosen depends upon what the program is expected to do and what facilities are available to the programmer.

The programming activity continues with coding of the logic described in the flowchart into statements in the language being used. These are usually written on coding paper designed for the particular language. These source language statements are then typed using a keyboard, line by line. The resulting group of lines form source program.

The translation phase begins with the loading of the translator and routine of the compiler into the computer memory. This routine reads the source program codes, interprets their meaning, and produces an object program on some machine readable output medium such as magnetic disk. A listing of the program is printed on the line printer or typewriter. This listing includes any error diagnostic, which the translator routine detects. The errors, which can be detected, are mainly textual errors involving improper use of the language. If errors are found, these must be corrected and the translation process repeated.

Programming is sometimes contrasted with coding which generally refers to the writing and debugging of programs for given program's specifications. The text of a program is sometimes referred to as code, and lines of program text are refereed to as lines of code, especially in the case of machine-language programs.

8.10 Debugging

When a program is compiled or executed it may produce a number of errors. Errors may become discouraged because of bugs, but this should not be the case. Debugging should be considered to be a part of programming.

Thus debugging is the process of checking the correctness of the program either manually or through facility of compiler program error checking. How, then to get rid of the bugs? When test data produces incorrect output, it is necessary to trace through the logic to find out how and where the program has failed. You can examine the values of memory variables by introducing additional PRINT or DISPLAY statements at selected points. Then use some variation of the dry run to trace through the code and see how these values are being produced. At the end, ensure that such statements added or removed for de-bugging purposes properly after the error has been corrected.

On inspecting the code, a few pointers may be helpful :

(a)   It is important to be able to approach the code with a fresh and open mind, even when looking at it for the last time. Never believe even yourself; it is surprising how easy it is to make assumptions. The code must be seen from the viewpoint of an obedient and "dumb" computer.

(b)   Only the output of a program is relevant while analyzing a failure. The error in the output is a direct indication of what has failed, and however impossible it may seem at first (or even second) glance, the error must exist at a relevant point.

(c)   In case of an elusive error, keep in mind that an error can escalate and show up at a point far from where it was caused. The total picture must, therefore, be re-examined at such times.

(d)   It sometimes helps to be able to "image" the problem, especially when it is connected with one of the input or output devices or with a file transfer. While considering each statement, try to image exactly what would be happening on the computer in response.

A higher-level language usually simplifies debugging. The coding is normally not as lengthy and logic of the program is easier to follow. The programmer first does desk checking of his program, tracing through the logic to see if it does what is intended. The program is then ready for a test run. If it does not run correctly, corrections are made in the source, and the program is translated again.

8.11   Types of Errors

In general, bugs can be detected during compilation while the second is detected during or after execution. If the rules of syntax are violated, then the program will not compile. On the other hand, the program may be syntactically perfect but there can be a logical error. Thus the three types of errors that can occur in a program are :

(a)   Syntax error, or syntactical errors,

(b)   Run-time errors, and

(c)   Logic errors, or logical errors.

Syntax Errors

Syntax errors occur when there is a violation in any of the rule of language formation. Errors causes by misunderstanding or misinterpreting the syntax and type rules of the programming language are trivial. Mistakes may arise due to applying rules of one higher language to another like a student who has learnt BASIC and FORTRAN first and now learning PASCAL may tend to apply rules of these two languages into the statements being written in PASCAL. A person habituated BASIC may tend to write the assignment statement MARK=5 instead of MARK: = 5 and PRINT instead of WRITELN of PASCAL. These errors are usually easy to correct because the compiler will point out where an error has occurred. The Pascal compiler produces these error messages while it is attempting to translate a Pascal program into machine language. Any grammatical mistake will cause problems when the translation is performed. The complier will attempt to produce a message indicating where the mistake is and what it believed the mistake to be.

Disk Checking

It's unusual for complex programs to run to completion on the first attempt. In fact, the time spent in DEBUGGING and testing often equals or exceeds the time spent in program coding. To reduce the number of errors, the programmer should carefully check the coding for accuracy before entering it into the computer. This desk checking process should include an examination of program logic and program completeness. For this, typical input data should be manually traced through the program processing paths to identify possible errors. After desk checking, an attempt is made to convert the source program into object program form. Compiler programs and interpreters contain error-diagnostic features, which detect (and print messages about) mistakes caused by the incorrect application of the language used to prepare the source program.

When changes have been made, in response to errors detected, a re-compilation can be ordered. This process may continue until all detected syntax errors have been remedied.

8.12 Testing

During the programming stage, each programmer or programming team will perform its own program testing to the specifications laid down by the designer. The completed programs are then passed on to the designer for further testing. He will be anxious not only to examine the delivered programs but also to prove their interfaces with the rest of the system. Testing will be performed by both desk checking comparing the program flowcharts with the original specifications and by running the program using test data.

Test data should be manually compiled and the results produced by the system compared with the appropriate clerical figures or the current computer system. For example, in a system designed to produce and print examination certificates, a sample of student's data should be taken and entered into the new computer system. The generated certificates can then be compared with their clerically produced counter parts and discrepancies investigated.

It is also important that the system correctly identifies errors, omissions and testing for these are especially critical. Common error tests include the input of :

- Oversize and undersize data items.
- Incorrect formats.

When testing, a program take care to select the test data so that it tests all cases, e.g. pick a set of data which will cover all possible selections. Large programs are very difficult to test completely once they are completed because of their complexity and the time needed to try all possible cases. If top-down programming is adopted it should be possible to test program modules thoroughly at each step along the way. Despite all these testing methods programs may still be faulty when they are tried out on the computer. Well-tested programs sometimes work for a while and then suddenly produce a fault. This may happen because some combination of circumstances has occurred which the program designer had not taken into account while designing the program.

The purpose of testing is to determine whether the results are correct. The testing procedure involves using the program to process input test data that will produce known results. The items developed for testing should include:

- Typical data, which will test the generally used program paths.
- Unusual but valid data, which will test the program paths used to handle exceptions.
- Incorrect, incomplete, or inappropriate data, which will test the program error handling capabilities.

A testing procedure that's often followed is to separately test different portions of a program. This helps to isolate detected errors to a particular program segment.

The use of a modular programming approach, of course, eases this procedure. Another technique that's often used is to entrust much of the testing to someone other than the programmer who wrote the code. A fresh outlook is often helpful, and errors that are missed by a programmer who is "too familiar" with the code may be easily picked up by someone else.

- It is good practice to test a program as it is being written and before it is tried out on the computer.
- How will the system be tested to ensure its readiness for use?
- How is the system to be implemented in terms of conversion?
- How is the system controlled for errors?

To centre heading on a line, count the number of characters on the heading, including spaces between words. Subtract this number from the number of available print positions on each line (80) to get the total number of blank spaces around the heading. Dividing this number by 2 gives the number of spaces that should be inserted in front of the heading.

Levels of Testing

One of the most difficult questions with regard to testing is how much is enough? Although the aim of testing is to reveal errors, it is likely that some will get through the testing process without being found. Also, experience shows that, while it is fairly easy to find say, 95 % of the errors in a piece of code, it becomes more and more costly and difficult to find and correct the remaining errors. This has led to something of a compromise between what is desirable and what is achievable in terms of programs correctness, and has led to a distinction between different "levels" of correctness.

The way most testing works is to input a set of values, then compare the expected results with the actual ones. If the output produced by a test run is correct it shows the program has correctly processed that set of data. Depending on the type of data input, we can identify three levels of program correctness – possible, probable and absolute.

- ***Possible correctness*** follows obtaining correct output for some arbitrary input. If the outcome of such a test is wrong, the program cannot possibly be correct.

- ***Probable correctness*** involves obtaining correct output for a number of carefully selected inputs. If all potentially problematic areas are checked in this way, the program is probably correct.

- ***Absolute correctness*** can be demonstrated only by a test that involves every possible combination of inputs. Such a test would take a huge amount of time; it is therefore not practicable.

Coding errors will not occur very often if you adopt a systematic approach. When they do occur, they almost invariably follow a misuse of the language facilities. This is usually due to an inadequate understanding of or familiarity with the languages in use. All programmers should ensure that they understand fully all aspects of the languages they use, rather than "muddle through" using sometimes an inappropriate subset.

Difference between Testing and Debugging

It is very easy to make mistakes when writing programs, and so programs often fail to work the first time they are tried. If a program has been well-designed the faults should be easier to find and correct. The program faults are called "bugs" and getting rid of these faults by making appropriate changes to the program is called debugging.

Debugging is often regarded as a "patching up job". In fact alterations made to programs in order to get rid of bugs are often called "patches" or "fixed". Treating debugging in this way is rather a risky way to do things, because in patching one bug, another bug may be introduced. A more sound approach to debugging is to return to the program design process, and all stages in programming, so that the previously unforeseen circumstances are wholly incorporated into the design.

Testing is part of the procedure that ensures the program corresponds with the original specification, and that it works in its intended environment. We have already come across some similar verification and validation techniques. Dry running the code helps to ensure its logical correctness, and inspections and walk-through are to confirm that no errors follow the transition from stage to stage, e.g. specification to design.

The difference between these activities and testing is that they are "static", while testing is "dynamic". Dynamic in this situation means the process uses executable code, rather than listings or documents while describing the code. Testing should form a major part of any verification and validation activity on any software project. Static methods can be used to very good effect, and contribute significantly to the discovery of errors at an early stage – but they can never replace dynamic testing.

Most programmers, asked to define testing, say something like "Testing is the process of checking a program to show there are no errors". This type of definition concentrates on errors being absent – implying that successful test is one that shows no errors, and a failed test is one that finds no error. However, this approach is wrong. The aim of testing is to find errors so that they can be corrected, resulting in a more reliable, and better quality of final program.

CHAPTER 9

Networks

9.1 Introduction

All computers, which are connected via a transmission media, are known as Computer Networks. Suppose a server, which is kept in office where all computers are connected together, means they can share their data and file. Fig. 9.1 shows the data transmission over the network in the office. We can say all interconnected collection of autonomous computer is termed as computer network. Two computers are said to be interconnected as they are able to exchange the information. Computer network started its journey by Telegraph Network & Telephone network

Some simple definitions of network are:

- A *computer network* is computers and devices connected together.
- A single computer is limited to its own hardware and software.
- The capabilities of a computer are increased when connected with other devices to form a computer network

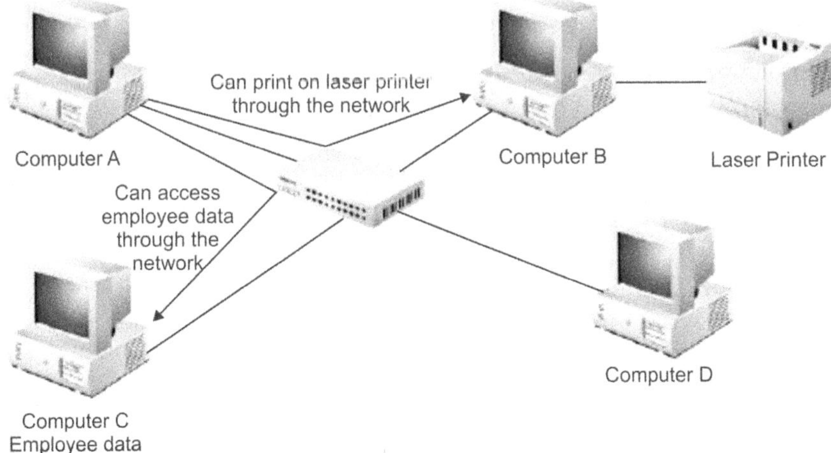

Fig. 9.1 Data Transmission over the Network in the Office.

In 1851 the first submarine cable was established between London and Paris. Eventually, networks of telegraph stations were established covering all the continents. In these networks a message or telegram would arrive at a telegraph station, and an operator would make a routing decision based on the destination address.

In 1875 Alexander Graham Bell invented **Telephone network,** which transmits voice signal. Nowadays this is known as modern telephone service. It is connection oriented service because they require setting up of connection before the actual transfer of information can take place.

The first Computer Network was the Semi-Automatic Ground Environment **(SAGE)** system developed between 1950 and 1956 for air defense system [Green 1984]. The system consisted of 23 computer networks, each network connecting radar sites, ground to air data links and other locations to a central computer. In the 1960s tree topology terminal oriented networks were developed to allow user terminals to connect to a single central shared computer.

The **ARPANET** (Advanced Project Research Network) was the first major effort at developing a network to interconnect computers over a wide geographical area. At the end of 1967 ARPA initiated a small contract with the Stanford Research Institute for the development of specifications for the necessary communications system. Elmer Shapiro was to be the key person on this study the first sites of the ARPANET were picked to provide either network support services or unique resources.

Advantages of Computer Networks:

- Sharing computers.
- Networked computers can share resources such as Printers, fax modems, scanners, hard disk, CD-ROMs, and DVDs. (Resource sharing).
- Networks also make computer management easier.
- Maximum utilization of resources.
- This reduces costs and the work of support staff.
- Computer networks can help to improved communications through groupware.
- E-mail, electronic calendars, collaborative writing, and video conferencing are available.
- Computer networks allow to be managed from one central location.

9.2   Types of Network

According to the capacity of network is divided into following categories:

- Server-Based Network
- Local Area Network (LAN)
- Wide Area Network (WAN)

- Metropolitan Area Network (MAN)
- Wireless Network
- Internet
- Internet work.

9.2.1 Server-Based Network

This type of the network belongs to Client Server Model . It consist of one powerful machine which is known as server and rest are known as Clients. This is commonly used TCP/IP protocol to transfer their data.

- The network has special high-powered server controls.
- The server is dedicated to running the network.
- Print and file servers, application servers, communication servers, and directory service servers are common.

9.2.2 Local Area Network (LAN)

A local area network (LAN) is a group of computers and associated devices that share a common communications line or wireless link and typically share the resources of a single processor or server within a small geographic area (for example, within an office building). Usually, the server has applications and data storage that are shared in common by multiple computer users. A local area network may serve as few as (for example, in a home network) or as many as thousands of users (for example, in FDDI network).

- Network computers are located relatively close to each other.
- They are generally limited to buildings owned by one organization.
- They operate at high speeds.
- They are low-cost networks

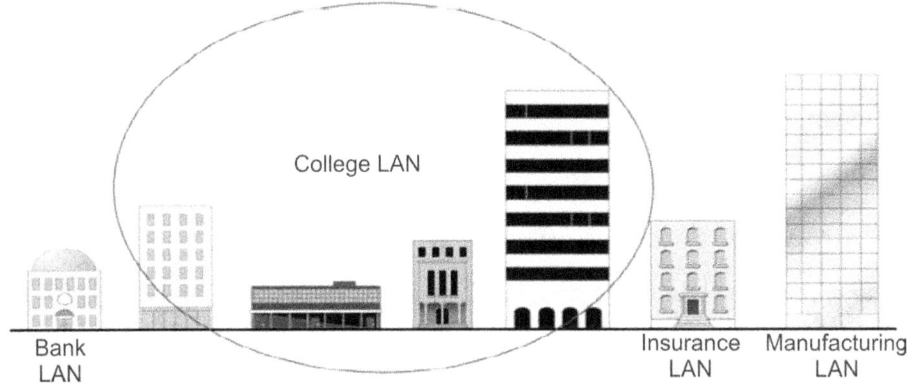

Fig. 9.2 Local Area Network (LAN).

FDDI

Ethernet is by far the most commonly used LAN technology. A number of corporations use the Token Ring technology. FDDI is sometimes used as a backbone LAN interconnecting Ethernet or Token Ring LANs. Another LAN technology, ARCNET once the most commonly installed LAN technology, is still used in the industrial automation industry.

Typically, a suite of application programs can be kept on the LAN server. Users who need an application frequently can download it once and then run it from their local hard disk. Users can order printing and other services as needed through applications run on the LAN server. A LAN server may also be used as a Web server if safeguards are taken to secure internal applications and data from outside access.

In some situations, a wireless LAN may be preferable to a wired LAN because it is cheaper to install and maintain.

9.2.3 Wide Area Network (WAN)

A WAN is a data communications network that covers a relatively broad geographic area and that often uses transmission facilities provided by common carriers, such as telephone companies. Typically, a WAN consists of two or more local-area networks (LANs). WAN technologies generally function at the lower three layers of the OSI reference model: the physical layer, the data link layer, and the network layer It connects computers and LANs over a larger geographical area. It crosses public thoroughfares such as roads, railroads, and water.

- Network computers are spread out over a larger area.
- They generally cross public thoroughfares.
- Public carriers often manage them.
- They operate at lower speeds.
- They are a higher-cost network

9.2.4 Metropolitan Area Network (MAN)

These Networks serve an area of 3 to 30 miles, approximately the area of a typical city. MAN supports high-speed disaster recovery systems, real-time transaction backup systems, interconnections between corporate data centers, Internet service providers, and government, business, medicine, and education (Fig. 9.3).

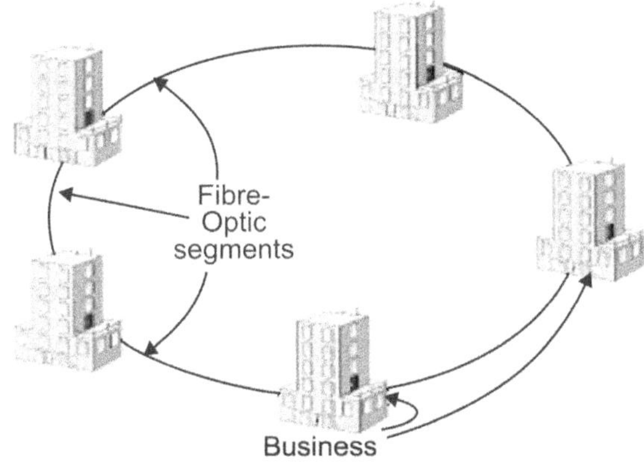

Fig. 9.3 Metropolitan Area Network (MAN).

9.2.5 Wireless Network

The term wireless networking refers to technology that enables two or more computers to communicate using standard network protocols, but without network cabling. A wireless network can also use an access point, or base station. In this type of network the access point acts like a hub, providing connectivity for the wireless computers. It can connect (or "bridge") the wireless LAN to a wired LAN, allowing wireless computer access to LAN resources, such as file servers or existing Internet Connectivity. An ad-hoc, or peer-to-peer wireless network consists of a number of computers each equipped with a wireless networking interface card. Each computer can communicate directly with all of the other wireless enabled computers. They can share files and printers this way, but may not be able to access wired LAN resources. Fig. 9.4 shows a wireless network, which can access from H/W access point.

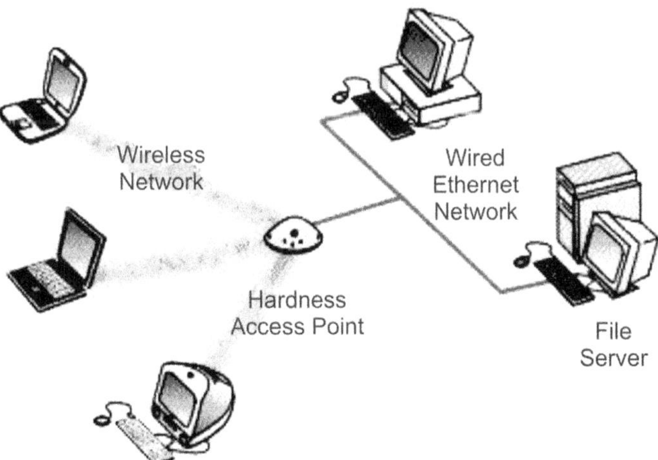

Fig. 9.4 showing Wireless Network.

9.2.6   Internet

The Internet uses high-speed data lines, called backbones, to carry data. Smaller networks connect to the backbone, enabling any user on any network to exchange data with any other user (Fig. 9.5). Every computer and network on the Internet uses the same protocols (rules and procedures) to control timing and data format.

- The World Wide Web is a part of the Internet, which supports hypertext documents, allowing users to view and navigate different types of data.

- A Web page is a document encoded with hypertext markup language (HTML) tags. HTML allows designers to link content together via hyperlinks.

- Every Web page has an address, a Uniform Resource Locator (URL).

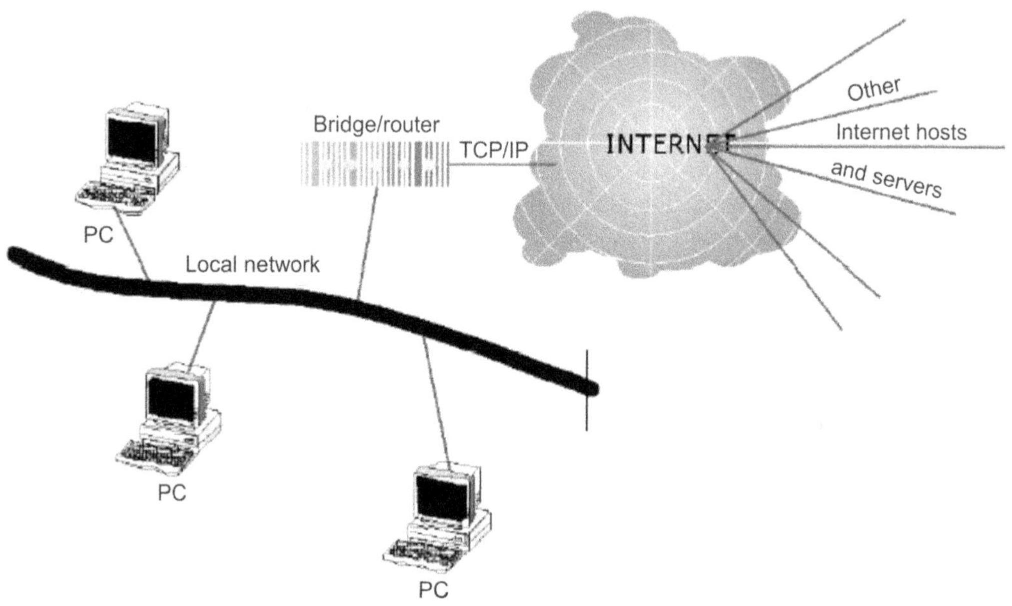

Fig. 9.5 Diagram of Internet.

9.2.7   Intranet

A network connected within university, college or any organization to transfer data between these organizations is known as Intranet. It is usually a connected collection of LANs. It is also known as Internet work. An *Internet work* is a collection of individual networks, connected by intermediate networking devices, which function as a single large network. Internet working refers to the industry, products, and procedures that meet the challenge of creating and administering Internet works. For example, a university having 4 Labs, i.e. Computer Lab, Physics Lab, Electronics Lab, Chemistry Lab, if they are connected from the LAN, that is known as intranet.

Some Features of Networking

Hosts : A computer system that is accessed by a user working at a remote location. Typically, the terms are used when there are two computer systems connected by modems and telephone lines. The system that contains the data is called the host, while the computer at which the user sits is called the remote terminal.

Node : In networks, it is a processing location. A node can be a computer or some other device, such as a printer. Every node has a unique network address, sometimes called a Data Link Control (DLC) address or Media Access Control (MAC) address.

Download : To copy data (usually an entire file) from a main source to a peripheral device. The term is often used to describe the process of copying a file from an online service or bulletin board service (BBS) to one's own computer.

Downloading can also refer to copying a file from a network file server to a computer on the network.

Upload : To transmit data from a computer to a bulletin board service, mainframe, or network. For example, if you use a personal computer to log on to a network and you want to send files across the network, you must upload the files from your PC to the network.

9.3 Advantages of Networks

The following advantages are particularly true for LANs, although they apply to MANs and WANs as well.

Sharing of peripheral devices : Laser printers, disk drives, and scanners are examples of peripheral devices. As you'll recall, a peripheral device is any piece of hardware that is connected to a computer. Any newly introduced piece of hardware is often quite expensive, as is the case with laser or color printers. To justify their purchase, companies want them to be shared by many users. Usually the best way to do this is to connect the peripheral device to a network serving several computer users.

Sharing of programs and data : In most organizations, people use the same software and need access to the same information. It could be expensive for a company to buy one copy of, say, a word processing program for each employee. The company will usually buy a network version of that program that will serve many employees.

Organistions also save a great deal of money by letting all employees have access to the same data on a shared storage device. This way the organization avoids such problems as some employees updating customer addresses on their own separate machines, while other employees remain ignorant of such changes.

Finally, network-linked employees can, using workgroup software, work together online on shared projects.

Better communications : One of the greatest features of networks is electronic mail, as we have seen. With e-mail everyone on a network can easily keep others posted about important information. Thus, the company eliminates the delays encountered with standard interoffice mail delivery or telephone tag.

Security of information : Before networks became commonplace, an individual employee might be the only one with particular information, stored in his or her desktop computer. If the employee was dismissed – or if a fire or flood demolished the office – no one else in the company might have any knowledge of that information. Today such data would be backed up or duplicated on a networked storage device shared by others.

Access to databases : Networks also enable users to tap into numerous databases, whether the private databases of a company or the public databases of online services.

9.4   Local Area Networks (LANs)

A computer network that spans a relatively small area. Most LANs are confined to a single building or group of building. However, one LAN can be connected to other LANs over any distance via telephone lines and radio waves. A system of LANs connected in this way is called a wide-area network (WAN).

Most LANs connect workstations and personal computer. Each node (individual computer) in LAN has its own CPU with which it executes programs, but it is also able to access data and devices anywhere on the LAN. This means that many users can share expensive devices, such as laser printers, as well as data. Users can also use the LAN to communicate with each other, by sending e-mail or engaging in chat sessions.

There are many different types of LANs. Ethernets being the most common for PCs. Apple Macintosh networks are based on Apple's Talk network system, which is built into Macintosh computers.

The following characteristics differentiate one LAN to another :

Topology : The geometric arrangement of devices on the network. For example, devices can be arranged in a ring or in a straight line.

Protocols : The rules and encoding specifications for sending data. The protocols also determine whether the network users a peer-to-peer or client/server architecture.

Media : Twisted-pair wire, coaxial cables, or fiber optic cables can connect Devices. Some networks do without connecting media altogether, communicating instead via radio waves.

LANs are capable of transmitting data at very fast rates, much faster than data transmitted over a telephone line; but the distances are limited, and there is also a limit on the number of computers that can be attached to a single LAN.

LANs may be client-server or peer-to-peer and include components such as cabling, network interface cards, operating system, other shared devices, bridges and gateways. The topology, or shape, of a network may take five forms: star, ring, bus, hybrid, FDDL

Although large networks are useful, many organizations need to have a local network – an in-house network-to tie together their own equipment. Here let's consider the following aspects of local area networks:

- Types of LANs
- Components of a LAN
- Topology
- Impact of LANs

9.4.1 Types of LAN

Client / Service architecture : Network architecture in which each computer of process on the network is either a client or a server. Servers are powerful computer or processors dedicated to managing disk drives (file servers), printers (print servers), or network traffic (network servers). Clients are PCs or workstations on which users run applications (Fig. 9.6).

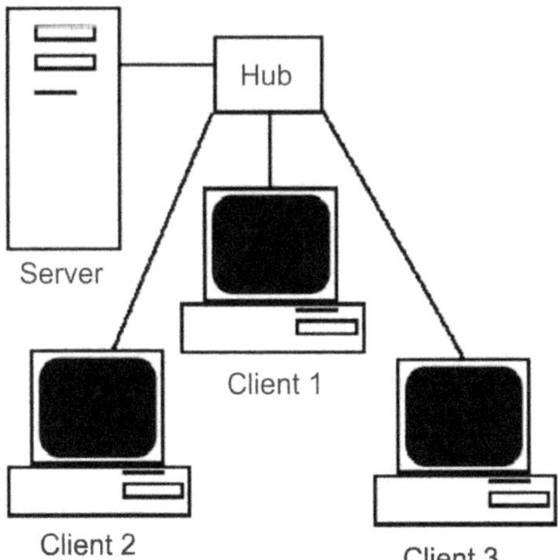

Fig. 9.6 Client / Server architecture.

In Peer-to-peer architecture, each workstation has equivalent capabilities and responsibilities (Fig. 9.7). This differs from client/server architectures, in which some computers are dedicated to serving the others. Peer-topeer networks are generally simpler and less expensive, but they usually do not offer the same performance under heavy loads.

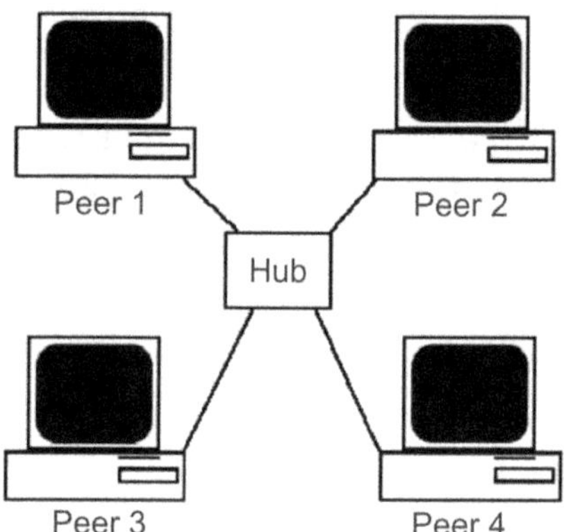

Fig. 9.7 Peer-to-peer architecture.

9.4.2 Components of LAN

Media or cabling system : In computer networks, media refer to the cables linking workstations together. There are many different types of transmission media, the most popular being twisted-pair wire, coaxial cable (the type of cable used for cable television), and fiber optic cable (cables based on higher propagation).

Computer with Network Interface card : More than one computer are required to make a network interface card often abbreviated as NIC, an expansion board you insert into a computer so the computer can be connected to a network. Most NICs are designed for a particular type of network, protocol, and media, although some can serve multiple networks. The most popular NIC protocol is Ethernet.

Ethernet : A local-area network (LAN) protocol developed by Xerox Corporation in co-operation with DEC and Intel in 1976. Ethernet uses a bus or star topology and supports data transfer rates of 10 Mbps. The Ethernet specification served as the basis for the IEEE 802.3 standard, which specifies the physical and lower software layers. Ethernet uses the CSMA/CD access method to handle simultaneous demands. It is one of the most widely implemented LAN standards.

A newer version of Ethernet, called 100Base-T (Fast Ethernet), supports data transfer rates of 100 Mbps. And the newest version, Gigabit Ethernet supports, data rates of 1 gigabit (1,000 megabits) per second.

Network Operating System (NOS) *:* An operating system that includes special functions for connecting computers and devices into a local-area network (LAN). Some operating systems, such as UNIX, have networking functions built in. The term network operating system, however, is generally reserved for software that enhances a basic operating system by adding networking features. For example, some popular NOS's for DOS and Windows systems include Novell Netware, Artisoft's LAN testic, Microsoft LAN Manager, and Windows NT.

Bridges *:* A device that connects two local-area networks (LANs), or two segments of the same LAN (Fig. 9.8). The two LANs being connected can be alike or dissimilar. For example, a bridge can connect an Ethernet with a Token-Ring network. Unlike routers, bridges are protocol-independent. They simply forward packets without analyzing and re-routing messages. Consequently, they're faster than routers, but also less versatile.

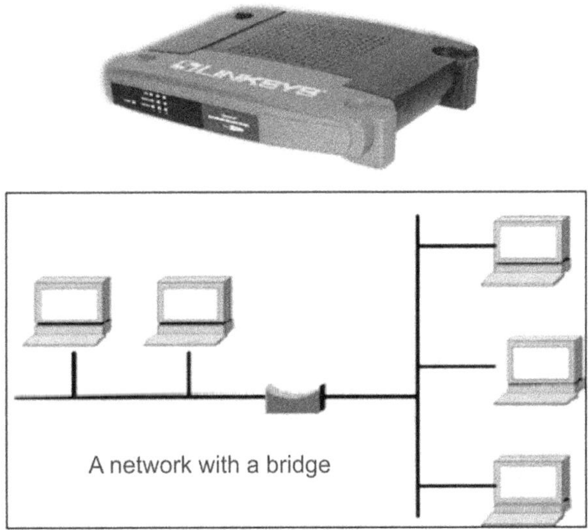

Fig. 9.8 Bridge.

HUB *:* A common connection point for devices in a network. Hubs are commonly used to connect segments of a LAN. A hub contains multiple ports. When a packet arrives at one port, it is copied to the other ports so that all segments of the LAN can see all packets.

A passive hub serves simply as a conduit for the data, enabling it to go from one device (or segment) to another. Intelligent hubs include additional features that enable an administrator to monitor the traffic passing through the hub and to configure each port in the hub. Intelligent hubs are also called manageable hubs.

A third type of hub, called a switching hub, actually reads the destination address of each packet and then forwards the packet to the correct port.

***Router* :** A device that connects two LANs (Fig. 9.9). Routers are similar to bridges, but provide additional functions, such as the ability to filter messages and forward them to different places based on various criteria.

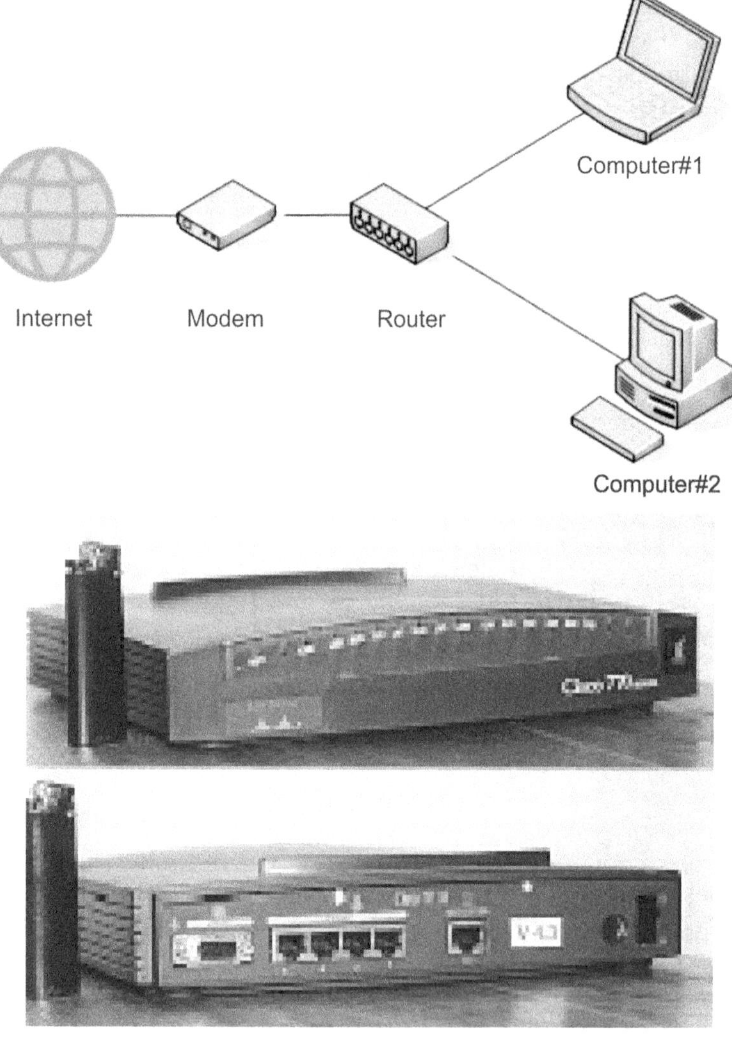

Fig. 9.9 Router.

Repeater : A network device used to regenerate or replicate a signal. Repeaters are used in transmission systems to regenerate analog or digital signals distorted by transmission loss. Analog repeaters frequently can only amplify the signal while digital repeaters can reconstruct a signal to near its original quality.

In a data network, a repeater can relay messages between sub-networks that use different protocols or cable types. Hubs can operate as repeaters by relaying messages to all connected computers. A repeater cannot do the intelligent routing performed by bridges and routers.

Gateway : In networking, a combination of hardware and software that links two different types of networks (Fig. 9.10). Gateways between e-mail systems, for example, allow users on different e-mail systems to exchange messages.

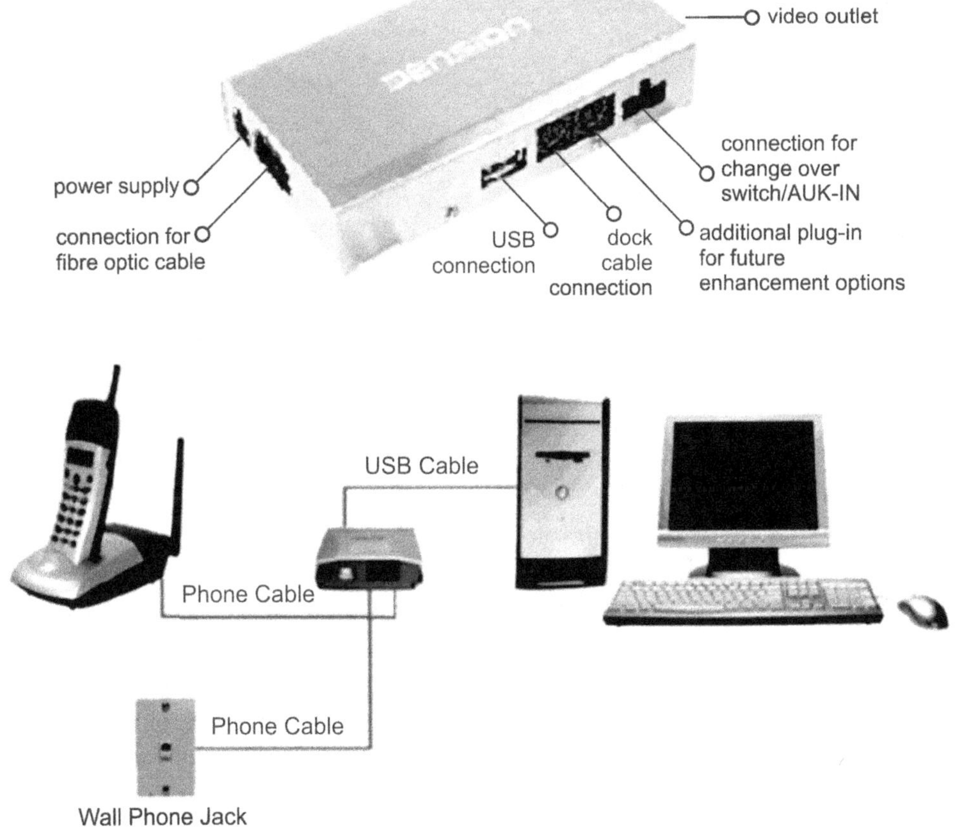

Fig. 9.10 Gateway.

9.4.3 Topology of LAN

The geometric arrangement of a computer system or the shape of a local-area network (LAN) or other communications systems is called topology. There are three principal topologies used in LANs.

Bus topology : In bus topology all devices are connected to a central cable, called the bus or backbone (Fig. 9.11). Bus networks are relatively inexpensive and easy to install for small networks. Ethernet systems use a bus topology.

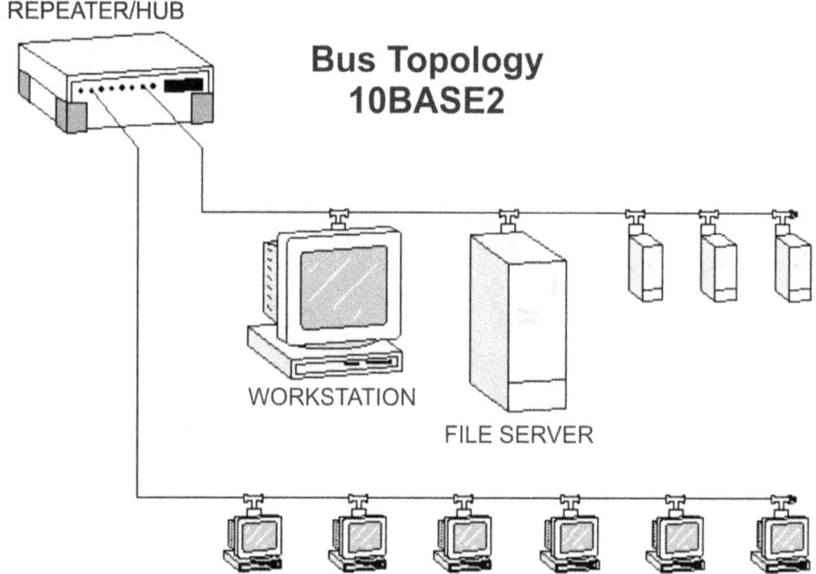

Fig. 9.11 Bus topology.

Advantages of Bus Topology

- ***Short cable length and simple layout :*** Because there is a single common data path connecting all nodes, the bus topology allows a very short cable length to be used. This decreases the installation cost, and also leads to a simple, easy-to-maintain wiring layout.

- ***Easy to extend :*** Additional nodes can be connected to an existing bus network at any point along its length. More extensive additions can be achieved by adding extra segments connected by a type of signal amplifier known as a repeater.

- ***Resilient architecture :*** The bus architecture has an inherent simplicity that makes it very reliable from a hardware point of view. There is a single cable through which all data passes and to which all nodes are connected.

Disadvantages

- ***Fault diagnosis is difficult*** : Although the simplicity of the bus topology means that there is very little that can go wrong, fault detection is not a simple matter. In most LANs based on a bus, control of the network is not centralized in any particular node. This means that detection of a fault may be performed from many points in the networks.

- ***Fault isolation is difficult*** : In the star topology, a defective node is easily isolated from the network by removing its connection at the center. If a node is faulty on a bus. it must be rectified at the point where the node is connected to the network. Once the fault has been located, the node can simply be removed. In the case where the fault is in the network medium it self, an entire segment of the bus must be disconnected.

- ***Nodes must be intelligent*** : Each node on the network is directly connected to the central bus. This means that some way of deciding who can use the network at any given time must be performed in each node. It tends to increase the cost of the nodes irrespective of whether this performed in hardware or software.

- ***Repeater configuration*** : When a bus-type network has its backbone extended using repeaters, reconfiguration may be necessary. This may involve tailoring cable lengths, adjusting terminators etc.

Ring topology : In ring topology all devices are connected to one another in the shape of a closed loop, so that each device is connected directly to two other devices, one on either side of it (Fig. 9.12). Ring topologies are relatively expensive and difficult to install, but they offer high bandwidth and can span large distances.

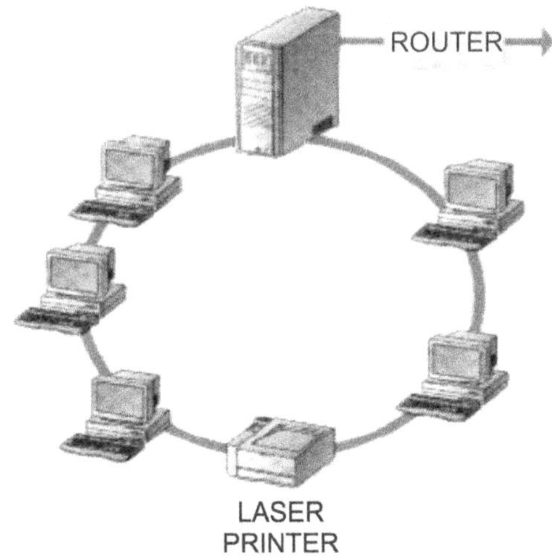

Fig. 9.12 Ring topology.

Advantages

- ***Short cable length*** *:* The amount of cabling involved in a ring topology is comparable to that of a bus and is small relative to that of a star. This means that fewer connections will be needed, which will in turn increase network reliability.

- ***No wiring closet space required*** *:* Since there is only one cable connecting each node to its immediate neighbors, it is not necessary to allocate space in the building for wiring closets.

- ***Suitable for optical fibers*** *:* Optical fibers offer the possibility of very high speed transmission. Because traffic on a ring travels in one direction, it is easy to use optical fibers as a medium of transmission. Also, since a ring is made up of nodes connected by short segments of transmission medium, there is a possibility of mixing the types used for different parts of the network.

Disadvantages

- ***Node failure causes network failure*** *:* The transmission of data on a ring goes through every connected node on the ring before returning to the sender. If one node fails to pass data through it, the entire network fails and no traffic can flow until the defective node has been removed from the ring.

- ***Difficult to diagnose faults*** *:* The facts the failure one node will affect all others has serious implications for fault diagnosis. It may be necessary to examine a series of adjacent nodes to determine the faulty one. This operation may also require diagnostic facilities to be built into each node.

- ***Network reconfiguration is difficult*** *:* The all or nothing nature of the ring topology can cause problems when one decides to extend or modify the geographical scope of the network. It is not possible to shut down a small section of the ring while keeping the majority of it working normally.

- ***Topology affects the access protocol*** *:* Each node on a ring has a responsibility to pass on data that is received. This means that the access protocol must take this into account. Before a node can transmit its own data, it must ensure that the medium is available for use.

Star topology *:* In a star topology several devices are connected to one centralized computer (Fig. 9.13). In this topology none of the other computer can communicate with each other if the central computer breaks down. All the transmission between with each other of the network is through the central computer. This topology is used in the case where centralized record keeping is necessary, like in banking sector.

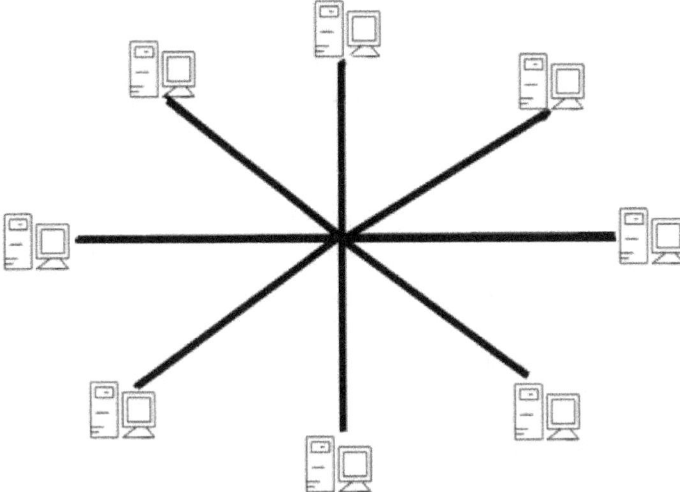

Fig. 9.13 Star topology.

The star topology has found extensive application in areas where intelligence in the network is concentrated at the central node. The tendency in the latest computer systems is away from host-based computing power, and the advent of microprocessor-based systems, where all nodes possess a high level of processing power have led to a fall off in the use of this topology. Nevertheless, the technology is well understood and it is currently the dominant configuration in traditional data communication.

Advantages

- ***Ease of service :*** That star topology has a number of concentration points, i.e. at the central node or at intermediate wiring closets. These provide easy access for service of reconfiguration of the network.

- ***One device per connection :*** Connection points in any network are inherently prone to failure. In the star topology, failure of a single concentration typically involves disconnecting one node from an otherwise fully functional network.

- ***Simple access protocols :*** Any given connection in a star network involves only the central node and one peripheral node. In this situation, contention for who has control of the medium for transmission purposes is easily solved.

- ***Centralised control/problem diagnosis :*** The fact that the central node is connected directly to every other node in the network means that faults are easily detected and isolated. It is a simple matter to disconnect failing nodes from the system.

Disadvantages

- ***Long cable length :*** Because each node is directly connected to the center, the star topology necessitates a large quantity of cable. While the cost of the cable is often small, congestion in cable ducts and maintenance and installation problems can increase costs considerably.

- ***Difficult to expand :*** The addition of a new node to a star network involves a connection all the way to the central node. Providing large numbers of redundant cables during the initial wiring usually caters for expansion. However, problems can arise if a longer cable length is needed or an unanticipated concentration of nodes is required.

- ***Central node dependency:*** If the central node in a star network fails, the entire network is rendered inoperable. This introduces heavy reliability and redundancy constraints on this node.

Tree topology : In tree topology all devices are linked in a hierarchical fashion (Fig. 9.14). This topology is also known as hierarchical topology. This topology is commonly used in the organisation where the headquarter communicate with regional officers and they communicated with branch officers and district officers, and so on.

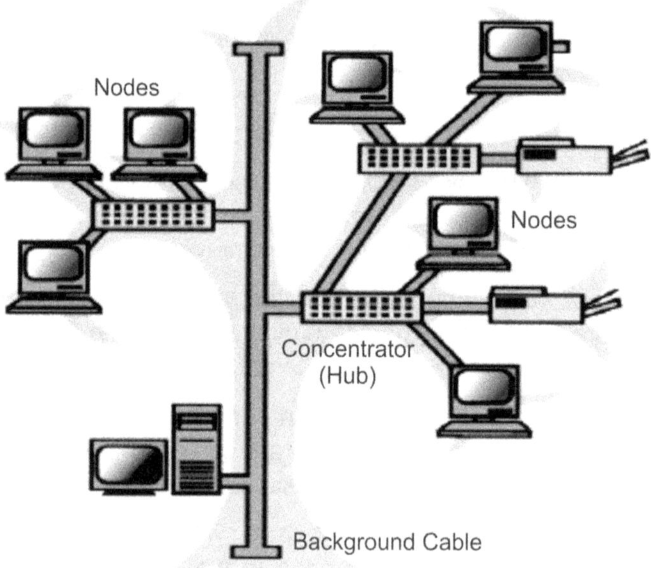

Fig. 9.14 Tree topology.

Advantages

- **_Easy to extend:_** _Because_ the tree is of its very nature, divided into subunits, it is easier to add new nodes or branches to it.

- **_Fault isolation :_** It is possible to disconnect whole branches of the network from the main structure. This makes it easier to isolate a defective node.

Disadvantages

- **_Dependent on the root :_** If the 'head end' device fails to operate, the entire network is rendered inoperable. In this respect the tree suffers from the same reliability problems as the star.

- **_Mesh Topology :_** In mesh topology point-to-point connections have between every device in the network (Fig. 9.15). Each device requires an interface on the network. Mesh topologies are not usually considered practical. In addition, unless each station frequently sends signals to all the other stations, an excessive amount of network bandwidth is wasted. However, mesh networks are extremely fault-tolerant, and each link provides guaranteed capacity.

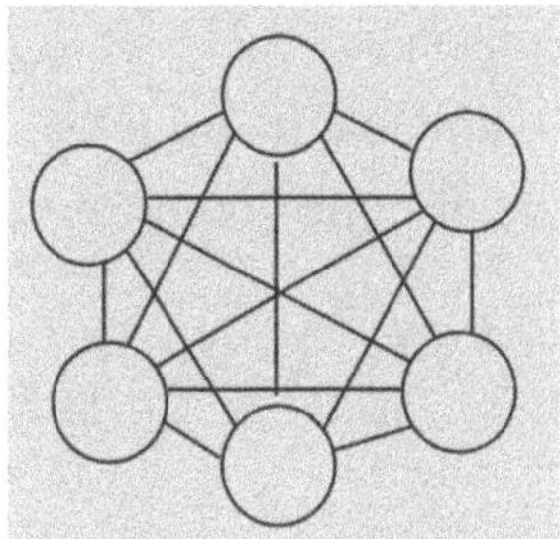

Fig. 9.15 Mesh topology.

Generally mesh topologies used in a hybrid network with just the largest or most important sites interconnected. For example, suppose your organization operates a WAN with 4 or 5 main sites and a large number of remote offices. Each main site has a mainframe and all or the mainframes must communicate to maintain a distributed main site to ensure continuous communications between the mainframes.

Advantages

- **_Units Affected by Media Failure:_** Mesh topologies resist media failure better than other topologies. Implementations that include more than two devices will always have multiple paths to send signals from one device to another. If one path fails, the transmission signals can be routed around the failed link.

- **_Ease of Troubleshooting:_** Mesh topologies are easy to troubleshoot because each medium link is independent of all others. You can easily identify faults and can isolate the affected link.

Disadvantages

- ***Ease to Instal*** *:* Mesh networks are relatively difficult to install because each device must be linked directly to all other devices. As the number of devices increase, the difficulty of installation increases geometrically.

- ***Ease of Reconfiguration:*** Mesh topologies are difficult to reconfigure for the same reasons that they are difficult to instal.

9.5   Factors Affecting Communications among Devices

Factors affecting how data is transmitted include the transmission rate (frequency and bandwidth), the line configuration (point-to-point or multipoint), serial versus parallel transmission, and the direction of transmission flow (Simplex, half-duplex, or full-duplex),

Several factors affect how data is transmitted. They include:

- Transmission rate – frequency and bandwidth
- Line configurations – point-to-point verses multipoint
- Serial versus parallel transmission
- Direction of transmission – simplex, half-duplex, and full-duplex
- Transmission mode – asynchronous versus synchronous
- Packet switching
- Multiplexing
- Protocols.

Transmission Rate *:* Transmission Rate is a function of two variables : frequency and bandwidth.

- ***Frequency*** *:* The amount of data that can be transmitted on a channel depends on the wave frequency – the cycles of waves per second. Frequency is expressed in hertz: one cycle per second equals one hertz. The more cycles per second, the more data that can be sent through that channel.

- ***Bandwidth*** *:* The amount of data that can be transmitted in a unit of time. For digital devices, the bandwidth is usually expressed in bits per second (bps) or bytes per second. For analog devices, the bandwidth is expressed in cycles per second, or Hertz (Hz).

The bandwidth is particularly important for I/O devices. For example, a bus with a low bandwidth can hamper a fast disk drive. This is the main reason that new buses, such as AGP, have been developed for the PC.

A twisted-pair telephone wire of 4000 hertz might send only 1 kilobyte of data in a second. A coaxial cable of 100 megahertz might send 10 megabytes. And a fiber optic cable of 200 trillion hertz might send 1 gigabyte.

Line Configurations: Point-to-point & Multipoint *: There are two principal line configurations, or ways of connecting communications lines: point-to-point and multipoint.

- ***Point-to-point*** *:* A point-to-point line directly connects the sending and receiving devices, such as a terminal with a central computer. This arrangement is appropriate for a private line whose sole purpose is to keep data secure by transmitting it from one device to another.

- ***Multipoint*** *:* A multipoint line is a single line that interconnects several communications devices to one computer. Often on a multipoint line only one communications device, such as a terminal, can transmit at any given time.

Serial & Parallel Transmission *:* Data is transmitted in two ways – serial and parallel.

Serial data transfer refers to transmitting data one bit a time. The opposite of serial is parallel, in which several bits are transmitted concurrently.

Parallel data transmission refers to processes that occur simultaneously. Printers and other devices are said to be either parallel or serial. Parallel means the device is capable of receiving more than one bit at a time (that is, it receives several bit in parallel). Most modern printers are parallel.

9.6 Direction of Transmission Flow

When two devices are in communication, data can be flow in three ways – simplex, half duplex, or full duplex. These are described as follows :

Simplex data transmission *:* This refers to transmission in only one direction (Fig. 9.16). Note the difference between simplex and half-duplex. Simplex refers to one-way communications where one party is the transmitter and the other is the receiver. An example of simplex communications is a simple radio, which you can receive data from stations but can't transmit data.

Half duplex data transmission *:* It refers to the transmission of data in just one direction at a time (Fig. 9.17). For example, a walkie-talkie is a half-duplex device because only one party can talk at a time. In contrast, a telephone is a full-duplex device because both parties can talk simultaneously.

Most modems contain a switch that lets you select between half-duplex and fullduplex modes. The correct choice depends on which program you are using to transmit data through the modem.

In half-duplex mode, each character transmitted is immediately displayed on your screen. (For this reason, it is sometimes called local echo – the local device echoes characters). In full-duplex mode, transmitted data is not displayed on your monitor until it has been received and returned (remotely echoed) by the other device.

Full duplex data transmission *:* This refers to the transmission of data in two directions simultaneously. For example, a telephone is a full-duplex device because both parties can talk at once.

Most modems have a switch that lets you choose between full-duplex and halfduplex modes. The choice depends on which communications program you are running. In full-duplex mode, data you transmit does not appear on your screen until it has been received and sent back by the other party. This enables you to validate that the data has been accurately transmitted. If your display screen shows two of each character, it probably means that modem is set to half-duplex mode.

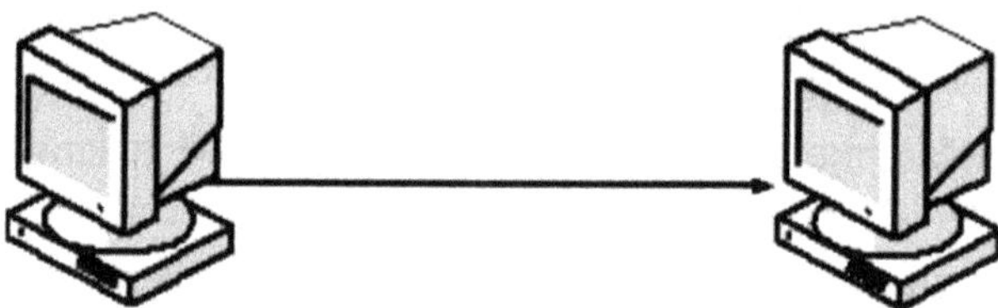

Fig. 9.16 Simplex data transmission.

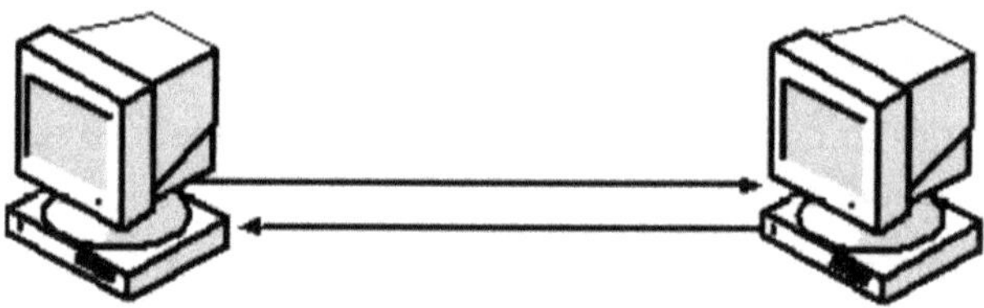

Fig. 9.17 Half-duplex data transmission.

9.7   Transmission Modes

Asynchronous mode *:* Asynchronous mode means not synchronized mode ; that is, the transmission not occurring at predetermined or regular intervals. The term asynchronous is usually used to describe communications in which data can be transmitted intermittently rather than in a steady stream. For example, a telephone conversation is asynchronous because both parties can talk whenever they like. If the communication were synchronous, each party would be required to wait a specified interval before speaking.

The difficulty with asynchronous communications is that the receiver must have a way to distinguish between valid data and noise. In computer communications, this is usually accomplished through a special start bit and stop bit at the beginning and end of each piece of data. For this reason, asynchronous communication is sometimes called start-stop transmission.

Synchronous mode *:* In this mode transmission occurs at regular intervals. The opposite of synchronous is asynchronous. Most communication between computers and devices is asynchronous – it can occur at any time and at irregular intervals. Communication within a computer, however, is usually synchronous and is governed by the microprocessor clock. Signals along the bus, for example, can occur only at specific points in the clock cycle.

Packet Switching *:* This refers to protocols in which messages are divided into packets before they are sent. Each packet is then transmitted individually and can even follow different routes to its destination. Once all the packets forming a message arrive at the destination, they are recompiled into the original message.

Most modern Wide Area Network (WAN) protocols, including TCP/IP, X.25, and Frame Relay, are based on packet-switching technologies. In contrast, normal telephone service is based on a circuit-switching technology in which a dedicated line is allocated for transmission between two parties. Circuit switching is ideal when data must be with most real-time data, such as live audio and video. Packet switching is more efficient and robust for data that can withstand some delays in transmission, such as e-mail messages and Web pages.

ATM *:* Short for asynchronous transfer mode, a network technology based on transferring data in cells or packets of fixed size. The cell used with ATM is relatively small compared to units used with older technologies. The small, constant cell size allows ATM equipment to transmit video, audio, and computer data over the same network, and assures that no single type of data hogs the line.

Current implementations of ATM support data transfer rates vary from 25 to 622 Mbps. This compares to a maximum of 100 Mbps for Ethernet, the current technology used for most LANs.

Some people think that ATM holds the answer to the Internet bandwidth problem, but others are skeptical. ATM creates a fixed channel, or route, between two points whenever data transfer begins. This differs from TCP/IP, in which messages are divided into packets and each packet can take a different route from source to destination. This difference makes it easier to track and bill data usage across an ATM network, but it makes it less adaptable to sudden surges in network traffic.

- ***Constant Bit Rate (CBR)*** specifies a fixed bit rate so that it is sent in a steady stream. This is a popular choice for voice and video conferencing data.

- ***Variable Bit Rate (VBR)*** provides a specified throughput capacity but data is not sent evenly. This is a popular choice for voice and video confining data.

- ***Unspecified Bit Rate (UBR)*** does not guarantee any throughput levels. This is used for applications, such as file transfer, that can tolerate delays.

- ***Available Bit Rate (ABR)*** provides a guaranteed minimum capacity but allows data to be busted at higher capacities when the network is free.

Multiplexing : To combine multiple signals (analog or digital) for transmission over a single line or media. A common type of multiplexing combines several low-speed signals for transmission over a single high-speed connection. The following are examples of different multiplexing methods.

- ***Frequency Division Multiplexing (FDM) :*** A multiplexing that uses different frequencies to combine multiple streams of data for transmission over a communications medium. FDM assigns a discrete carrier frequency to each data stream and then combines many modulated carrier frequencies transmission (Fig. 9.18). For example, television transmitters use FDM to broadcast several channels at once.

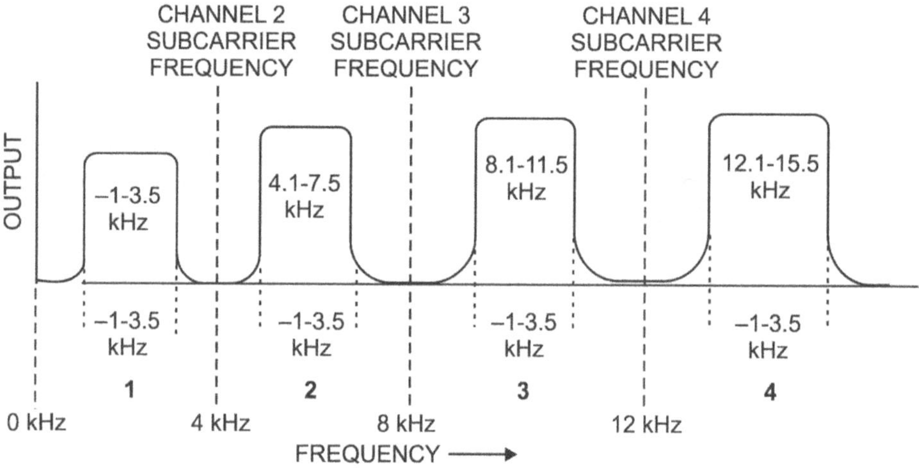

Fig. 9.18 Multiplexing.

- ***Time Division Multiplexing (TDM) :*** A type of multiplexing that combines data streams by assigning each stream a different time in a set. TDM repeatedly transmits a fixed sequence of time over a single transmission channel (Fig. 9.19). Within T. Carrier systems, such as T-1 and T-3, TDM combines Pulse Code Modulated (PCM) Streams created for each conversation of data stream.

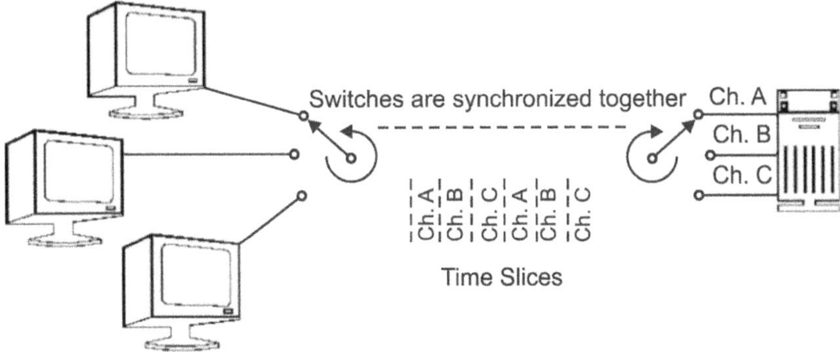

Fig. 9.19 Time Division Multiplexing.

- ***Statistical Time Division Multiplexing (STDM)** :* Time slots are assigned to signals dynamically to make better use of bandwidth.

- ***Wavelength Division Multiplexing (WDM)** :* A type of multiplexing developed for use on optical fiber. WDM modulates each of several data streams onto a different part of the light spectrum. WDM is the optical equivalent of FDM.

***Multiplexor** :* A communications device that multiplexes (combines) several signals for transmission over a single medium. A demultiplexor completes the process by separating multiplexed signals from a transmission line. Frequently a multiplexor and demultiplexor are combined into a single device capable of processing both outgoing and incoming signals. A multiplexor is sometimes called a mux.

***Concentrator** :* A type of multiplex that combines multiple channels onto a single transmission medium in such a way that all the individual channels can be simultaneously active. For example, ISPs use concentrators to combine their dial-up modem connections onto faster T-1 lines that connect to the Internet.

Concentrators are also used in local-area networks (LANs) to combine transmissions from a cluster of nodes. In this case, the concentrator is often called a hub or MAU. Information frame is not regenerated. Additions or deletions of stations of the ring can be disruptive, if the changes are not managed property.

9.8 Wide Area Network

As the name suggest, WAN spread across countries and continents, satellite being the transmission media. A wide area network is a network that links separate geographical locations. A WAN can be public system or can also use most other types of circuit including satellite networks, value added networks (VANS/VADS).

The network can be a private system made up from a network of circuits leased from the local telephone company or setup public system as virtual private networks. A virtual private network is one which operates in the same way as a private network but which uses public switched services for the transmission of information. The main distinguishing feature between a WAN and LAN is that the LAN is under the complete control of the owner, where as the WAN needs the involvement of another authority. LAN are also able to handle very high data transfer rates at low cost because of the limited area covered, LANs have a lower error rate than WANs.

9.8.1 Types of Wide Area Networks

The essential purpose of WAN, regardless of the size or technology used is to link separate locations in order to move data around. A WAN allows these locations to access shared computer resources and provides the essential infrastructure for developing widespread distributed computing systems. The different types of WAN are:

Public Networks: Public networks are those networks, which are installed and run by the telecommunications authorities and are made available to any organisation or individual who subscribe it.

Public Switched Telephone Network (PSTN): The features of the PSTN are its low speed, the analog nature of transmission, a restricted bandwidth and its widespread availability. The PSTN is most useful in wide area data communication systems as an adjusted to other mechanism.

Public Switched Data Networks (PSDN): The term PSDN refers a number of technologies, although currently it is limited to public packet switched network available to the public. The main features of all PSDNs are their high level of reliability and the high quality of the connections provided. PSDN is very popular for connecting public and private mail system to implement electronic mail services with other companies.

Value Added Services (VANS/VADS): In value added services the provider of such services must process, store and manipulate the data that are carried onto the network, that is, add value to it. The technique can be used in specific type of business in which it is advantageous to be able to share information with other companies in the secure line. Electronic data interchange (EDI) is one area for value added services in which two trading partners exchange trading documents.

Integrated Service Digital Network (ISDN): The ISDN is a networking concept providing for integration of voice, video and data services using digital transmission media and combining both circuit and packet switching techniques. The motivating force behind ISDN is that telephone networks around the world have been making a transition towards utilizing digital transmission facilities for many years.

Private Network: The basic technique used in all forms of private WAN is to use private circuits to link the locations to be served by the network. Between these fixed points the owner of the network has complete freedom to use the circuits in anyway they want. They can use the circuits to carry large quantities of data or high-speed transmission.

9.9   Transmission Media

Magnetic Media :

One of the most common way to transport data from one computer to another is to write them onto magnetic tape or floppy disks, physically transport the tape or disks to the destination machine. While this method is not as sophisticated as using a geo-synchronous communication satellite, it is often much more cost-effective, especially for applications in which high bandwidth or cast per bit transported is the key factor.

A simple calculation makes this point clear. An industry slandered 6250 bpi magnetic tape can hold 180 megabytes. A station wagon or light truck can easily transport 200 tapes at one time. Suppose the source and destination machines are an hour's due apart. The effective data rate between these two machines is then 288000 megabits in 3600 sec or 80 Mbps. No wide area network transfer in this order of magnitude of this bandwidth. Few local networks can even match it for a bank with gigabytes of data to be backed up daily on a second machine it is likely that no other transmission technology can even begin to approach magnetic tape for performance or cost-effectiveness.

Twisted Pair :

Although the bandwidth characteristics of magnetic tape are excellent, the delay characteristics are poor. Transmission time is measured in minutes or hours not milliseconds. For many application an online connection is needed. The oldest and still most common transmission medium is twisted pair (Fig. 9.20).

UTP Cable (4-pair)

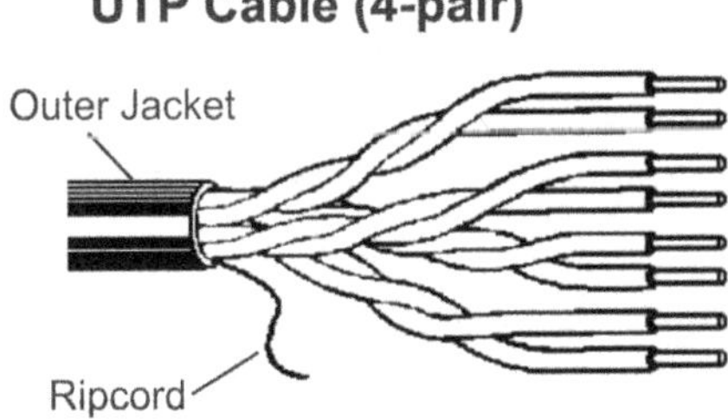

Fig. 9.20 Twisted Pair.

A twisted pair consists of two insulated copper wires, typically about 1 mm thick. The wires are twisted together in a helical form. Just as a DNA molecule. The twisted form is used to reduce electrical interference to similar pairs close by. The most commonly used application of twisted pair is telephone system.

Coaxial Cable :

Another common transmission medium is the co-axial cable (known to its many funds as just "Core") (Fig. 9.21). Two kinds of coaxial cable are widely used. One kind 50-ohm cable is used for analog transmission.

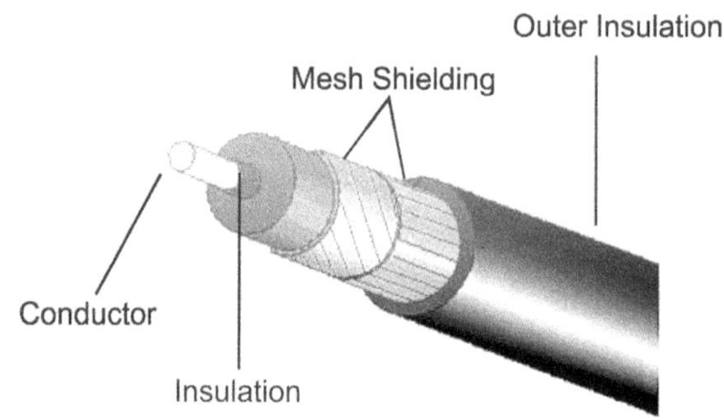

Fig. 9.21 Coaxial Cable.

The construction of the coaxial cable gives it a good combination of high bandwidth and excellent noise immunity. The bandwidth possibly depends on the cable length. For 1 km cables a data rate of 10 Mbps is feasible. Coaxial cables are used for local area networks and for long distance transmission within the telephone system.

There are two ways to connect computers to a coaxial cable. The first way is to the cable cleanly and insert a T junction a connector that reconnects the cable but also provide a third wire leading off to the computer. The second way is to use a vampire tap, which is a hole of exceedingly priercing depth and width drilled into due cable, terminating in the core. Into this hole is secured a special connector that achieves the same goal as a T-junction, but without the need to cut the cable in two.

Inserting a T-junction requires cutting the cable; if the hole is drilled too deep it may break the core into unconnected pieces. If it is not deep enough the connection may give inter milder errors.

The cable used for empire tops are the thickest and more expensive than the cable used width T-junctions.

The other kind of coaxial cable system uses analog transmission in standered cable television cabling. It is called broadband. Though the term broad comes from the telephone world, where it refers to anything wider than 4 KHz, in the computer networking used "broadband", it means any cable network using analog transmission.

Since broadband networks are use standered cable television technology, the cables can be used up to 300 MHz and can run for nearly 100 km due to the analog signaling which is much critical than digital signaling. This transmits digital signals and analog network. Each interface must contain electronics to convert the outgoing bit stream to an analog signal, and the incoming analog signal to a bit stream.

Broadband systems are normally divided into multiple channels, frequently the 6 MHz channels used for television broadcasting. Each channel can be used for analog television's high quality audio, or a digital bit stream at, say 3 Mbps, independent of other channels. Television and data can be mixed on the some cable.

One key difference between base band and broadband is that broadband systems need analog amplifiers to strengthen the signal periodically. This amplifier only transits signals in one direction. So a computer outputting a packet will not be able to reach computer from it if an amplifier lies between them. To get around this problem two types of broadband systems have been developed – cable and single cable systems.

Fiber Optics

Recent developments in optical technology have mode it possible to transmit data by pulse of light. A light pulse can be used to signal a 1 bit, the absence of a pulse signals a 0 bit. Visible light has a frequency of about 10 MHz, so the bandwidth of an optical transmission system is potentially enormous.

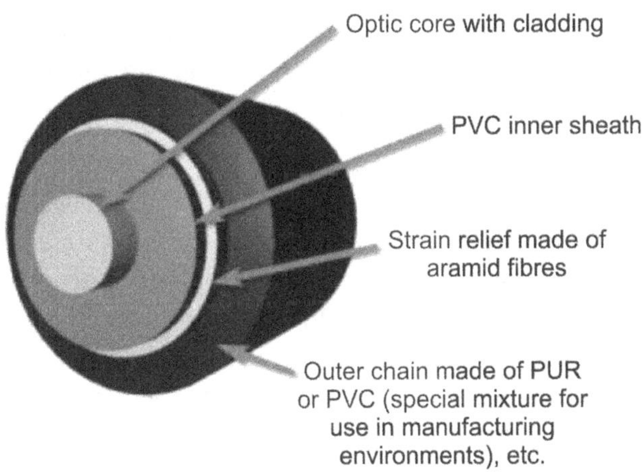

Fig. 9.20 Fiber Optics.

An optical transmission system has three components : the transmission medium, the light source, and the detector. The transmission medium is an ultra thin fiber of glass or fused silica. The light source is either an LED (Light Emitting Diode) or a laser diode, which unit light pulses when an electrical current is applied. The detector is a photodiode, which generates an electrical pulse when light falls on it. By attaching an LED or lesser diode to one end of an optical fiber and a photodiode to the other, we have a unidirectional data transmission system that accepts an electrical signal, concerts and transmits it by light pulses and then reconverts the output to an electrical signal at the receiving end.

This transmission system is based on an interesting principle of physics. When a light way passes from one medium to another, for example, from fused silica to air, it is refracted at the silica air boundary. Here we see a light ray incident on the boundary at an angle a1 emerging at one angle b1. The amount of refraction depends on endurance properties of the two media. For angles of incidence above a certain critical value the light is reflected back into the silica. Thus a light ray incident at or above the critical angle is trapped inside the fiber and can propagate for many kilometers with virtually no loss.

Fiber optics links are being installed for long distance telephone lines in many countries. Fibers can also form the basis for lanes although the technology is more complex. The basic problem is that which ampire taps can be made on fiber LAN's by fusing the incoming fiber from the computer with the LANs fiber. The process of making a tap is very tricky and substantial light is lost. Two types of interfaces are used. A passive interface consists of two fused onto the main fiber. One tap has an LED or laser diode at the end of it and other has a photodiode. The tap itself is completely passive and is thus extremely reliable because a broken LED or photodiode does not break the ring. If one computer does not break the ring, it just takes one computer offline.

Two other interface type is the active repeater. The incoming light is connected to an electrical signal, regenerated to full strength if it has been weakened, and retransmitted as light. The interface width the computer is an ordinary copper wire that comes into the signal regenerator. In this design each interface has a fiber running from its transmitter to a silica cylinder, with due incoming fibers fused to one end of the cylinder. Similarly fibers fused to the other end of the cylinder are run to each of the receivers. Whenever an interface of a light pulse occurs, it is diffused inside the passive star to illuminate all the receivers, thus achieving broadcast. In effect the passive star performs a Boolean OR of all the incoming signals and transmits the result out on all lines.

Since the incoming energy is decided among all the outgoing lines the number of nodes in the network is limited by the sensitivity of the photodiodes. It is instructive to compare coaxial cable to fiber optics. Fiber provides externally high bandwidth with little power loss; it can run for long distances between repeaters.

ISDN

For last more than a century, the primary international communication infrastructure has been the telephone system. This system was designed for analog voice transmission and is proving inadequate for modern communication needs such as data transmission facsimile and video. User demands for these and other services have led to an international undertaking to replace a major portion of the worldwide telephone system with an allowanced digital system by the early part of the twenty-first century. This new system, called ISDN (Integrated services digital network), has its primary goal the integration of voice and non-voice services.

SERVICES

The key service will continue to be voice although many enhancements will be added. For example many corporate managers have an intercom button on their telephone that rings their recreations instantly. One ISDN feature is telephones with multiple buttons for instant called setup to arbitrary telephones anywhere in world. Another feature is telephones that display the caller's telephone number, name and address. A more sophisticated feature allows the telephone to be connected to a computer, so that the caller's database record is displayed on the screen as the call comes in.

They allow users to connect their ISDN terminal or computer to any other one in the world. At present such connections are frequently impossible internationally due to incomputable national telephone systems. Connections may also involve three or more parties, along with the possibility of a broadcast. It may also involve three or more multinational corporations sending an electronic message, say, about changes in the retirement policy to all employers over the age of 60.

9.10   OSI Reference Model

Computer network is also called NETWORK. Besides physically connecting computer and communication devices, network system serves the important function of establishing a cohesive architecture that allows a variety of equipment to transfer information in a near-seamless fashion. A popular architecture is Open System Interconnection (OSI). It is a standard description for new messages, which should be transmitted between any two points in a telecommunication network.

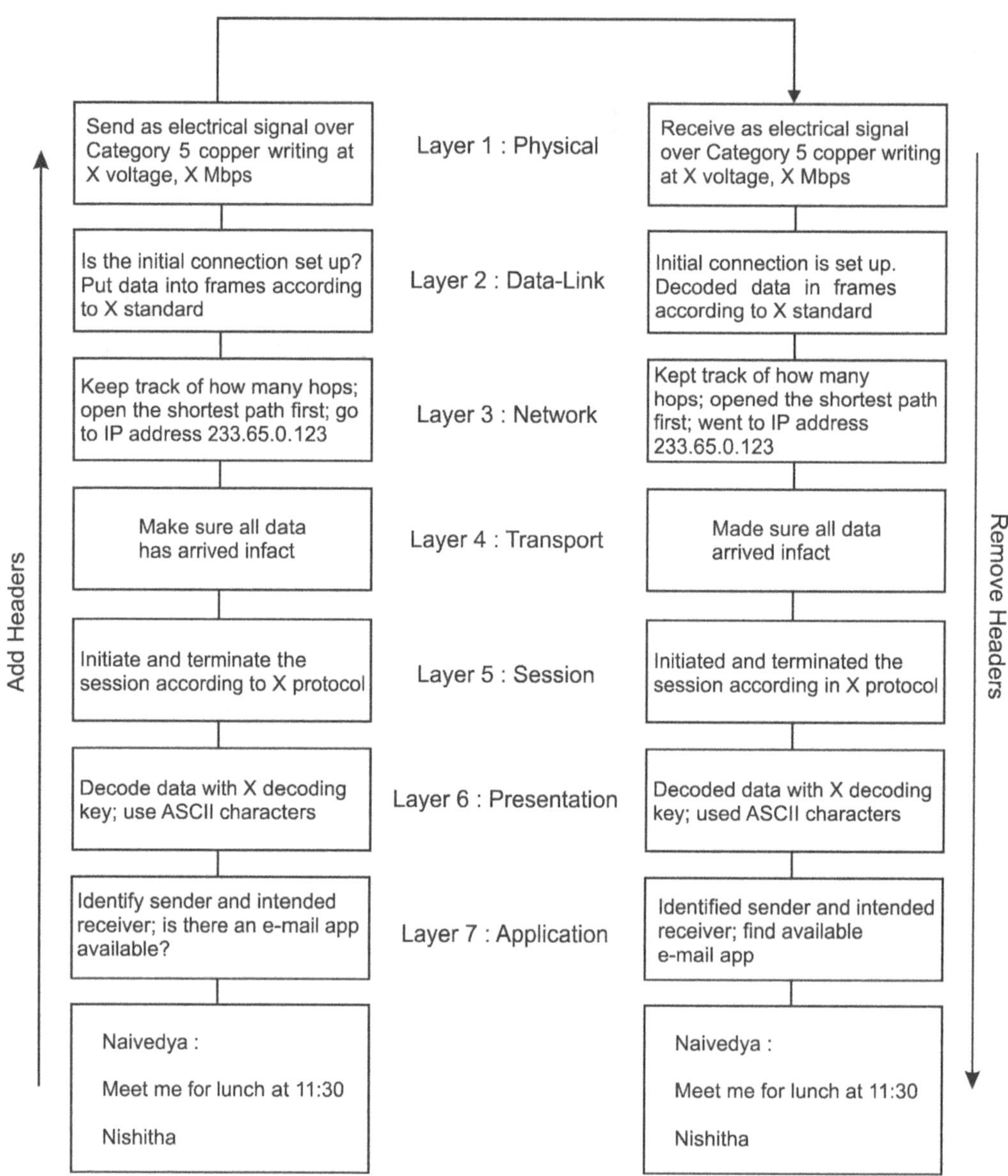

Fig. 9.21 OSI Reference Model.

The main idea in OSI is that the process of communication between two and users in a telecommunication network can be divided into layers, with each layer adding its own set of special, related functions. Each communicating user is at a computer equipped with these seven layers of functions. So, in a given message between users, there will be a flow of data through each layer at one end down through the layers in that computer and at the other and when the messages arrives another flow of data up through the layers in the receiving computer and ultimately to the end user. The actual programming and hardware that furnishes these seven layers of function is usually a combination of the computer operating system, applications.

Application Layer (Layer – 7) : Applications software is that which carries out useful functions on behalf of the user. This software may well need access to network services. This top layer defines the language and syntax that program uses to communicate with other programs. Application layer represents the purpose of communicating in the first place. At this layer the communication partners are identified, quality of service is identified, user authentication, privacy are considered and constraints on data syntax are identified.

Presentation Layer (Layer – 6) : This layer defines how the system provides files and services in a uniform way to applications. This layer can in some ways be considered the function of the operating system. When data is transmitted between different types of computer system, the presentation layer negotiates and manages the way data is represented and encoded. For example, it provides a common denominator between ASCII and EBCDIC machines as well as between different floating point and binary formats. This layer is also used for encryption and decryption.

Session Layer (Layer 5) : This layer sets up, coordinates, and terminates conversations, exchanges and dialogs between the applications at each end. It deals with session and connection coordination. This layer manages network connections on behalf of the high-level layers.

It is responsible for 'logging in' and users authentications. It provides coordination's of the communications in an orderly manner. It determines one way or two-way communications and manages the dialogue between both parties. For example, making sure that the previous request has been fulfilled before the next one is sent. It also marks significant parts of the transmitted data with checkpoints to allow for fast recovery in the event of a connection failure.

Transport Layer (Layer–4) : It is responsible for constructing streams of data packets, sending and checking for correct delivery. This layer manages the end-to-end control and error checking. It ensure complete data transfer. The transport layer is responsible for overall end-to-end validity and integrity of the transmission. The lower data link layer is only responsible for delivering packets from one made to another. Thus, if a packet gets lost in a router somewhere in the enterprise internet, the transport layer will detect it.

Network Layer (Layer-3) : Network layer from individual packets from data supplied by the transport layer. The network layer establishes the route between the sending and receiving stations. The node-to-node function of the data link layer is extended across the entire internet-work, because the routable protocol contains a network address in an addition to a station addresses. This layer handles the routing of the data. This layer is the switching function of the dial-up telephone system as well as the functions performed by routable protocol such as IP. If all stations are contained within a single network segment, then the routing capability in this layer is not required.

Data Link Layer (Layer-2) *:* Also called line layer of media access. Controls access to the physical network hardware. This layer provides error control and synchronization for the physical level and does bit-stuffing for strings of access of 5. It furnishes transmission protocol knowledge and management. The data link is responsible for node-to-node validity and integrity of the transmission. The transmitted bits are divided into frames. The data link layer, which packages the data units into frames, is divided into two sub layers:

- *LLC (Local Link Control) Top sub layer:* Establishes and maintains links between communicating devices. It also responsible for frame error connection and hardware address.

- *MAC (Media Access Control) Bottom sub layer:* Controls how devices share a media channel. There are two main methods.

   (i) With connection, all devices attached to the network can transmit whenever they have something to communicate.

   (ii) With token passing, computers on the network cannot transmit on to the network cable until they are given a frame or token.

Physical Layer (Layer-1) *:* The physical layer is responsible for passing bits onto and receiving them from the connecting medium. This layer conveys the bit stream through the network at the electrical and mechanical level. It provides the hardware means of sending and receiving data on a carrier. Physical layer includes hardware, wires, plugs and sockets, signal generators etc. This layer has no understanding of the meaning of the bits, but deals with the electrical and mechanical characteristic of the signals and signaling methods.

CHAPTER 10

Data Structure

10.1 Data Structure

In computer science, a data structure is a way of storing data in a computer so that it can be used efficiently. Often a carefully chosen data structure will allow a more efficient algorithm to be used. The choice of the data structure often begins with the choice of an abstract data structure. A well-designed data structure allows a variety of critical operations to be performed, using as little resources as possible – both execution time and memory space.

Different kinds of data structures are suited to different kinds of applications, and some are highly specialized to certain tasks. For example, B-trees are particularly well-suited for implementation of databases, while routing tables rely on networks of machines to function.

In the design of many types of programs, the choice of data structures is a primary design consideration, as experience in building large systems has shown that the difficulty of implementation and the quality and performance of the final result depend heavily on choosing the best data structure. After the data structures are chosen, the algorithms to be used often become relatively obvious. Sometimes things work in the opposite direction – data structures are chosen because certain key tasks have algorithms that work best with particular data structures. In either case, the choice of appropriate data structures is crucial.

This insight has given rise to many formalised design methods and programming languages in which data structures, rather than algorithms, are the key organizing factors. Most languages feature some sort of module system, allowing data structures to be safely reused in different applications by hiding their verified implementation details behind controlled interfaces. Object-oriented programming languages such as C++ and Java in particular use objects for this purpose.

Since data structures are so crucial to professional programs, many of them enjoy extensive support in standard libraries of modern programming languages and environments, such as C++'s Standard Template Library, the Java API, and the Microsoft .NET framework.

The fundamental building blocks of most data structures are arrays, records, discriminated unions, and references. There is some debate about whether data structures represent implementations or interfaces. How they are seen may be a matter of perspective. A data structure can be viewed as an interface between two functions or as an implementation of methods to access storage that is organized according to the associated data type. (Fig. 10.1).

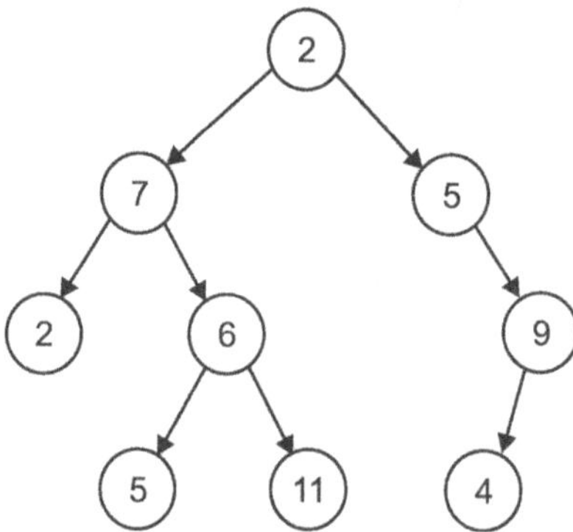

Fig. 10.1 A binary tree, a simple type of branching linked data structure.

10.2   List of Data Structures

The following is a list of data structures. For a wider list of terms, see list of terms relating to algorithms and data structures.

Linear data structures
   Array
      Dynamic array
      Parallel array
   List
      Linked list
      Skip list
      Unrolled linked list
      V List
      Associative array (a.k.a. dictionary or map)
      Hash table
      Stack
      Queue
         Priority queue
         D-queue

Tree data structures

    M-Way Tree

      B-tree

  Binary search trees

    Self-balancing binary search trees

      AVL tree

      Red-black tree

      Scapegoat tree

      Splay tree

Graph data structures

Disjoint-set data structure

Graph-structured stack

10.3   Linear Structure

The most common organization for components is a linear structure. A structure is linear if it has these 2 properties:

Property P1

Each element is `followed by' at most one other element.

Property P2

No two elements are `followed by' the same element.

An array is an example of a linearly structured data type. We generally write a linearly structured data type like this: A->B->C->D (this is one value with 4 parts).

•*Counter example 1 (violates P1)* : A points to B and C B<-A->C N.L

•*Counter example 2 (violates P2)* : A and B both point to C A->C<-B

Dropping Constraint P1 : If we drop the first constraint and keep the second, we get a tree structure or hierarchy: no two elements are followed by the same element.

This is a very common structure too, and is extremely useful. We'll study it in considerable detail.

Counter example 1 is a tree, but counter example 2 is not.

More complex example :

A is followed by B C D B by E F, C by G. We are not allowed to add any more arcs that point to any of these nodes (except possibly A - see cyclic structures).

Dropping both P1 and P2 :

If we drop both constraints, we get a graph. In a graph, there are no constraints on the relations we can define.

10.4   Cyclic Structure

All the examples we've seen are acyclic. This means that there is no sequence of arrows that leads back to where it started. Linear structures are usually acyclic, but cyclic ones are not uncommon.

Example of cyclic linear structure: A B C D A

Trees are virtually always acyclic.

Graphs are often cyclic, although the special properties of acyclic graphs make them an important topic of study.

Example : Add an edge from G to D, and from E to A

10.5   Stack

Stack is one of the most useful concepts of data structure in Computer Science.

A stack is an ordered collection of items into which new items can be inserted and from which items may be deleted at only beginning of the list, shown in Fig. 10.2.

<table>
<tr><td>E</td></tr>
<tr><td>D</td></tr>
<tr><td>C</td></tr>
<tr><td>B</td></tr>
<tr><td>A</td></tr>
</table>

Fig. 10.2 Stack Containing Stack terms.

In computer science, a stack is a data structure that works on the principle of Last In First Out (LIFO). This means that the last item put on the stack is the first item that can be taken off, like a physical stack of plates. A stack-based computer system is one that is based on the use of stacks, rather than being register based.

The stack method of expression evaluation was first proposed by early German computer scientist F.L. Bauer, who received the IEEE Computer Society Pioneer Award in 1988 for his work on Computer Stacks.

10.5.1 Operations

The two main operations applicable in the stack are :

*Push : an item is put on top of the stack, increasing the stack size by one. As stack size is usually limited, this may provoke a stack overflow if the maximum size is exceeded.

*pop : the top item is taken from the stack, decreasing stack size by one. In the case where there was no top item (i.e. the stack was empty), a stack underflow occurs.

Some environments that rely heavily on stacks may provide additional operations, for example:

*dup : the top item is popped and pushed again twice, so that an additional copy of the former top item is now on top, with the original below it.

*peek : check the topmost item. This is also called top operation in many articles.

*Swap or exchange: the two topmost items are exchanged.

*Rotate : the three topmost items exchange places in a rotary fashion. Two variants of this operation are possible, most often called left and right rotate.

10.5.2 Empty Stack

If a stack contains a single item and stack is popped, the resulting stack contains no items it is called the empty stack. Although the push operation is applicable to any stack, the pop operation cannot be applied to the empty stack because such a stack has no elements to pop. Therefore, before applying the Pop operator to a stack, we must ensure that the stack is not empty. The operation empty(s) determines whether or not a stack (S) is empty. If the stack is empty, empty(s) returns the value TRUE; otherwise it returns the value FALSE.

10.5.3 Abstract Data Type Stack

Before discussions the ADT stack, we define system stack. System stack is used by a program at run time to process function causes. Whenever a function is invoked, the program creates a structure, referred to as an activation record or a stack frame and places it on top of the system stack. Initially the activation record for the invoked function contains only a pointer to the previous stack frame and return address. The previous stack frame pointer points to the stack frame of the invoking function; the return address contains the location of the statement to be executed after the function terminates. Since only one function executes at any given time, the function whose stack frame is on top of the system stack is chosen. If this function invokes another function, the local variables and the parameters of the invoking function are added to its stack frame. A new stack frame is created for the invoked function and placed terminates, its stack frame is removed and the processing of the invoking function, which is again on top of the stack, continues.

Since all functions are stored similarly in the system stack, it makes no difference if the invoking function calls itself. That being a recursive call requires no special strategy; the run time program simply creates new stack frame for each recursion call. However, recursion can consume a significant portion of the memory allocated to the system stack, it could consume the entire available memory.

The representation of a stack as an abstract data type is straightforward :

abstract typ def <<elt type>> stack (elt type);

abstract empty (s)

stack (eltype) s;

post condition empty = = (lens(s)= =0);

abstract eltype pop(s)

stack (eltype)s;

precondition empty (s)= =false;

   Pop = = first (s)

   S = = sub (s,1, len (s) −1);

abstract push (s, elt)

Stack (eltype)s;

eltype elt;

Post condition S = = <elt> +s;

10.5.4   Applications

Now that we have defined a stack and have indicated the operations that can be performed on it, let us see how we may use the stack in problem solving. Consider a mathematical expression that includes several sets of nested parentheses :

$$5\text{-}(A\ (A + B)\ /\ (X - 3) + B)\ /\ (4 - 2.5)$$

We want to ensure that the parentheses are nested correctly; than, we check it :

1. There are an equal number of right and left parentheses.

2. Every right parenthesis is preceded by a matching left parenthesis.

    Expressions such as

   ((X+Y or X+Y(/Violate Condition 1 and

    expressions such as

   (X+Y (-Z or (X+Y))-(X+Z /Violate Condition 2)

To solve this problem, think of each left parenthesis as opening a scope and each right parenthesis as closing a scope.

The two conditions that must hold if the parentheses in an expression from an admissible pattern are as follows:

1. The parentheses count at the end of the expression is O. This implies that no scopes have been left open or that exactly as many right parentheses as left parentheses have been found.

2. The parentheses count at each point in the expression is non-negative. This implies that no right parenthesis is connected for which a matching left parenthesis had not previously been encountered.

```
6-((X+Y)*X)
    12   1 0
((A+B)
12    1
2+3 (

    1
) X+Y (-Z
-1      0
```

10.5.5　Expression Evaluation and Syntax Parsing

Calculators employing reverse-polish notation use a stack structure to hold values. Expressions can be represented in prefix, postfix or infix notations. Conversion from one form of the expression to another form needs a stack. All compilers use stack for parsing the syntax of expressions, program blocks etc. before translating into low level code. Most of the programming languages are context free languages and they can be parsed with stack-based machines. Note that natural languages are context sensitive languages and power of stack is not enough to interpret their meaning.

Runtime Memory Management

A number of computer languages are stack-oriented, meaning they define most basic operations (adding two numbers, printing a character) as taking their arguments from the stack, and placing any return values back on the stack. For example, PostScript has a return stack and an operand stack, and also has a graphics state stack and a dictionary stack.

The Forth programming language uses two stacks; one for argument passing and one for subroutine return addresses. The use of a return stack is extremely commonplace, but the somewhat unusual use of an argument stack for a human readable programming language is the reason it is referred to as a stack-based language.

Many virtual machines are also stack-oriented: p-Code machine, Java virtual machine.

Almost all computer environments use a special stack (the "function stack") to hold information about procedure/function nesting. They follow a runtime protocol between callers and called to save arguments and return value on the stack. The value of stack becomes more critical to support the nested function calls.

Solving search problems

Many search problems need exhaustive or optimal search of the entire solution space. Exhaustive search solutions include backtracking. Optimal search exploring methods include branch and bound solutions. All these problems need a stack space to remember what has been noticed, but not explored yet. Only alternative to use stack is to use recursion and let the compiler do the remembering for you. The examples of such problems are simple inorder traversal of tree, depth first traversal of a graph, a crossword puzzle or even playing a chess game. Some of these problems can be solved by alternative data structures like queue, when the order of traversal is not important.

10.5.6   Infix, Postfix and Prefix

This section examines a major algorithm that illustrates the different types of states and various operations and functions defined upon them. The example is also an important topic of computer science in its own right.

Consider the Product of X and Y. We think applying the operator "X" to operands X and Y and write it as X*Y. This particular representation is called infix. There are two alternate notations for expressing the product of X and Y using the symbols X, Y and*. These are

        XY Prefix   XY Postfix

The 'Pre-,' "Post," and 'in-" refer to the relative position of the operator with respect to the operands. In prefix notation the operator precedes the two operands, in postfix notation the operator follows the two operands, and in infix notation the operator is between the two operands.

We consider binary operation. For these operators the following is the order of precedence (highest to lowest):

1. Exponentiation ($\uparrow$), unary (-), unary +, NOT

2. Multiplication (*), division (/), mod, AND (&&)

3. Addition (+), Subtraction (-), or (!)

4. <, <=, =,<>, >=

We give the following examples of converting from infix to postfix and prefix that you understand each of these examples before proceeding to the remainder of this section.

1   X and Y OR NOT (A>B)

	Postfix	**Prefix**
T1 = A>B	AB>	>AB
X and Y or NOT T1		
T2 = NOT TI	TI NOT	NOT TI
T3 = X and Y	XY and	and XY
T4 = T3 OR T2	T3T2 OR	OR T3T2
	T3T1 NOT OR	OR T3 NOT T1
	XY AND AB> NOT OR	OR and XY NOT >AB

Take another example:

B↑B * C - D + E|F/G+H

			Postfix	**Prefix**
T1	=	B ↑ B	BB↑	↑BB
T2	=	T1*C	T1C*	*T1C
T3	=	E|F/G	EFIG/	|E/FG
T4	=	T2-D	T2D-	-T2D
T5	=	T4+T3	T4T3+	+T4T3
T6	=	T5+H	T5H+	+T5H
			T4T3+H+	++T4T3H
			T2D-EFIG/+H+	++-* TIC D|E/FG
			TIC * D-EF|G/+H+	++ - * ↑ BBCD|E/FG
			BB ↑ C * D-EF|G/+H+	

Converting an Expression from Infix to Postfix

Procedure play an important role in transforming infix to postfix, let us assume the existence of a function (op1,op2), where op1 and op2 are characters representing operators. This function returns TRUE if op1 has precedence over op2 when op1 appears to the left of op2 in an infix expression without parentheses. Pred (op1,op2) returns FALSE otherwise.

The algorithm to convert an infix string without parentheses into a postfix string as follows:

```
Opstk=the empty stack;
While (not end of input)
{
        symb=next input character;
            if (symb is an operand add symb to postfix string)
            else
                {
                while (! Empty (opstk) &&prcd(stacktop(opstk),symb))
                {
                topsymb = pop(opstk)
                add topsymb to the postfix string;
                        } /*end while*/
                        push (opstk, symb);
                        } /*end else*/
            }/* end while*/
            /* output any remaining operators */
            while (empty (opstk))
            {
                topsymb = pop(opstk);
                add topsymb to the postfix string;
                add topsymb to the postfix string;
                }/*endwhile*/
```

We illustrate this algorithm with example:

Example 1 : A + B * C

The contents of symb, the postfix string, and opstk are shown after scanning each symbol. Opstk is shown with its top to the right

S. No.	Symb	Postfix string	Opstk
1	A	A	
2	+	A	
3	B	AB	+
4	*	AB	+ *
5	C	ABC	+*
6		ABC	+
7		ABC *	+

Lines 1, 3 and 5 correspond to the scanning of an operand; therefore, the symbol (symb) is immediately placed on the postfix string. In line 2 an operator is scanned and the stack is found to be empty and the operator is therefore placed on the stack. In line 4, the precedence of the new symbol (*) is greater than the precedence of symbol on the top of the stack (+), therefore the new symbol is pushed onto the stack. In steps 6 and 7, the input string is empty, and the stack is therefore popped and its contents are placed on the postfix string.

Modified algorithm to convert any infix string into a postfix string is as follows:

```
Opstk=the empty stack;
While (not end of input)
{
symb=next input character;
        if (symb is an operand add symb to postfix string)
        else
{
while (! Empty (opstk) &&prcd(stacktop(opstk),symb))
{
topsymb = pop(opstk)
add topsymb to the postfix string;
} /*end while*/
    If (empty (opstk) II symb!=')')
    Push (opstk, symb);
    Else /* pop the open parenthesis and discard it */
    Top symb=pop (opstk);
while (empty (opstk))
{
    topsymb = pop(opstk);
    add topsymb to the postfix string;
    add topsymb to the postfix string;
    }/*endwhile*/
```

Example 2 : (X+Y)*Z

Symb	postfix string	opstk
(		(
X	X	(
+	X	(+
Y	XY	(+
)	XY	+
*	XY+	*
Z	XY+Z*	

In this example, when right parenthesis is encountered the stack is popped until a left parenthesis is encountered, at which point both parenthesis are discarded. Using parenthesis to force an order of precedence different than the default, the order of appearance of the operators.

10.6 Array

In computer programming, an array, also known as a vector or list, is one of the simplest data structures. Arrays hold a series of data elements, usually of the same size and data type. Individual elements are accessed by index using a consecutive range of integers, as opposed to an associative array. Some arrays are multidimensional, i.e. they are indexed by a fixed number of integers, for example by a tuple of four integers. Generally, one- and two-dimensional arrays are the most common.

Most programming languages have arrays as a built-in data type. Some programming languages (such as C, Fortran, and J) generalize the available operations and functions to work transparently over arrays as well as scalars, providing a higher-level manipulation than most other languages, which require loops over all the individual members of the arrays.

10.6.1   Uses

Although useful in their own right, arrays also form the basis for several more complex data structures, such as heaps, hash tables, and VLists, and can be used to represent strings, stacks and queues. They also play a minor role in many other data structures. All of these applications benefit from the compactness and locality of arrays.

One of the disadvantages of an array is that it has a single fixed size, and although its size can be altered in many environments, this is an expensive operation.

Dynamic arrays or growable arrays are arrays which automatically perform this resizing as late as possible, when the programmer attempts to add an element to the end of the array and there is no more space. To average the high cost of resizing over a long period of time, they expand by a large amount, and when the programmer attempts to expand the array again, it just uses more of this reserved space.

In the C programming language, one-dimensional character arrays are used to store null-terminated strings, so called because the end of the string is indicated with a special reserved character called a null character.

Some applications where the data are the same or missing for most values of the indices, or for large ranges of indices, space is saved by not storing an array at all, but having an associative array with integer keys. There are many specialized data structures specifically for this purpose, such as Patricia tries and Judy arrays. Example applications include address translation tables and routing tables.

10.6.2 Multi-dimensional Arrays

Ordinary arrays are indexed by a single integer. Also useful, particularly in numerical and graphics applications, is the concept of a multi-dimensional array, in which we index into the array using an ordered list of integers, such as in a [3,1,5]. The number of integers in the list used to index into it is always the same and is referred to as the dimensionality of array, and the bounds on each of these are called the dimensions of array. An array with dimensionality k is often called k-dimensional.

One-dimensional arrays correspond to the simple arrays discussed thus far; two-dimensional arrays are a particularly common representation for matrices. In practice, the dimensionality of an array rarely exceeds three.

Mapping a one-dimensional array into memory is obvious, since memory is logically itself a one-dimensional array. When we reach higher-dimensional arrays, however, the problem is no longer obvious. Suppose we want to represent this simple two-dimensional array:

A few common representations include:

Row-major order. Used most notably by statically declared arrays in C. The elements of each row are stored in order.

1 2 3 4 5 6 7 8 9

Column-major order. Used most notably in Fortran. The elements of each column are stored in order.

1   5   7   2   4   8   3   6   9

Arrays of arrays. Multi-dimensional arrays are represented by one-dimensional arrays of references to other one-dimensional arrays. The sub arrays can be either the rows or columns.

The first two forms are more compact and have potentially better locality of reference, but are also more limiting; the arrays must be rectangular, meaning that no row can contain more elements than any other. Arrays of arrays, on the other hand, allow the creation of ragged arrays, also called jagged arrays, in which the valid range of one index depends on the value of another, or in this case, simply that different rows can be different sizes. Arrays of arrays are also of value in programming languages that only supply one-dimensional arrays as primitives.

In many applications, such as numerical applications working with matrices, we iterate over rectangular two-dimensional arrays in predictable ways. For example, computing an element of the matrix product AB involves iterating over a row of A and column of B simultaneously. In mapping the individual array indexes into memory, we wish to exploit locality of reference as much as we can. A compiler can sometimes automatically choose the layout for an array so that sequentially accessed elements are stored sequentially in memory; in our example, it might choose row-major order for A, and column-major order for B. Even more exotic orderings can be used, for example if we iterate over the main diagonal of a matrix.

10.6.3   Advantages and Disadvantages

Arrays permit efficient constant time, random access but not efficient insertion and deletion of elements. Linked lists have the opposite trade-off. Consequently, arrays are most appropriate for storing a fixed amount of data that will be accessed in an unpredictable fashion, and linked lists are best for a list of data that will be accessed sequentially and updated often with insertions or deletions.

Another advantage of arrays that has become very important on modern architectures is that iterating through an array has good locality of reference, and so is much faster than iterating through (say) a linked list of the same size, which tends to jump around in memory. However, an array can also be accessed in a random way, as is done with large hash tables, and in this case this is not a benefit.

Arrays also are among the most compact data structures; storing 100 integers in an array takes only 100 times the space required to store an integer, plus perhaps a few bytes of overhead for the whole array. Any pointer-based data structure, on the other hand, must keep its pointers somewhere, and these occupy additional space. This extra space becomes more significant as the data elements become smaller. For example, an array of ASCII characters takes up one byte per character, while on a 32-bit platform, which has 4-byte pointers, a linked list requires at least five bytes per character. Conversely, for very large elements, the space difference becomes a negligible fraction of the total space.

10.6.4   Types of Array

Dynamic array

A dynamic array, growable array, resizable array, dynamic table, or array list is a data structure, an array that is automatically expanded to accommodate new objects if filled beyond its current size. It may also automatically de-allocate some of its unused space to save memory. They have become a popular data structure in modern mainstream programming languages, supplied with most standard libraries. Note that in this article, a dynamic array is not the same thing as a dynamically allocated array, which is just an ordinary fixed-size array whose size is selected at runtime.

One of the main disadvantages of a simple array is that it has a single fixed size, and although its size can be altered in some environments (for example, with C's realloc function), this is an expensive operation that may involve copying the entire contents of the array. Dynamic arrays automatically perform this resizing as late as possible, when the programmer attempts to add an element to the end of the array and there is no more space. However, if we add just one element to the array each time it runs out of space, the cost of the resizing operations rapidly becomes prohibitive. To deal with this, we instead resize the array by a large amount, such as doubling its size. Then, the next time we need to enlarge the array, we just expand it into some of this reserved space. The amount of space we have allocated for the array is called its capacity, and it may be larger than its current logical size. Here's how the operation adding an element to the end might work:

```
function insertEnd(dynarray a, element e) {
if a.size = a.capacity {
    resize a to twice its current capacity
    a.capacity = a.capacity × 2
}
a[a.size] := e
a.size := a.size + 1
}
```

Performance

In most ways, the dynamic array performs similar to an array, with the addition of new operations to add and remove elements from the end :

*Getting or setting the value at a particular index.

*Iterating over the elements in order.

*Add an element to the end.

*Remove an element from the end.

*Dynamic arrays benefit from many of the advantages of arrays, including good locality of reference and data cache utilization, compactness (low memory use), and random access. They usually have only a small fixed additional overhead for storing information about the size and capacity. This makes dynamic arrays an attractive tool for building cache-friendly data structures.

The main disadvantage of dynamic arrays compared to normal arrays is that when they grow they reserve a great deal of space (linear space in fact) that may never be used. This becomes especially problematic when there are a large number of such arrays. There are variants however, which waste only space at any time.

Global array

The Global Arrays toolkit provides an efficient and portable "shared-memory" programming interface for distributed-memory computers. Each process in a MIMD parallel program can asynchronously access logical blocks of physically distributed dense multi-dimensional arrays, without need for explicit cooperation by other processes. Unlike other shared-memory environments, the Global Array model exposes to the programmer the non-uniform memory access (NUMA) characteristics of the high performance computers and acknowledges that access to a remote portion of the shared data is slower than to the local portion. The locality information for the shared data is available, and a direct access to the local portions of shared data is provided.

Global Arrays have been designed to complement rather than substitute for the message-passing programming model. The programmer is free to use both the shared-memory and message-passing paradigms in the same program, and to take advantage of existing message-passing software libraries. Global Arrays are compatible with the Message Passing Interface (MPI).

Parallel array

In computing, a parallel array is a simple data structure for representing arrays of records. It keeps a separate, homogenous array for each field of the record, each having the same number of elements. Then, objects located at the same index in each array are implicitly the fields of a single record. Pointers from one object to another are replaced by array indices. This contrasts with the normal approach of storing all fields of each record together in memory. For example, one might declare an array of 100 names, each a string, and 100 ages, each an integer, associating each name with the age that has the same index.

Example

```
int ages[ ] =    {0,    27    23        4      25};
char *names[ ] = {"None", "Mike", "Billy", "Tom", "Stan"};
int parent[ ] = {0 /*None*/, 4/*Tom*/, 2/*Mike*/, 0 /*None*/, 4/*Tom*/};
for(i = 1; i <= 4; i++) {
    printf("Name: %s, Age: %d, Parent: %s \n",
        names[i], ages[i], names[parent[i]]);
}
```

Advantages

- They can be used in languages, which support only arrays of primitive types and not of records (or perhaps don't support records at all).

- Parallel arrays are simple to understand and use, and are often used where declaring a record is more trouble than its worth.

- They can save a substantial amount of space in some cases by avoiding alignment issues. For example, one of the fields of the record can be a single bit, and its array would only need to reserve one bit for each record, whereas in the normal approach many more bits would "pad" the field so that it consumes an entire byte or a word.

- If the number of items is small, array indices can occupy significantly less space than full pointers, particularly on architectures with large words.

- Sequentially examining a single field of each record in the array is very fast on modern machines, since this amounts to a linear traversal of a single array, exhibiting ideal locality of reference and cache behavior.

Disadvantages

- They have significantly worse locality of reference when visiting the records sequentially and examining multiple fields of each record, which is the norm.
- They obscure the relationship between fields of a single record.
- They have little direct language support (the language and its syntax typically express no relationship between the arrays in the parallel array.)
- They are expensive to grow or shrink, since each of several arrays must be reallocated.

Sparse array

A sparse array in computing is an array where only very few indices are used in practice. Arrays are data structures used in programming languages. They map integer positions, or indices, less than the array's length, to values. A typical implementation allocates space for the entire array, even if only a few indices are ever used. If the sparsely is known in advance, more space-efficient implementations can be used; only allocating space for the entries that are actually used.

Associative array

In computing, an associative array, also known as a map, lookup table, or dictionary, is an abstract data type very closely related to the mathematical concept of a function with a finite domain. Conceptually, an associative array is composed of a collection of keys and a collection of values, and each key is associated with one value. The operation of finding the value associated with a key is called a lookup or indexing, and this is the most important operation supported by an associative array.

The relationship between a key and its value is sometimes called a mapping or binding. For example, if the value associated with the key "bob" is 7, we say that our array maps "bob" to 7.

From the perspective of a programmer using an associative array, it can be viewed as a generalization of an array. While a regular array maps integers to arbitrarily typed objects (integers, strings, pointers, and, in an OO sense, objects), an associative array maps arbitrarily typed objects to arbitrarily typed objects. (Implementations of the two data structures, though, may be considerably different.)

The operations that are usually defined for an associative array are :

Add: Bind a new key to a new value

Reassign: Bind an old key to a new value

Remove: Unbind a key from a value and remove it from the key set

Lookup: Find the value (if any) that is bound to a key.

Examples

One can think of a telephone book as an example of an associative array, where names are the keys and phone numbers are the values. Another example would be a dictionary where words are the keys and definitions are the values.

10.7   Queue

A queue is a linear list in which additions are made only at one end of the list (the 'rear') and deletions only at the other end (the 'front'). This is a first in, first out (FIFO) list since it is clear that an element, once added to the rear of the list, can be removed when and only when all earlier additions have been removed.

When a receptionist makes a list of the names of patients who arrive to see a doctor, adding each new name at the front of the list and crossing the top name off the list as a patient is called in, her list of names has the structure of a queue. The word 'queue' is also used in many other everyday examples. Such as the queue of traffic at a road junction, but it should be noted that in many cases (the traffic queue is one), the example is not true queue.

A queue is a linear list where additions and deletions may take place at either end of the list, but never in the middle. A queue, which is both input-restricted and outputrestricted, must be either a stack or a queue.

10.7.1   Operations on Queue

Similar to stack operations, operations that define a queue are given below:

1. Create a queue

2. Check whether a queue is empty

3. Check whether a queue is full

4. Add item in the rear of queue (in queue)

5. Remove item from front of queue (dequeue).

10.7.2   Circular Queue

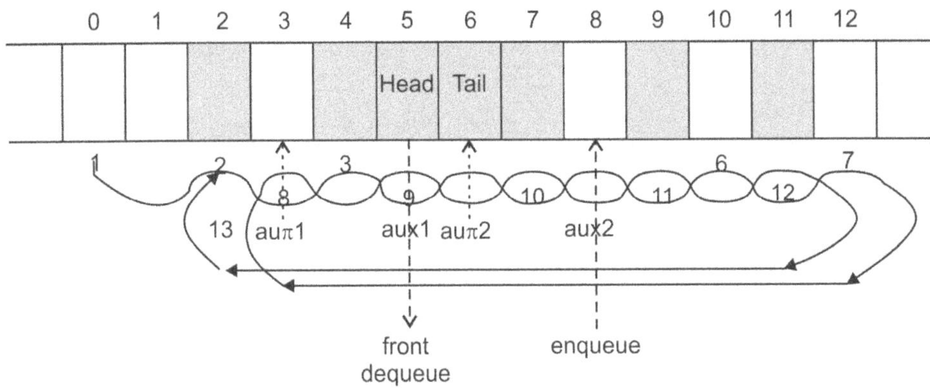

Fig. 10.3 Circular Queue.

Now if we try to insert, an overflow may occur even though some cells are free. To avoid this drawback, we can arrange the elements in a circular fashion. It is then called a circular array representation. We may depict a circular queue as given in Fig.10.3.

10.7.3   Insertion and Deletion in a Circular Queue

Procedure Q INSERT (var Q : Q type; element type);

Var

      New rear : integer;

      begin with Q do

         begin

         if Rear = Max

         then New rear = 1

         else new Rear = Rear +1

         If new Rear = Front

      then Q over flow

      else begin

         Rear = New Rear;

         queue [Rear] = X;

         then Front = Rear

         end

      end

```
end
Procedure queue Delete (var q : qtype; var x : element type);
begin
        with Q do
if Rear = 0
        the under flow
else begin
        X : queue [Front];
        if Front = Rear then
            begin
                Front :=0
                Rear :=0
            end
        else
        if Front = Max then Front :=1
        else Front :=Front +1;
        end
end
```

10.7.4 Applications

Queues are important in simulation models. They serve roles : as repetitive for scheduled events, as holding areas for entities through the system.

In a computer network, messages from one computer to another are generally created as asynchronously. These messages therefore need to be buffered until the receiving computer is ready for it. These communication buffers make extensive use of queues by storing these messages in a queue. Also, the messages need to be sent to receiving computer in the same order in which they are created, i.e. First in First out order.

The following example implements a communication buffer queue with messages of type char.

```
define EMPT       0
define MAX        10
define ALWAYS   1
define RING       "1007"
enum status {SUCCESS, FULL };
```

```
typedef char Data;
typedef data[Max];
struct-q-ptr-def
{
      int q-insert
      int q-remove
};
type def struct q-ptr-def q-PTR;
enum status insert – q(q2, q-Ptr xq-Ptr, Data message)
{
      int new-pos;
      if ((new-pos=q-Ptr-q-insert+1)=MAX)
      new-pos=0;
      if (new-pos==q-ptr q-remove)
          return (FULL);
      q-pt q-insert=new-pos;
      q[q-ptr-q-insert]=message;
          return (SUCCESS);
      }
      DATA remove-q(Qq, q-ptr*q-ptr)
      {
          DATA message
      if (q-ptr-q-remove = = q-ptr-q-insert)
      return (EMPT);
      if (q-ptr-q-remove+=1)=MAX)
      q-ptr-q-remove=0;
      message=q[q-ptr-q-remove];
      return (message);
      }
      main ( )
      { Q q;
          Q-PTR q-ptr;
          q-ptr q-insert = 0;
          q-ptr q-remove=0;
```

```
            while (ALWAYS)
    }
        {   case '1':
            print f("In Enter \"1\"to Add message in queue");
            print f("In Enter \"2\"to Remove message in queue");
            print f("In Enter \"3\"to Exit in");
            print f(" Enter message to queue in");
            if (inser-q(q,+q-ptr, get chs) ==FULL
            print f ("In queue FULL");
            break;
    Case '2':
            Printf ("Removed message is :%C"; remove-q(q,q1-ptr));
    break
    Case '3'
            exit ( );
            default:
                print (RING);
                break;
        }
    }
```

10.7.5   Priority Queue

The priority queue is a data structure in which the intrinsic ordering of the elements dues determines the results of its basic operations. There are two types of priority queues:

1. Ascending priority queue   2. Descending priority queue

An ascending priority queue is a collection of items into which items can be inserted arbitrarily and from which only the smallest item can be removed.

A descending priority queue is similar but allows deletion of any largest item.

10.8   Lists

Lists, like arrays, are used to store ordered data. A list is a linear sequence of data objects of the same type. Real-life events such as people waiting to be served at a bank counter or at a railway reservation counter may be implemented using list structures. In computer science, lists are extensively used in data base management systems, process managament, operating system, editors etc.

We shall discuss lists, linked lists such as singly, doubly and circularly linked lists, and their implementations, using arrays and using pointers.

In computer science, a list is usually defined as an instance of an abstract data type (ADT) formalizing the concept of an ordered collection of entities. For example, an ADT for un-typed, multiple lists may be specified in terms of a constructor and their operations.

In practice, lists are usually implemented using arrays or linked lists of some sort; due to lists sharing certain properties with arrays and linked lists. Informally, the term list is sometimes used synonymously with linked list. A sequence is another name, emphasizing the ordering and suggesting that it may not be a linked list.

10.8.1 Base Terminology

A linear list is an ordered set consisting of a variable number of elements to which addition and deletion can be made. A linear list displays the relationship of physical adjacency.

The first element of a list is called head of list and the last element is called tail of list.

The next element to the head of list is called its Successor. The previous element to the tail of the list is called its Predecessor. A head does not have a predecessor and tail does not have successor. Any other element of list has both one successor and one predecessor.

10.8.2 Characteristics

Lists have the following properties:

- The size and contents of lists may or may not vary at runtime, depending on implementations.

- Random access over lists may or may not be possible, depending on implementations.

Equality of lists:

In mathematics, sometimes equality of lists is defined simply in terms of object identity: two lists are equal if and only if they are the same object.

In modern programming languages, equality of lists is normally defined in terms of structural equality of the corresponding entries, except that if the lists are typed, then the list types may also be relevant.

Lists may be typed. This implies that the entries in a list must have types that are compatible with the list type. It is common that lists are typed when they are implemented using arrays.

10.8.3　Operations on the Lists

Following are some of the basic operations that may be performed on a list :

Create a list

Check for an empty list

Search for an element in a list

Search for a predecessor or a successor of an element of a list

Delete an element from a list

Add an element at a specified location of a list

Retrieve an element from a list

Update a list

Sort a list

Print a list

Determine the size or number of elements

Delete a list

More complex operations may be performed on a list. However a complex operation would generally turn out to be a combination of two or more of the above basic operations.

10.8.4　Specification

With the specification of collection complete, let's turn to lists. Our specification of list is a small extension of collection, taking into account the two special properties lists have that ordinary collections don't, namely (refer to handout) :

1. In a list, there is a linear order (called followed by, or next) defined on the elements: every element (except for one, called the last element) is followed by one other element, and no two elements are followed by the same element. There is exactly one element in a list (the first element) that does not follow after any element.

2. It is possible to access individual elements of a list. Having a window on the list provides this access; when we define the abstract type List, we will also have to define window.

The implications of list i.e. a special kind of collection are two-fold:

- Any operation that is applicable to a collection is applicable to a list. A list is a collection.

- However, lists are special kinds of collections – they have two special properties. We have to add extra post-conditions to the operators in order to say how these properties are affected by the operations.

INSERT:

if C is a list: V is the first element in C'.

DELETE:

if C is a list: it is the first occurrence of V in C that is deleted.

JOIN:

if C1 and C2 are both lists: in C1' the elements of C1 and C2 are in their original order, and the elements of C1 are before the elements of C2.

MAP :

if C is a list: if E1 occurs before E2 in C, then the call P(E1) is made before the call P(E2).

To complete our specification we just have to specify what a window is, how windows are affected by the above list operations, and what operations can be performed on windows.

A window is always associated with an individual element of a list; there is no concept of an empty window, or of a window that gives access to several elements.

We say that the window is on the element. A window allows us only to look at an element, not to change it.

Unlike the textbook definition we do not specify how many windows there will be for a given list. There could be none, there could be many.

A window is not to be confused with a list element. An element exists whether or not there is a window on it; if we have a window on an element and then we move or destroy the window, the element is unaffected. There can be several distinct windows all on the same element at the same time.

Of course, you shouldn't confuse windows with pointers in C. Window is an abstract type, which we are in the process of specifying. It might be possible to implement this abstract type with C pointers, but it might not; and even if it is possible, it may not be the best way to implement the abstract type. The question of how to implement windows is a separate issue from defining what a window is.

How are windows affected by the list operations? For example, if we create a window on the first element of L and then insert a new value into L, is the window now on the new first element, or does it stay attached to the element it was on before the insert? Our general answer is: if a window is on element E then it stays on element E unless explicitly moved. E.g., when we JOIN two lists, the windows all stay on their elements.

The operations on windows are specified in the handout:

CREATE_WINDOW

    input: L (a list), W (a window).

    output: W'.

    preconditions: L is not empty, W is undefined.

    postconditions: W' is on the first element in L. Storage is allocated as needed.

DESTROY_WINDOW

    input: W (a window).

    output: W'.

    preconditions: none.

    postconditions: W' is undefined. As much space is reclaimed as is possible.

Destroying a window does not affect the element or list that the window was on. But what is about the opposite? Suppose we have a window on element E in list L and we delete E, or destroy L. What happens to the window? This is an important part of the specification. The two main possibilities are:

1. When an element is deleted, or a list is destroyed, all the associated windows are destroyed automatically.

2. Deleting an element or destroying a list causes the associated windows to become invalid but the space they consume remains allocated.

Option (1) is the better choice, but it is also the harder to implement: it requires every list element to keep track of all the windows that are on it. This is not difficult, but for sake of simplicity we will take option (2). What this means is that the user is responsible for destroying the windows he creates, and for keeping track of whether a window is valid or not.

IS_LAST

    input: W (a window).

    output: boolean.

    preconditions: W is defined.

    postconditions: true if W is on the last element in a list, false otherwise.

GET_VALUE

    input: W (a window).

    output: V (a value of a list element).

    preconditions: W is defined.

    postconditions: V is the value of the element W is on.

MOVE_FORWARD

> input: W (a window).

> output: W'.

> preconditions: W is not on the last element of a list.

> postconditions: W' is on the element that follows the element W was on.

This is the only operation that moves a window. There are other useful ones we could have included - MOVE_BACKWARD, for example.

SPLIT

> input: L1, L2 (lists), W (a window).

> output: L1' and L2'.

> preconditions: W is a window into L1, L2 is undefined.

> postconditions: L2' = the elements of L1 following the one W is on, their order

> unchanged. If W is on the last element, L2' is empty. L1' = the elements of

L1

> up to and including the one W is on, their order unchanged.

Example of SPLIT:

SPLIT (L1, L2, W) would produce:

What about other windows that might be on elements of L1? Following our general rule, SPLIT does not affect them: they are on the same elements after SPLIT as they were before.

We are now finished the specification phase of our design for the abstract data types collection and list. The next design phase addresses the implementation of the data type. This is a design process, too, and it is concerned almost exclusively concerned with the type definitions:

> will something be a record, or an array, or a linked data structure?

> how many pointers will there be, where should they point?

> etc...

10.8.5   Implementation of Lists

We will not consider in any detail the code that implements the operations. The reason is this: once the C type definitions have been decided upon, the code for the operations is completely determined - the specification tells us what they must do, and the type definitions tell us on what specific data objects they must operate. Filling in the code requires no further decisions, just careful attention to detail. So you see the decisions about the type definitions are very important they determine how simple and efficient our code will be.

An Implementation

In LISP lists are the fundamental data type and can represent both program code and data. In most dialects, the list of the first three prime numbers could be written as (list 2, 3, 5). In several dialects of LISP, including Scheme, a list is collection of pairs, consisting of a value and a pointer to the next pair (or null value).

The standard way of implementing lists, originating with LISP, is to have each element of the list contain both its value and a pointer indicating the location of the next element in the list. This results in either a linked list or a tree, depending on whether the list has nested sub lists, although LISP implementation (such as the LISP used for the Symbolic 3600) often use "compressed lists" which are arrays.

Some languages may instead implement lists using other data structures, such as arrays. However, it is generally assumed that elements can be inserted into a list in constant time, while access of a random element in a list requires linear time; this is to be contrasted with an array (or vector), for which the time complexities are reversed.

Lists can be manipulated using iteration or recursion. The former is often preferred in non-tail-recursive languages, and languages in which recursion over lists is for some other reason uncomfortable. The latter is generally preferred in functional languages, since iteration is associated with arrays and often regarded as imperative. Because in computing, lists are easier to realize than sets, and finite set in mathematical sense can be realized as a list with additional restrictions, that is, duplicate elements are disallowed and such that order is irrelevant. If the list is sorted, it speeds up determining if a given item is already in the set but in order to ensure the order, it requires more time to add new entry to the list.

Time efficiency

We would like all our operations to be constant time type (except for MAP, DELETE, and DESTROY, which cannot possibly be constant time type).

Space efficiency

No maximum limit on list size: dynamic allocation of memory for elements (nodes).*Pointers consume memory; they are usually 32 bits, which is 4 times the size of a character and, in many systems, twice the size of an integer. This can be a significant overhead, so we'd like to minimize the number of pointers we have per element, while still having enough to permit all our operations to be constant time. It turns out that we can get away with one pointer per element. This is possible because of our choice of primitives: for example, if we had a command for moving backwards, we'd need two pointers per element.

10.8.6 Linked List

What are the drawbacks of using sequential storage to represent stacks and queues? One major drawback is that a fixed amount of storage remains allocated to the stack or queue even the structure is actually using a smaller amount or possibly no storage at all. Further, no more than that fixed amount of storage may be allocated, thus introducing the possibility of overflow.

In a sequential representation, the items of a stack or queue are implicitly ordered by the sequential order of storage. Thus, if q items [X] represent an element of a queue, the next element will be q items [X+1]. Suppose that the items of a stack or a queue were explicitly ordered, that is, each item contained within itself the address of the next item. Such an explicit ordering gives rise to a data structure pictured in Fig. 10.4, which is known as a linear linked list. Each item in the list is called a node and contains two fields, an information field and a next address field. The information field holds the actual element on the list. The next address field contains the address of the next node in the list.

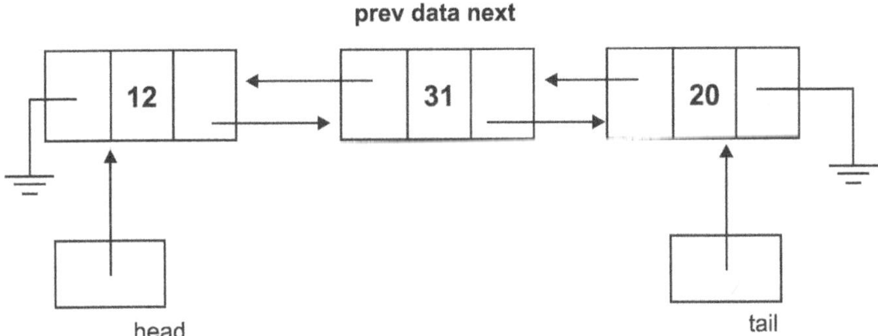

Fig. 10.4 Linear linked list.

Such an address, which is used to access a particular node, is known as a pointer. The next address field of the last node in the list contains a special value, known as null, which is not a valid address. This null pointer is used to signal the end of a list.

The list with no nodes on it is called the empty list or the null list. The value of the external pointer list to such a list is the null pointer. A list can be initialized to the empty list by the operation list = null.

In computer science, a linked list is one of the fundamental data structures used in computer programming. It consists of a sequence of nodes, each containing arbitrary data fields and one or two references ("links") pointing to the next and/or previous nodes. A linked list is a self-referential data type because it contains a pointer or link to another data of the same type. Linked lists permit insertion and removal of nodes at any point in the list in constant time, but do not allow random access. Several different types of linked list exist: singly linked lists, doubly linked lists, and circularly linked lists.

Linked lists can be implemented in most languages. Languages such as LISP and Scheme have the data structure built-in, along with operations to access the linked list. Procedural languages such as C, C++, and Java typically rely on mutable references to create linked lists.

Allen Newell, Cliff Shaw and Herbert Simon at RAND CORPORATION as the primary data structure developed linked lists in 1955-56 for their Information Processing Language. The authors, to develop several early artificial intelligence programs, including the Logic Theory Machine, the General Problem Solver, and a computer chess program, used IPL. Reports on their work appeared in IRE Transactions on Information Theory in 1956, and several conference proceedings from 1957-1959, including Proceedings of the Western Joint Computer Conference in 1957 and 1958, and Information Processing (Proceedings of the first UNESCO International Conference on Information Processing) in 1959. The now-classic diagram consisting of blocks representing list nodes with arrows pointing to successive list nodes appears in "Programming the Logic Theory Machine" by Newell and Shaw in Proc. WJCC, February 1957. Newell and Simon were recognized with the ACM Turing Award in 1975 for having "made basic contributions to artificial intelligence, the psychology of human cognition, and list processing".

The problem of machine translation for natural language processing led Victor Yngve at Massachusetts Institute of Technology (MIT) to use linked lists as data structures in his COMIT programming language for computer research in the field of linguistics.

A report on this language entitled "A programming language for mechanical translation" appeared in Mechanical Translation in 1958.

John McCarthy created LISP, standing for list processor, in 1958 while he was at MIT and in 1960 he published its design in a paper in the Communications of the ACM, entitled "Recursive Functions of Symbolic Expressions and Their Computation by Machine, Part I". One of LISP's major data structures is the linked list.

By the early 1960s, the utility of both linked lists and languages, which use these structures as their primary data representation, was well established. Bert Green of the MIT Lincoln Laboratory published a review article entitled "Computer languages for symbol manipulation" in IRE Transactions on Human Factors in Electronics in March 1961, which summarized the advantages of the linked list approach. A later review article, "A Comparison of list-processing computer languages" by Bobrow and Raphael, appeared in Communications of the ACM in April 1964.

Several operating systems developed by Technical Systems Consultants (originally of West Lafayette Indiana, and later of Raleigh, North Carolina) used singly linked lists as file structures. A directory entry pointed to the first sector of a file, and succeeding portions of the file were located by traversing pointers. Systems using this technique included Flex (for the Motorola 6800 CPU), mini-Flex (same CPU), and Flex9 (for the Motorola 6809 CPU). A variant developed by TSC for and marketed by Smoke Signal Broadcasting in California, used doubly linked lists in the same manner.

The TSS operating system, developed by IBM for the System 360/370 machines, used a double linked list for their file system catalogue. The directory structure was similar to Unix, where a directory could contain files and/or other directories and extend to any depth. A utility flea was created to fix file system problems after a crash, since modified portions of the file catalog were sometimes in memory when a crash occurred. Problems were detected by comparing the forward and backward links for consistency. If a forward link was corrupt, and if a backward link to the infected node was found, the forward link was set to the node with the backward link. A humorous comment in the source code where this utility was invoked stated "Everyone knows a flea caller gets rid of bugs in cats".

SINGLY LINKED LIST

The simplest kind of linked list is a singly linked list (or slist for short), which has one link per node. This link points to the next node in the list, or to a null value or empty list if it is the final node (Fig. 10.5).

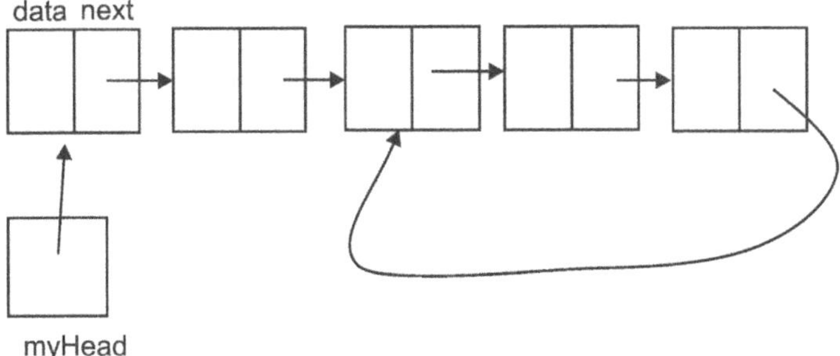

Fig. 10.5 A Singly-linked list.

10.8.7   Operation on Link List

Let us see how an insertion algorithm works for inserting an element in a linked list.

1. Check if list is empty, return of yes.
2. Search for the element after which the insertion is to be done.
3. Create a memory space for element to be inserted.
4. Assign the data value to its data field.
5. Assign its pointer to pointer of the success elements searched at step 2.
6. Assign pointer of the element searched at step 2 to this new element created.

Deletion from a list

Deletion of an element from a single linked list requires the following :

1. List to be checked for empty list.
2. Search for the element with key value same as the element to be deleted.
3. Its pointer to next element be saved and later assigned to next element of predecessor of the element searched at step 2.
4. Despise the memory space held by the deleted element.

Examples of List operations

We illustrated push and pop operations for lists, with some simple examples. The first example is to delete all occurrences of the number 4 from a test. The list is traversed in a search for nodes that contain 4 in their info fields. Each such node must be deleted from list. But to delete a node from a list, its predecessor must be known. For these reason two pointers, p and q are used. p is used to traverse the list, and q always points to the predecessor of p. The algorithm makes use of the pop operation to remove nodes from the beginning of the list.

```
q=null;
p=list;
while (p!=null)
{
    if (info (p)==4)
    if (q==null)
    {   /* remove first node of the list */
    x=pop (list);
    p=list;
    }
```

else

{ /*   delete the node after q and move up p*/

    p=next (p);

    delafter (q x);

    }   /* end if */

else

    {   /* continue traversing the list */

q=p;

p=next (p);

}   /*end if */

}   /* end while */

The practice of using two pointers, one following the other, is very common in working with lists. This technique is used in the next example as well. Assume that a list is ordered so that smaller items precede larger ones. Such a list is called an ordered list. It is desired to insert an item x into this list in its proper place. The algorithm to do so makes use of its proper place. The algorithm to do so makes use of the push operation to add a node in the middle of the list.

q=null;

for (p=list; p!=null && x> info (p); p=next(p)

    q=p;

    /* at this point, a node containing x must be inserted */

    if (q==null) /* insert at the head of the list */

    push (list,x);

    else

    insafler (q x);

10.8.8   Multi-Linked Lists

Doubly-linked list

A more sophisticated kind of linked list is a doubly-linked list or two-way linked list. Each node has two links: one points to the previous node, or points to a null value or empty list if it is the first node; and the other points to the next, or points to a null value or empty list if it is the final node (Fig. 10.6).

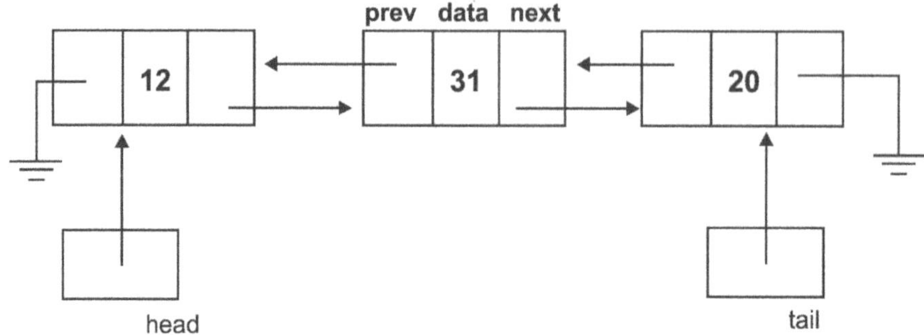

Fig. 10.6 Doubly-linked list.

In some very low-level languages, Xor-linking offers a way to implement doublylinked lists using a single word for both links, although the use of this technique is usually discouraged.

Doubly-linked lists are a special case of multi-linked lists; it is special in two ways :

*Each node has just 2 pointers

*The pointers are exact inverses of each other.

In a general multi-linked list, each node can have any number of pointers to other nodes, and there may or may not be inverses for each pointer.

Example 1 : Multiple Orders of One Set of Elements

The standard use of multi-linked lists is to organize a collection of elements in two different ways. For example, suppose my elements include the name of a person and his/her age, e.g.,(FRED, 19) (MARY, 16) (JACK,21) (JILL, 18).

I might want to order these elements alphabetically and also order them by age. I would have two pointers – NEXT-alphabetically, NEXT-age – and the list header would have two pointers, one based on name, the other on age.

Inserting into this structure is very much like inserting the same node into two separate lists. In multi-linked lists, it is quite common to have back-pointers, i.e. inverses of each of the forward links; in our example, this would mean that each node had four pointers.

Example 2: Sparse Matrices

A second very common use of multi-linked lists is sparse matrices. A sparse matrix is a matrix of numbers, as in mathematics, in which almost all the entries are zero.

These arise frequently in engineering applications. The use of a normal Pascal array to store a sparse matrix is extremely wasteful of space – in an N x N sparse matrix typically only about N elements are non-zero. For example:

```
X = 1 2 3

----------

Y=1  |  0     88    0
Y=2  |  0     0     0
Y=3  |  27    0     0
Y=4  |  19    0     66
```

We can represent this by having linked lists for each row and each column. Because each node is in exactly one row and one column, it will appear in exactly two lists – one row list and one column. So it needs two pointers: Next-in-this-row and Next-in this-column. In addition to storing the data in each node, it is normal to store the coordinates (i.e. the row and column data is in the matrix). Operations that set a value to zero cause a node to be deleted, and vice versa. As with any linked list in practice it is common for every pointer to have a corresponding back pointer.

10.8.9   Circular Lists

In a circularly linked list, the first and final nodes are linked together. This can be done for both singly and doubly-linked lists. To traverse a circular linked list, you begin at any node and follow the list in either direction until you return to the original node. Viewed another way, circularly-linked lists can be seen as having no beginning or end. This type of list is most useful for managing buffers for data ingest, and in cases where you have one object in a list and wish to see all other objects in the list.

Singly-circularly-linked list

In a singly-circularly-linked list, each node has one link, similarly to an ordinary singly-linked list, except that the next link of the last node points back to the first node. As in a singly-linked list, new nodes can only be efficiently inserted after a node we already have a reference to. For this reason, it's usual to retain a reference to only the last element in a singly linked list, as this allows quick insertion at the beginning, and also allows access to the first node through the last node's next pointer.

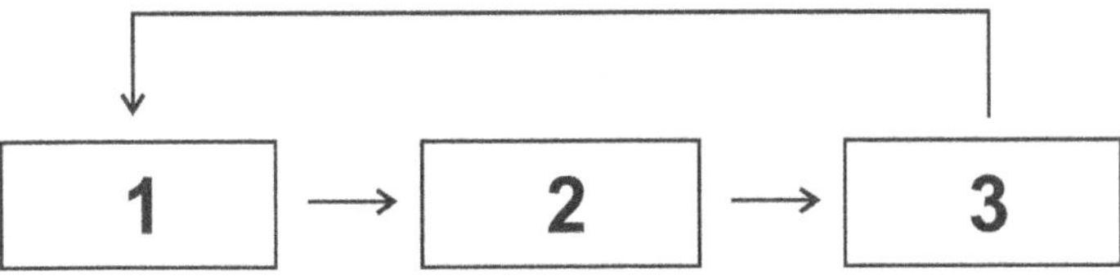

Fig. 10.7 Singly-circularly-linked list.

Doubly-circularly-linked list

In a doubly-circularly-linked list, each node has two links, similar to doubly-linked list, except that previous link of the first node points to the last node and the next link of the last node points to the first node. As in doubly-linked lists, insertions and removals can be done at any point with access to any nearby node.

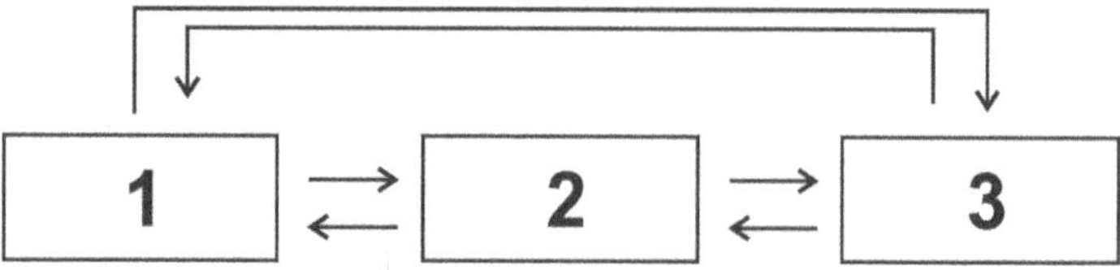

Fig. 10.8 Doubly-circularly-linked list.

Circular lists are usually preferable to non-circular ones, for two reasons:

- They provide easy access to both ends of a list: notice that we do not need the first pointer in the header, because we can easily reach the first node with L->last->next.

- The code for processing a circular list is often simpler than the code for processing a non-circular list – mainly because you don't have to constantly check if the next node is defined – it is always defined.

At the implementation level, however, circularity does create one very tricky case that is a very common source of bugs, and that is a singleton list. When there is only one node in a circular list, it points to itself as the next node. You have to think carefully to handle this correctly.

Suppose that a small change is made to the structure of a linear list, so that the next field in the last node contains a pointer back to the first node rather than the null pointer. Such a list is called a circular list and is illustrated in Fig. 10.7. From any point in such a list, it is possible to reach any other point in the list. If we begin at a given node and traverse the entire list, we ultimately end up at the starting point. A circular list does not have a natural "first" or "last" node. We must, therefore, establish a first and last node by convention. One useful convention is to let the external pointer to the circular list to the last node, and to allow the following node to be the first node, as illustrated in Fig. 10.8.

10.8.10 The Josephus Problem

Let us consider a problem that can be solved in a straightforward manner by using a circular list. This problem is known as the Josephus Problem.

The input to the program is the number n and a list of names, which is the clockwise ordering of the circle, beginning with the soldier from whom the count is to start. The last input line contains the string 'end' indicating the end of the input. The program should print the names in the order that they are eliminated and the name of the soldier who escapes.

For example, suppose that n=4 and that there are five soldiers named J, K, L, M, N. We count four soldiers starting at J so that M is eliminated first. We then begin by N and count N and back to J, K so that L is eliminated next. Then we count M, N and back to J, K (L is already been eliminated) and finally M, N, J. So that N is the one who escapes.

Clearly, a circular list in which each node represents one soldier is a natural data structure to use in solving this problem. To delete node from the list finally, when only one node remains on the list the result is determined.

The Algorithm might be as follows:

read (n);

read (name);

while (name!=EWD)

{

      insert name on the circular list

      read (name);

}   /* end while */

which (there is more than one node on the list)

{

      count through n-1 nodes on the list;

      print the name in the n node

      delete the n node

}   /* end while */

10.8.11 Applications of Linked Lists

Linked lists are used as a building block for many other data structures, such as stacks, queues and their variations.

The "data" field of a node can be another linked list. By this device, one can construct many linked data structures with lists; this practice originated in the LISP programming language, where linked lists are a primary (though by no means the only) data structures, and is now a common feature of the functional programming style.

Sometimes, linked lists are used to implement associative arrays, and are in this context called association lists. There is very little good to be said about this use of linked lists; they are easily outperformed by other data structures such as self-balancing binary search trees even on small data sets (see the discussion in associative array). However, sometimes a linked list is dynamically created out of a subset of nodes in such a tree, and used to traverse that set more efficiently.

10.8.12 Linked Lists vs. Arrays

Linked lists have several advantages over arrays. Elements can be inserted into linked lists indefinitely, while an array will eventually either fill up or need to be resized, an expensive operation that may not even be possible if memory is fragmented. Similarly, an array from which many elements are removed may become wastefully empty or need to be made smaller.

Further memory savings can be achieved, in certain cases, by sharing the same "tail" of elements among two or more lists — that is, the lists end in the same sequence of elements. In this way, one can add new elements to the front of the list while keeping a reference to both the new and the old versions — a simple example of a persistent data structure.

On the other hand, arrays allow random access, while linked lists allow only sequential access to elements. Singly linked lists, in fact, can only be traversed in one direction. This makes linked lists unsuitable for applications where it's useful to look up an element by its index quickly, such as heap sort. Sequential access on arrays is also faster than on linked lists on many machines due to locality of reference and data caches. Linked lists receive almost no benefit from the cache.

Another disadvantage of linked lists is the extra storage needed for references, which often makes them impractical for lists of small data items such as characters or Boolean values. It can also be slow, and with a naïve allocate, wasteful, to allocate memory separately for each new element, a problem generally solved using memory pools.

A number of linked list variants exist that aim to ameliorate some of the above problems. Unrolled linked lists store several elements in each list node, increasing cache performance while decreasing memory overhead for references. CDR coding does both these as well, by replacing references with the actual data referenced, which extends off the end of the referencing record.

A good example that highlights the pros and cons of using arrays vs. linked lists is by implementing a program that resolves the Josephus problem. The Josephus problem is an election method that works by having a group of people stand in a circle.

Starting at a predetermined person, you count around the circle n times. Once you reach nth person, take them out of the circle and have the members close the circle. Then count around the circle the same n times and repeats the process, until only one person is left. That person wins the election. This shows the strengths and weaknesses of a linked list vs. an array, because if you view the people as connected nodes in a circular linked list then it shows how easily the linked list is able to delete nodes (as it only has to rearrange the links to the different nodes). However, the linked list will be poor at finding the next person to remove and will need to recursive through the list till it finds that person. An array, on the other hand, will be poor at deleting nodes (or elements) as it cannot remove one node without individually shifting all the elements up the list by one. However, it is exceptionally easy to find the nth person in the circle by directly referencing them by their position in the array.

10.8.13 Doubly-Linked vs. Singly-Linked

Double-linked lists require more space per node (unless one uses XOR-linking), and their elementary operations are more expensive; but they are often easier to manipulate because they allow sequential access to the list in both directions. In particular, one can insert or delete a node in a constant number of operations given only address of that node. Some algorithms require access in both directions. On the other hand, they do not allow tail sharing, and cannot be used as persistent data structures.

10.8.14 Circularly-Linked vs. Linearly-Linked

Circular-linked lists are most useful for describing naturally circular structures, and have the advantage of regular structure and being able to traverse the list starting at any point. They also allow quick access to the first and last records through a single pointer (the address of the last element). Their main disadvantage is the complexity of iteration, which has subtle special cases.

10.8.15 Linked-List Operations

When manipulating linked lists in-place, care must be taken to not to use values that you have invalidated in previous assignments. This makes algorithms for inserting or deleting linked list nodes somewhat subtle. This section gives pseudo code for adding or removing nodes from singly-, doubly-, and circularly-linked lists in-place. Throughout we will use null to refer to an end-of-list marker or sentinel, which may be implemented in a number of ways.

Singly-linked lists

Our node data structure will have two fields. We also keep a variable first node, which always points to the first node in the list, or is null for an empty list.

```
record Node {
    data // The data being stored in the node
    next // A reference to the next node; null for last node
}
record List {
    Node firstNode // points to first node of list; null for empty list
}
```

Traversal of a singly-linked list is easy, beginning at the first node and following each next link until we come to the end :

```
node := list.firstNode
while node not null {
    (do something with node.data)
    node := node.next
}
```

The following code inserts a node after an existing node in a singly-linked list. The diagram shows how it works. Inserting a node before an existing one cannot be done; instead, you have to locate it while keeping track of the previous node.

```
function insertAfter(Node node, Node newNode) { // insert newNode after node
    newNode.next := node.next
    node.next := newNode
}
```

Inserting at the beginning of the list requires a separate function. This requires updating firstNode.

```
function insertBeginning(List list, Node newNode) { // insert node before current first
node
    newNode.next : = list.firstNode
    list.firstNode := newNode
}
```

Similarly, we have functions for removing the node after a given node, and for removing a node from the beginning of the list. The diagram demonstrates the former. To find and remove a particular node, one must again keep track of the previous element.

```
function removeAfter(Node node) { // remove node past this one
    obsoleteNode := node.next
    node.next := node.next.next
    destroy obsoleteNode
}
function removeBeginning(List list, Node node) { // remove first node
    obsoleteNode := list.firstNode
    list.firstNode := list.firstNode.next // point past deleted node
    destroy obsoleteNode
}
```

Notice that remove Beginning () sets list first Node to null when removing the last node in the list.

Since we can't iterate backwards, efficient "insert before" or "remove before" operations are not possible.

Doubly-linked lists

With doubly linked lists there are even more pointers to update, but also less information is needed, since we can use backwards pointers to observe preceding elements in the list. This enables new operations, and eliminates special-case functions. We will add a per field to our nodes, pointing to the previous element, and a last Node field to our list structure, which always points to the last node in the list. Both list First Node and list Last Node is null for an empty list.

10.9 Trees

In computer science, a tree is a widely used computer data structure that emulates a tree structure with a set of linked nodes. Each node has zero or more child nodes, which are below it in the tree (in computer science, unlike in nature, trees grow down, not up). A node that has a child is called the child's parent node. A child has at most one parent; a node without a parent is called the root node (or root). Nodes with no children are called leaf nodes.

In graph theory, a tree is a connected acyclic graph. A rooted tree is such a graph with a vertex singled out as the root (Fig. 10.9). In this case, any two vertices connected by an edge inherit a parent-child relationship. An acyclic graph with multiple connected components or a set of rooted trees is sometimes called a forest.

There are many different ways to represent trees; common representations represent the nodes as records allocated on the heap with pointers to their children, their parents, or both, or as items in an array, with relationships between them determined by their positions in the array (e.g., binary heap).

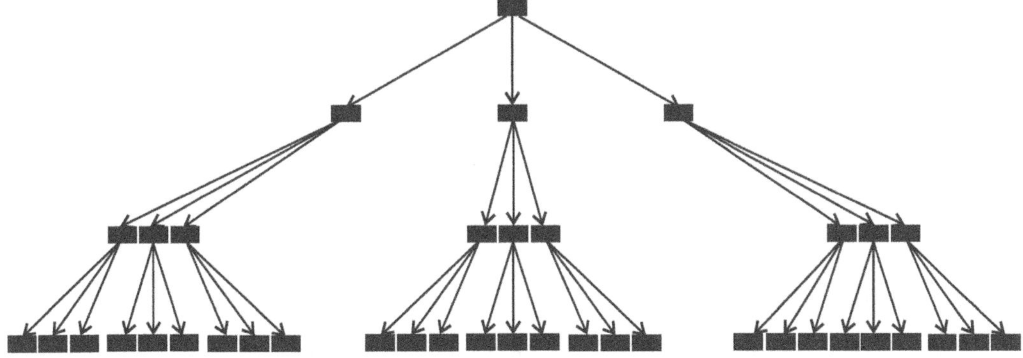

Fig. 10.9 Tree

10.9.1   Definition of Trees

Trees are as common and important as lists. There are many variations of trees like lists – binary search trees, balanced trees, and heaps are the main ones we will look at.

Recall that a list is a collection of components in which :

1. Each component (except one, the first) has exactly 1 predecessor.

2. Each component (except one, the last) has exactly 1 successor.

A tree is very similar: it has property (1) but (2) is slightly relaxed.

Each component has some number of successors.

If there is a limit on the number of successors that a node can have, the tree is called a general tree.

If there is a maximum number M of successors for a node, then the tree is called an M-ary tree. In particular, a binary (2-ary) tree is a tree in which each node has 0, 1, or 2 successors.

The unique node with no predecessor is called the root of the tree. A node with no successors is called a leaf – there will usually be many leaves in a tree. The successors of a node are called its children; the unique predecessor of a node is called its parent. If two nodes have the same parent, they are called brothers or siblings. In a binary tree, the two children are called the left and right.

10.9.2   Common Operations on Trees

*Enumerating all the items;

*Searching for an item;

*Adding a new item at a certain position on the tree;

*Deleting an item;

*Removing a whole section of a tree (pruning);

*Adding a whole section to a tree (grafting);

*Finding the root for any node.

10.9.3   Common Uses for Trees

*Manipulate hierarchical data;

*Make information easy to search;

*Manipulate sorted lists of data.

10.9.4   Drawing Trees

The root is at the top; below it are its children. An arc connects a node to each of its children: we sometimes draw arrow heads on the arc, but they are optional because the direction parent->child is always top->bottom.

Then, we continue in the same manner, the children of each node are drawn below the node.

In general, each child of a node is the root of a tree "within the big tree". For example, B is the root of a little tree (B,D,E), so is C. These inner trees are called sub trees. The sub trees of a node are the trees whose roots are the children of the node, e.g. the sub trees of A are the sub trees whose roots are B and C. In a binary tree, we refer to the left sub tree and the right sub tree.

10.9.5　Path in a Tree

A path is any linear subset of a tree, e.g. A-B-E and C-F are paths. The length of a path could be counted as either the number of nodes or the number of edges on the path – we will count the nodes; e.g. A-B-E has length 3. But be careful: There is no agreed definition! The textbook defines path length as the number of edges.

There is a unique path from the root to any node. Simple as this property seems, it is extremely important: All our algorithms for processing trees will depend upon it. The depth or level of a node is the length of this path. When you draw a tree, it is very useful if all the nodes in the same level are drawn as a neat horizontal row. The depth or height of a tree is the maximum depth of the nodes in the tree.

10.9.6　Ordered Trees

There are two basic types of trees. In an unordered tree, there is no distinction between the various children of a node – none is the "first child" or "last child". A tree in which such distinctions are made, is called an ordered tree, and data structures built on them are called ordered tree data structures. Ordered trees are by far the most common form of tree data structure.

A simple example is binary tree.

Binary search trees are one kind of ordered trees, and there is a one-to-one mapping between binary trees and general ordered trees.

A tree is ordered if there is some significance to the order of the sub trees. For example, consider this tree:

If this is a family tree, there could be no significance to left and right. In this case, the tree is unordered, and we could redraw the tree exchanging sub trees without affecting the meaning of the tree. On the other hand, there may be some significance to left and right – maybe the left child is younger than the right... or (as is the case here) may be the left child has the name that is earlier in the alphabet. Then, the tree is ordered and we are not free to move around the sub trees.

For now, we will restrict ourselves to ordered trees. Like lists, ordered N-ary trees have a nice recursive structural definition:

10.9.7   Structural Definition of Binary Trees

A binary tree is either empty or it has 3 parts:

- a value
- a left sub tree
- a right sub tree

Whenever a data structure has a recursive definition like this, most of the 'properties' of the data structure can be computed in a recursive manner, which exactly mirrors the definition.

For example, here is a function to compute the number of nodes in a binary tree:

```
int size(binary_tree *t)

{

return is_empty(t) ? 0 : 1 + size(t->left) + size(t->right);

}
```

With lists we had an alternative to recursion – we could scan through a list as easily with normal loops (while, do ... while) as with recursion. This is not true for trees. It is possible to scan through a tree non-recursively, but it is not nearly as easy as scanning recursively.

10.9.8   Tree Traversal

To traverse a data structure is to process, however you like, every node in the data structure exactly once. e.g. we can talk about "traversing a list", which means going through the list and processing every node once. We had a special name for this : map. For a specific data structure, we talk about the different orders in which it might be traversed. For a list there are two common traversal orders: first-to-last (the most common) and last-to-first. The general recursive pattern for traversing a (non-empty) binary tree is this : At node N you must do these three things :

*(L) recursively traverses its left sub tree. When this step is finished, you are back at N again.

*(R) recursively traverses its right sub tree. When this step is finished, you are back at N again.

*(N) actually process N itself.

We may do these things in any order and still have a legitimate traversal. If we do (L) before (R), we call it left-to-right traversal; otherwise we call it right-to-left traversal.

Pre-Order Traversal

do (N) before anything else.

Post-Order Traversal

do (N) after everything else.

In-Order, or Infix Order, Traversal

do (N) in between the two sub trees.

Let us look at what order the nodes will get processed given this tree:

Using Left-To-Right traversal:

For example, suppose we were writing out the nodes of the tree:

```
void print_tree(binary_tree *t)
{
if (! is_empty(t)) {
    print_tree(t->left); /* L */
    print_tree(t->right); /* R */
    printf("%d\n",t->value); /* N */
}
}
```

The preceding diagrams show us the order in which the nodes will get written :

- Pre-Order : A-B-D-C-E-F Root Left Right

- In-Order : B-D-A-E-C-F Left Root Right

- Post-Order : D-B-E-F-C-A Left Right Root

10.9.9   Binary Trees

A binary tree is a tree, which is either empty or consists of a root node and two disjoint trees called the left sub tree and right sub tree.

In a binary tree, no node can have more than two children (Fig. 10.10).

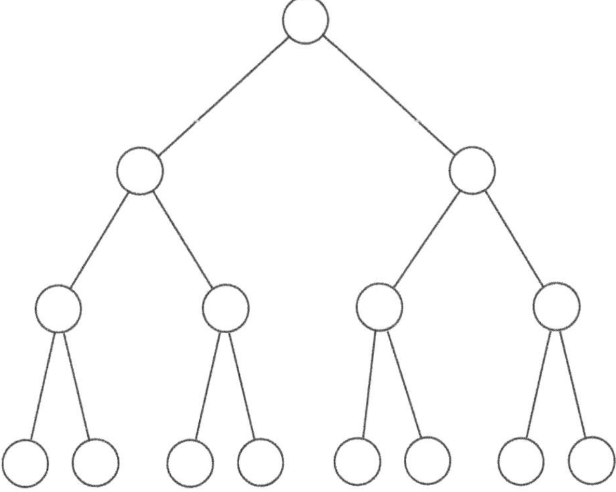

Fig. 10.10 A binary tree.

Properties of binary tree:

1. A binary tree with N internal nodes has maximum of (N+1) external nodes: Root is considered as an internal node.

2. The external path length of any binary tree with N internal nodes is 2N greater than the internal path length.

The height of a full binary tree with N internal nodes is about log2 N.

A full binary tree or a complete binary tree is a binary tree in which all internal nodes have same degree and all leaves are at the same level.

Linked lists most commonly represent binary trees. Each node can be considered as having 3 elementary fields: a data field left pointer, pointing to left sub tree and right pointer pointing to the right sub tree.

10.9.10 Binary Search Tree

In computer science, a binary search tree (BST) is a binary tree where every node has a value, every node's left sub tree contains only values less than or equal to the node's value, and every node's right sub tree contains only values that are greater than or equal. (Depending on the application of the binary search tree, equal values may not be allowed in either the left or right sub tree). This requires that the values have a linear order. New nodes are added as leaves (Fig. 10.11). Sort algorithms and search algorithms exist for binary search trees. The values of a binary search tree can be retrieved in ascending order using an in-order traversal.

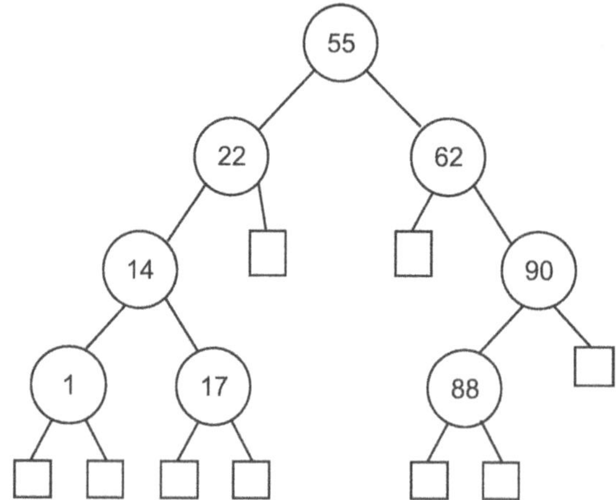

Fig. 10.11 Binary Search Tree

A binary search tree, BST, is an ordered binary tree T such that either it is an empty tree or :

Each value in its left sub tree is less than the root value,

Each data value in its right sub tree is greater than the root value, and

Left and right sub trees are again binary search trees.

Operations

Searching

The algorithm/pseudo-code is :

Tree-Search(x,k)

1. if x=Null or k=key[x]
2. then return x
3. if k < key[x]
4. then return Tree-Search(left[x],k)
5. else return Tree-Search(right[x],k)

```
def search_binary_tree(treenode, value) :
    if treenode is None: return None # failure
    left, nodevalue, right = treenode.left, treenode.value, treenode.right
    if nodevalue > value :
        return search_binary_tree(left, value)
    elif value > nodevalue :
        return search_binary_tree(right, value)
    else :
        return nodevalue
```

This operation requires O(log n) time in the average case, but needs Ù(n) time in the worst-case, when the unbalanced tree resembles a linked list.

10.9.11 B-Tree

In computer science, B-trees are tree data structures that are most commonly found in databases and file systems. B-trees keep data sorted and allow amortized logarithmic time insertions and deletions. B-trees generally grow from the bottom up as elements are inserted, whereas most binary trees grow down.

The idea behind B-trees is that internal nodes can have a variable number of child nodes within some pre-defined range. As data are inserted or removed from the data structure, the number of child nodes varies within a node and so internal nodes are coalesced or split so as to maintain the designed range. Because a range of child nodes is permitted, B-trees do not need re-balancing as frequently as other self-balancing binary search trees, but may waste some space. The lower and upper bounds on the number of child nodes are typically fixed for a particular implementation (Fig. 10.12). For example, in a 2-3 B-tree (often simply 2-3 tree), each internal node may have only 2 or 3 child nodes. A node is considered to be in an illegal state if it has an invalid number of child nodes.

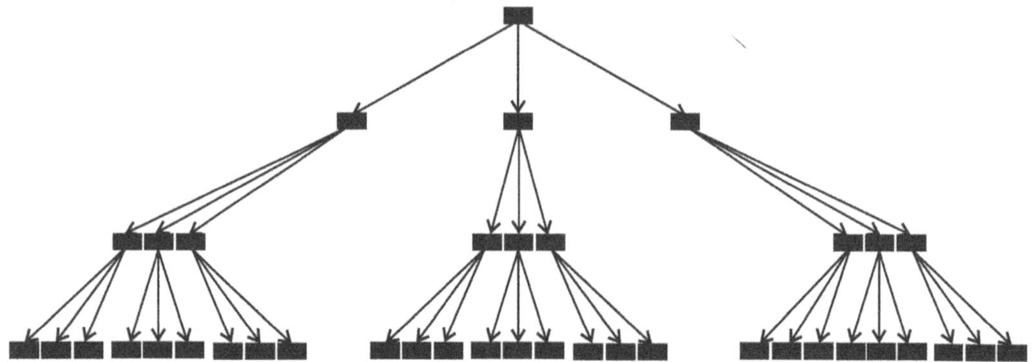

Fig. 10.12 B Tree.

B-trees have substantial advantages over alternative implementations when node access times far exceed access times within nodes. This usually occurs when most nodes are in secondary storage such as hard drives. By maximizing the number of child nodes within each internal node, the height of the tree decreases, balancing occurs less often, and efficiency increases. Usually this value is set such that each node takes up a full disk block or an analogous size in secondary storage.

The B-tree's creator, Rudolf Bayer, has not explained what the B stands for. The most common belief is that B stands for balanced, as all the leaf nodes are at the same level in the tree. B may also stand for Bayer, or for Boeing, because he was working for Boeing Scientific Research Labs.

Algorithms

Search

Search is performed in the typical manner, analogous to that in a binary search tree. Starting at the root, the tree is traversed top to bottom, choosing the child pointer whose separation values are on either side of the value that is being searched.

Binary search is typically used within nodes to determine this location.

Insertion

For a node to be in an illegal state, it must contain a number of elements which are outside of the acceptable range.

1. First, search for the position into which the node should be inserted. Then, insert the value into that node.

2. If no node is in an illegal state then the process is finished.

3. If some node has too many elements, split it into two nodes. Continue this process recursively up the tree. If you split the root node, create a new root node. You must select the minimum and maximum number of elements such that the minimum is no more than one half of (the maximum plus one) in order for this to work.

4. First, search for the value, which will be deleted. Then, remove the value from the node, which contains it.

5. If no node is in an illegal state then the process is finished.

6. If some node is in an illegal state then there are two possible cases:

   *Its sibling node, a child of the same parent node, can transfer one or more of its child nodes to the current node and return it to a legal state. If so, after updating the separation values of the parent and the two siblings the process is finished.

   *Its sibling does not have an extra child because it is on the lower bound. In that case both siblings are merged into a single node and we recurse onto the parent node, since it has had a child node removed. This continues until the current node is in a legal state or the root node is reached, upon which the root's children are merged and the merged node becomes the new root!

10.9.12 AVL Tree/Height Balanced Tree

A binary tree of height h is completely balanced or balanced if all leaves occurs at nodes of level h or h-1 and all nodes at levels lower than h-1 have two children. According to this definition, the tree given below is balanced, because all leaves occur at level 3 considering at level 1 and all nodes at levels 1 and 2 have two children.

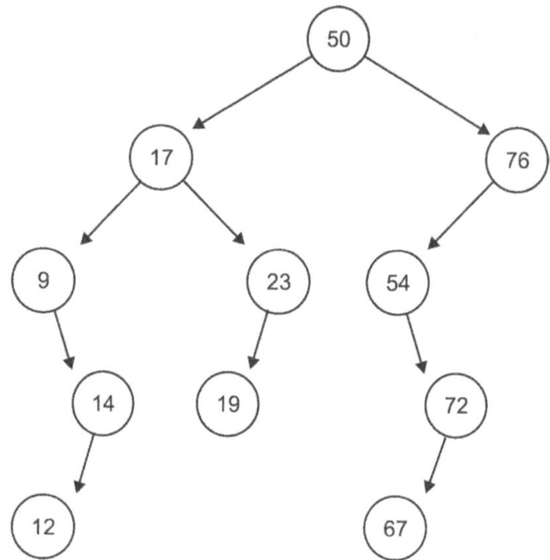

Fig. 10.13 AVL Tree.

More precisely a tree is height balanced if, for each node in the tree, the height of the left sub tree differs from the height of the right sub tree.

An almost height balance tree is called an AVL tree. AVL tree may or may not be perfectly balanced tree (Fig. 10.13).

Details of Rotation And Insertion, Sketch of Deletion, For AVL Trees

- Tree Rotation: The General Algorithm
- General Insertion Algorithm
- Deletion of a Node From an AVL Tree

Tree Rotation : The General Algorithm :

Step 1 : The pivot node is the deepest node at which there is an imbalance. The rotator node is the root of the pivot's taller sub tree.

Step 2 : There may be more nodes above the pivot's parent. Step 3 prunes the rotators 'inside' sub tree, i.e. the one on the pivot's side.

Step 3 : Which of the rotator's sub trees is the inside sub tree, which is the outside? It depends on whether the rotator is the left or right child of the pivot. If the rotator is the right child (as in this picture), the inside sub tree is its left sub tree and the outside sub tree is its right sub tree. On the other hand, if the rotator is the left child, the inside sub tree is its right sub tree and the outside sub tree is its left sub tree.

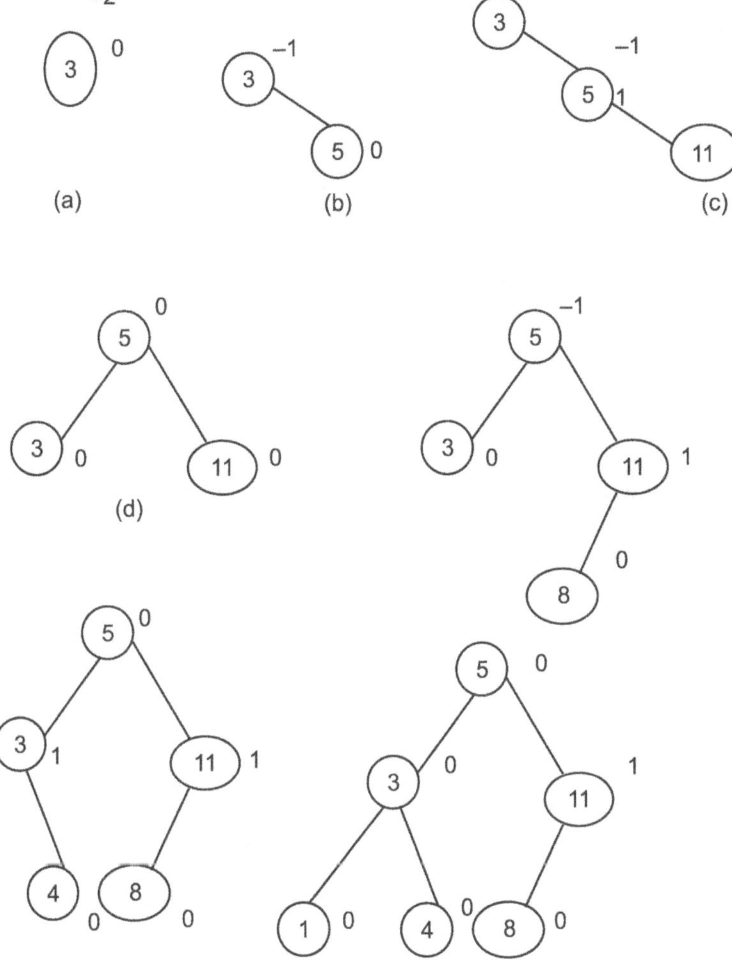

Step 4 : Join the pruned inside sub tree to the pivot (in the place where the rotator had been).

Step 5 : Join the pivot to the rotator (in the place where inside had been).

Step 6 : Join the rotator to the pivot's (original) parent (in the place where the pivot had been).

Following these steps, the result of the rotation is this: the rotator has rotated up, the pivot has rotated down on the other side, and the inside sub tree has jumped across to join the pivot:.

General Insertion Algorithm

1. Do a normal BST insert.

2. If the tree is balanced, you are finished. Otherwise do 3-4.

3. Starting at the newly inserted node, work your way up the tree until you find the first node whose sub trees' heights differ by 2. This node is the pivot, the root of its taller sub tree is the rotator.

4. It is necessarily the case that the new value was inserted in one of the rotator's sub trees. If it was inserted in the rotator's outside sub tree, then this sub tree will be taller than inside, and a single rotation (of the rotator) will correct the imbalance. Otherwise you must first rotate the root of the rotator's inside sub tree up into the rotator's position (the rotator does down the other side), and then rotate the node that replaced the rotator up into the pivot's position.

Deletion of a Node From an AVL Tree

The inverse of the INSERT operation is the DELETE operation : given a value X and an AVL tree T, delete the node containing X and rebalance the resulting tree, if necessary. It turns out that DELETE is considerably more complex than INSERT.

To illustrate the additional complexity, recall that to insert a new value into an AVL tree, we never need to do more than 2 rotations in order to restore the tree's balance. We can use rotations to restore the balance when we do a deletion, too, but in some cases we may have to do a rotation at every level of the tree (O(logN) rotations in the worst case).

Here is a tree that causes this worse case # of rotations (we're deleting X). At every node, the left sub tree is one shorter than the right sub tree (numbers shown are height of sub trees).

10.9.13   M-Way Search Trees

A binary search tree has one value in each node and two sub trees. This notion easily generalizes to an M-way search tree, which has (M-1) values per node and M sub trees. M is called the degree of the tree. A binary search tree, therefore, has degree 2.

In fact, it is not necessary for every node to contain exactly (M-1) values and have exactly M sub trees. In an M-way sub tree, a node can have anywhere from 1 to (M-1) values, and the number of (non-empty) sub trees can range from 0 (for a leaf) to 1+(the number of values). M is thus a fixed upper limit on how much data can be stored in a node.

The values in a node are stored in ascending order, V1 < V2 < ... Vk (k <= M-1) and the sub trees are placed between adjacent values, with one additional sub tree at each end. We can thus associate with each value a `left' and `right' sub tree, with the right sub tree of Vi being the same as the left sub tree of V(i+1). All the values in V1's left sub tree are less than V1 ; all the values in Vk's sub tree are greater than Vk; and all the values in the sub tree between V(i) and V(i+1) are greater than V(i) and less than V(i+1).

In our examples, it will be convenient to illustrate M-way trees using a small value of M. But we should bear in mind that, in practice, M is usually very large. Each node corresponds to a physical block on disk, and M represents the maximum number of data items that can be stored in a single block. M is maximized in order to speedup processing: to move from one node to another involves reading a block from disk – a very slow operation compared to moving around a data structure stored in memory.

The algorithm for searching for a value in an M-way search tree is the obvious generalization of the algorithm for searching in a binary search tree. If we are searching for value X and are currently at node consisting of values V1...Vk, there are four possible cases that can arise :

1. If X < V1, recursively search for X in V1's left sub tree.
2. If X > Vk, recursively search for X in Vk's right sub tree.
3. If X=Vi, for some i, then we are done (X has been found).
4. The only remaining possibility is that, for some i, Vi < X < V(i+1). In this case, recursively search for X in the sub tree that is in between Vi and V(i+1).

For example, suppose we were searching for 68 in the tree above. At the root, case (2) would apply, so we would continue the search in V2's right sub tree. At the root of this sub tree, case (4) applies, 68 is between V1=55 and V2=70, so we would continue to search in the sub tree between them. Now case (3) applies, 68=V2, so we are done. If we had been searching for 69, exactly the same processing would have occurred down to the last node. At that point, case (2) would apply, but the sub tree we want to search in is empty. Therefore, we conclude that 69 is not in the tree.

Other algorithms for binary search trees – insertion and deletion – generalize in a similar way. As with binary search trees, inserting values in ascending order will result in a degenerate M-way search tree; i.e. a tree whose height is O(N) instead of O(logN). This is a problem because all the important operations are O(height), and it is our aim to make them O(logN). One solution to this problem is to force the tree to be height-balanced; we sketched this last lecture for binary search trees and now we will examine it in detail for M-way search trees.

10.9.14   Threaded Binary Tree

We consider the linked representation of a binary tree T. Approximately half of the entries in the pointer fields LEFT and RIGHT will contain null elements. Replacing the null entries to it other type of information may more efficiently use this space. Specifically we will replace certain null entries by special pointers, which point towards higher in tree. These special pointers are called threads, and binary tree that must be distinguished are called threaded trees.

In a threaded tree threads must be distinguished in some way from ordinary pointers. The threads in diagram of a threaded tree must be distinguished by dotted lines. In computer memory an extra 1 bit TAG field may be used to distinguish thread from ordinary pointer or alternatively threads may be denoted by negative integers, when ordinary pointers are denoted by positive integers.

Threading may choose a one-way threading or two-way threading. Accordingly in one-way threading of T, a thread will appear in the right facts of anode and will point to the next node in the nodes traversal of T and in the two-way threading of T, a thread will also appear in the left field of the first node and the right pointer of the last node.

There is an analysis one-way threading of a binary tree T which corresponds to the preorder traversal of T. On the other hand, there is no threading of T which corresponds to the post-order traversal of T.

10.10   Graph

A graph is a set of objects called vertices (or nodes) connected by links called edges (or arcs), which can be directed (assigned a direction). Typically, a graph is designed as a set of dots (the vertices) connected by lines (the edges).

Structures that can be represented, as graphs are ubiquitous, and many problems of practical interest can be represented by graphs. The link structure of a website could be represented by a directed graph: the vertices are the web pages available at the website and there's a directed edge from page A to page B if and only if A contains a link to B. The development of algorithms to handle graphs is therefore of major interest in computer science.

Assigning a weight to each edge can extend a graph structure. Graphs with weights can be used to represent many different concepts; for example if the graph represents a road network, the weights could represent the length of each road. Another way to extend basic graphs is by making the edges to the graph directional (A links to B, but B does not necessarily link to A, as in webpages), technically called a directed graph or digraph. A digraph with weighted edges is called a network.

Networks have many uses in the practical side of graph theory network analysis (for example, to model and analyze traffic networks or to discover the shape of the internet, see Applications below). However, it should be noted that within network analysis, the definition of the term "network" may differ, and may often refer to a simple graph.

One of the first results in graph theory appeared in Leonhard Euler's paper on Seven Bridges of Königsberg, published in 1736. It is also regarded as one of the first topological results in geometry; that is, it does not depend on any measurements. This illustrates the deep connection between graph theory and topology.

In 1845, Gustav Kirchhoff published his Kirchhoff's circuit laws for calculating the voltage and current in electric circuits.

In 1852, Francis Guthrie posed the four-colour problem, which asks if it is possible to colour, using only four colours, any map of countries in such a way as to prevent two bordering countries from having the same colour. This problem, which was only solved a century later in 1976 by Kenneth Appel and Wolfgang Haken, can be considered the birth of graph theory. While trying to solve it, mathematicians invented many fundamental graph theoretic terms and concepts.

Definition

A Graph G consists of a set of vertices (nodes) and a set E of edges (arcs). We write:

G = (V,E) is a finite and non-empty set of vertices. E is a set of pairs of vertices;

these pair is called edges. Therefore,

V(G), read as V of G is set of vertices,

E(G), read as E of G is set of edges,

And edge e = (v,w) is a pair of vertices v and w.

A graph may be pictorially represented as : (Fig. 10.14)

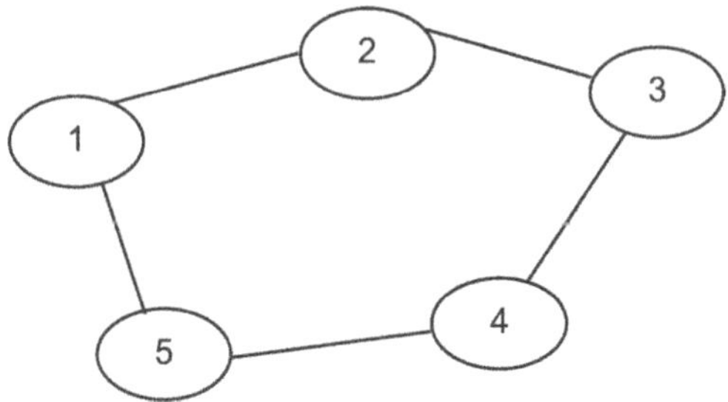

Fig. 10.14 A Graph.

If we write (1,5) and (5,1) it means ordering of vertices is not significant in an in-directed graph. Thus, the sequence so generated is V2, V8, V3, V5, V6, V7. Here, we need a query instead of stack to implement it.

10.11 Sorting

GENERAL SORTING STRATEGY (RECURSIVE)

A sorting algorithm is an algorithm whose input is any list and whose output is a list (or a change in the given list) that is sorted and has the same elements as the given list.

Most well-known sorting algorithms are based on this general strategy. Given a list L,

- If L has zero or one element, then it is already sorted, so nothing need be done;
- Otherwise,

    1. Divide in L into two smaller lists, L1 and L2.

    2. Recursively sort each of the smaller lists. Result : L1 and L2 are now sorted.

    3. Combine L1 and L2. The result is a sorted version of the original list. How do we combine L1 and L2? As just discussed there's only one way to do so and produce a sorted list. We MERGE them.

This strategy works no matter how we do step (1). The pieces can be any size; they could be the same size, or they could be of very different sizes; and it does not matter which elements of L we put together or in what order we put them into the pieces.

We can divide up and scramble up the elements any way we like, and we will still sort L. In fact, we could even divide L into more than two pieces, we could divide it into 3, or 7, or whatever.

The one thing we must avoid is having one of the pieces equal to L; if this happens we would have an infinite loop. But that is the only thing we have to avoid.

We will now look at three specific versions of this general strategy : Merge Sort, Insertion Sort and Quick Sort.

10.11.1   Merge Sort

Although the general strategy uses MERGE to put the pieces back together, there is a specific version of the general strategy called Merge Sort. The defining feature of Merge Sort is that in step (1), the given list is divided into two equal size pieces (or as near equal as possible).

There are various ways of dividing L into 2 equal pieces. We will illustrate the algorithm by putting the first half of L in one piece and the second half of L in the other piece. We proceed until we're down to singleton or empty lists, which are always sorted, then we work our way back up the recursion by MERGING together the short lists into larger ones (which replace the list that we started with at that level).

The slowest step in this algorithm is the MERGE operation. Earlier we looked at two special cases of MERGE - INSERT and JOIN. How can we change the way we do step (1) – SPLIT L into pieces, so that we can use INSERT or JOIN instead of MERGE?

Merge sort divides the array into two halves which are sorted recursively and then merged to form a sorted whole. The array is divided into equal-sized parts (up to truncation) so there are log2(N) levels of recursion.

It is interesting to compare quick sort with merge sort; the former has a pre-order structure and the latter a post-order structure. In fact there is also a bottom-up, breadthfirst merge sort.

```
function merge(int inA[], int lo, int hi, int opA[])
/* sort (input) inA[lo..hi] into (output) opA[lo..hi] */
{ int i, j, k, mid;
if(hi > lo) /* at least 2 elements */
    { int mid = (lo+hi)/2; /* lo <= mid < hi */
    merge(opA, lo, mid, inA); /* sort the ... */
    merge(opA, mid+1, hi, inA); /* ... 2 halfs */
    i = lo; j = mid+1; k = lo; /* and merge them */
    while(true)
    { if( inA[i] <= inA[j] ) /* ? smaller ? */
        { opA[k] = inA[i]; i++; k++;
        if(i > mid) /* copy rest */
        { for( ; j <= hi; j++)
            { opA[k]=inA[j]; k++; }
            break;
        }
      }
    else
    { opA[k] = inA[j]; j++; k++;
    if(j > hi) /* copy rest */
    { for( ; i <= mid; i++)
        { opA[k]=inA[i]; k++; }
        break;
        }
      }
    }/*while */
  }/*if */
}/*merge */
function mergeSort(int a[], int N) /* wrapper routine */
/* NB sort a[1..N] */
    { int i; int b[N];
    for(i=1; i <= N; i++) b[i]=a[i];
    merge(b, 1, N, a);
```

Complexity

Time

The best, average and worst case time-complexities of the (basic) algorithm are all the same, O(N*log(N)).

Space

The space complexity of the recursive algorithm is O(N+log(N)), N for the "workingspace array" and log(N) for the stack space.

A naive non-recursive translation would still use O(N+log(N)) space, log(N) being for an explicit stack. However, because the array sections vary in a simple and systematic way, there is a non-recursive version that does not need any stack and requires O(N) space only (but there again, log(N)<<N, if N is large).

There are in fact in-situ merging algorithms that only use O(1) space but they are difficult!

Stability

Merge sort is stable if written carefully, it is a matter of a `<=' versus a `<'.

Once upon a time, computer programs were written in Fortran* and entered on punched cards, about 2000 cards to a tray. Fortran code was typed in columns 1 to 72 of each card, but columns 73-80 could be used for a card number. If you ever dropped a large deck of cards you were really in the pool, unless the cards had been numbered in columns 73-80. If they had been numbered you were saved+: They could be fed into a card-sorting machine and restored to their original order.

The card-sorting machine was the size of three or four large filing cabinets. It had a card input hopper and ten output bins, numbered 0 to 9. It read each card and placed it in a bin according to the digit in a particular column, e.g. column 80. This gave ten stacks of cards, one stack in each bin. The ten stacks were removed and concatenated, in order: stack 0, then 1, 2, and so on up to stack 9. The whole process was then repeated on column 79, and again on columns 78, 77, etc., down to column 73, at which time your deck was back in its original order!

Note that the cards are sorted on the least significant digit (column 80) first and on the most significant digit (column 73) last. Think about it!

```
function pass(a, N, dig) // e.g. in JavaScript      //A C 1
// pre: a[1..N] is sorted on digits [dig-1..0]          l o 9
// post: a[1..N] is sorted on digits [dig..0]            g m 9
{ var counter = new Array(11); // for digit occurrences   p 9
var temp = new Array();              //D .
var i, d;                            //S S
                                     // c
```

```
for( d = 0; d <= 9; d++ ) counter[d] = 0; // i
for( i = 1; i <= N; i++ ) counter[ digit(a[i], dig) ] ++;
for( d = 1; d <= 9; d++ ) counter[d] += counter[d-1];

for( i = N; i >= 1; i-- )
{ temp[ counter[ digit(a[i], dig) ] -- ] = a[i]; }

for( i = 1; i <= N; i++ ) a[i] = temp[i];
}//pass

function radixSort(a, N)
{ var p;
for( p=0; p < NumDigits; p++ )
pass(a, N, p);
}//radixSort

// e.g. number = 1066
// digit 3^ ^digit 0
```

10.11.2   Insertion Sort

In order to use INSERT instead of MERGE, it is clear what we have to do. We have to divide L so that one of the pieces is a singleton. This is easy, for example, just separate the head of L from its tail. Knowing that this piece is a singleton, we also can delete the recursive call that sorts it. This leads to the algorithm:

1. Divide L into two pieces, its HEAD and its TAIL.
2. Recursively sorts the TAIL.
3. INSERT the HEAD into the sorted TAIL.

This is called Insertion Sort.

Example: Given L = [56,35,42,29]:

1. HEAD = 56. TAIL = [35,42,29].
2. Recursively sort the TAIL. Result = [29,35,42]. (The details of this step are given below.)
3. INSERT 56 into [29,35,42]. Result = [29,35,42,56].

Step (2) is a recursive call, so it follows the same pattern, except for this computation, L = [35,42,29].

1. HEAD = 35. TAIL = [42,29].
2. Recursively sorts the TAIL. Result = [29,42].
3. INSERT 35 into [29,42]. Result = [29,35,42].

So, we have succeeded in replacing the MERGE operation in step (3) with an INSERT operation, which is quite a bit more efficient. However, we have made a major sacrifice in efficiency in order to do this. Merge Sort happens to be one of the fastest sorting algorithms known; its speed is entirely due to the fact that it cuts the given list L into two equal size pieces. Insertion Sort gives up this source of efficiency, and as a result, it is much less efficient for large lists. We will see how to analyze the efficiency of algorithms later.

10.11.3 Quick Sort

The idea behind Quick Sort is to replace the MERGE operation in step 3 with the very much faster JOIN operation. If this could be done, while still splitting the list more or less in half in step (1), we would have an algorithm that is clearly faster than Merge Sort. How can we change the way we do step (1) – SPLIT L into pieces – so that we can use JOIN instead of MERGE? This is the secret to Quick Sort.

When is it safe to JOIN two sorted lists L1 and L2?

When everything in L1 is smaller than everything in L2.

So that's how we cut our list in two. Pick a number, CUTOFF, and put all the elements less than CUTOFF into L1 and all the ones bigger than CUTOFF into L2.

How shall we choose the CUTOFF value? Does it matter?

We must keep 3 things in mind when we choose CUTOFF:

1. Its value must be fairly cheap to compute.
2. It must not be bigger than, or smaller than, all the values in the given list. Why? If it were, then one of the pieces would be identical to L and we'd be in an infinite loop.
3. Ideally, roughly half the values in L will be smaller than CUTOFF. Cutting-in-half will make Quick Sort very efficient.

Considering (2) and (3), the very best choice for CUTOFF is the median value in the given list. By definition the median of a list is the value in the list which is larger than exactly half the values in the list.

Let's illustrate Quick Sort with the list (above) [56,29,35,42,15,41,75,21], assuming that the median is chosen for splitting. At this point I'll also add one little wrinkle –

Quick Sort actually splits the list into three pieces :

• L1 = {elements with keys strictly less than CUTOFF}

• LC = {elements with keys equal to CUTOFF}

• L2 = {elements with keys strictly greater than CUTOFF}

L1 and L2 are sorted recursively. Then, we join L2 to LC and then join the result to L1.

- L = [56,29,35,42,15,41,75,21]

- LC = [35] • L1 = [15,21,29], which happens to be sorted by a fluke.
- L2 = [56,42,41,75]

Recursively sort L1:

- L = [15,21,29]
- LC = [21]
- L1 = [15]. This is a singleton; so next recursive call will return it unchanged.
- L2 = [29] (ditto).
- JOIN: L1' LC L2' = [15,21,29]

We obtain L1' = [15,21,29].

Recursively sort L2.

- L = [56,42,41,75]
- LC = [42]
- L1 = [41]. This is a singleton; so next recursive call will return it unchanged.
- L2 = [56,75]. Recursively sort L2.
- L = [56,75]
- LC = [56]
- L1 = [], so next recursive call will return it unchanged.
- L2 = [75], singleton, recursive call won't change it.
- JOIN: L1' LC L2' = [56,75]

L2' = [56,75]

- JOIN: L1' LC L2' = [41,42,56,75]

We obtain L2' = [41,42,56,75]

JOIN L1' LC L2' = [15,21,29, 35 ,41,42,56,75]

Quick sort is very efficient if you use the median as the CUTOFF value, because the list is always split into two equal size pieces. But now we must consider, how efficiently can we compute the median of a list? There is no obvious way to do this quickly – in fact, all the obvious methods require you to sort the list! This obviously is no good – we are trying to use the median to do the sorting, so we can't sort the list in order to compute the median! There are some complex algorithms that do better than this, but in practice people do not use the median, they use something else that is easier to compute:

- The first element in the list.
- The mean (or average).
- The "median of 3". The way this is computed is to extract three elements from the list and use the middle of these 3 values as the CUTOFF.

What can go wrong? It can happen with these techniques that one of the pieces is empty – the CUTOFF value is removed from the list, and the other piece contains all the other values. For example, suppose you were unlucky and always used the smallest element in the list as the CUTOFF. L1 has all the elements smaller than this – there are none! In this case, called the worst case, Quick Sort is about the same efficiency as Insertion Sort.

Quick Sort is usually used with arrays. In this case, there is a special version of Quick Sort that sorts the array in place, i.e. without using any extra memory (normally you would create L1 and L2 by copying the values out of L into them, so you'd need enough space for two whole copies of L). This is done by a complex method of shuffling around the values within the array: the basic idea is not too difficult to understand, but the code itself is very tricky.

Quick Sort partitions the array into two sections, the first of "small" elements and the second of "large" elements. It then sorts the small and large elements separately.

Ideally, partitioning would use the median of the given values, but the median can only be found by scanning the whole array and this would slow the algorithm down.

In that case, the two partitions would be of equal size; in the simplest versions of Quick Sort an arbitrary element, typically the first element, is used as an estimate (guess) of the median.

```
quicksort(int a[], int lo, int hi)
/* sort a[lo..hi] */
{ int left, right, median, temp;
if( hi > lo ) /* i.e. at least 2 elements, then */
{ left=lo; right=hi;
  median=a[lo]; /* NB. just an estimate! */

    while(right >= left) /* partition a[lo..hi] */
    /* a[lo..left-1]<=median and a[right+1..hi]>=median */
    { while(a[left] < median) left++;
    /* a[left] >= median */

    while(a[right] > median) right--;
    /* a[left] >= median >= a[right] */
    if(left > right) break;
    //swap:
    temp=a[left]; a[left]=a[right]; a[right]=temp;
    left++; right--
```

```
    }
    /* a[lo..left-1]<=median and a[right+1..hi]>=median
       and left > right */
    quicksort(a, lo, right);// divide and conquer
    quicksort(a, left, hi);
    }
  }/*quicksort*/

    function quick(a, N)
    /* sort a[1..N], N.B. 1 to N */
    { quicksort(a, 1, N); }
    Complexity
```

Time

In the best case, the partitions are of equal size at each recursive call, and there are then log2(N) levels of recursive calls. The whole array is scanned at each level of calls, so the total work done is O(N*log(N)).

The average time complexity is also O(N*log(N)).

The worst-case time complexity is log2(N). This occurs when the estimate of the median is systematically always poor, e.g. on already sorted data, but this is very unlikely to happen by chance.

Space

As coded above the best- and average-case space-complexity is O(log(N)), for the stack-space used.

The worst-case space-complexity is O(N), but it can be limited to O(log(N)) if the code is modified so that the smaller half of the array is sorted first (and an explicit stack, or the tail-recursion optimisation, used).

In that case, the best-case space-complexity becomes O(1) [-- Andrew Clausen '05], "gcc -O2 does tail-recursion optimization, but -O1 doesn't."

Stability

Quick sort is not stable.

Testing

It is very easy to make errors when programming Quick Sort. The basic idea is simple but the details of the manipulation of the "pointers" hi, lo, left, right, is very easily messed up – this is the voice of bitter experience!

10.11.4 Two Way Merge Sort

Merge sort is also of one `divide and conquer' class of algorithms. The basic idea into this is to divide the list into a number of sub lists, sort each of these sub lists and merge them to get a single sorted list. The recursive implementation of 2-way merge sort divides the list into 2 sorts sub lists and then merges them to get the sorted list. This is also called concatenate sort. Merge sort is the best method for sorting linked lists in random order. The total computing time is of the order 0 (n log2 n).

The disadvantage of this is it requires two arrays of the same size and type for the merge phase.

If T1 (j) < T2 (i)

then select T1 (j) and write into NT.

else select T2 (x) and write into NT.

CHAPTER 11

Programming Language 'C'

11.1 Introduction

C is a general purpose, structured programming language, which can be used to write very concise source codes for commercial and scientific applications. It is an outgrowth of two earlier languages called Basic Combined Programming Language (BCPL) and B. It was originally developed by Dennis Retchie at bell Laboratories.

C was largely confined to use within Bell Laboratories untill 1978, when Brain Kernighan and Ritchie published a definitive description of C language. This description is commonly referred as 'K&RC'.

Following the publication of K&R description computer professionals, impressed with its many desirable feature, began to promote the use of the language. The language becomes more and more popular till mid 1980's. Several compiler and interpreters are written for different computers and different uses. Many commercial software which were earlier written in some other languages, were re-written in C because of its power and efficiency.

11.1.1   Importance

C is chracterised by the ability to write very concise source program, due in part to the large number of operators included within the language. It has a relatively small instruction set. The compiler combines the capability of an assembly language with the feature of a high level language and therefore it is well suited for both system software and application software.

Program written in C are efficient and fast. It is many times faster then BASIC.

An important characteristic of C is that it is highly portable. The reason for this is that C relegates most computer dependent futures to its library function. These library functions are relatively standard and· each individual library function is generally accessed in the same manner from one version of C to another. So the C programs written for one computer can be run on another computer with little or no alteration.

C language is well suited for structured programming, thus requiring the user to think of a problem in terms of function modules or blocks. A proper collection of these modules would make a complete program. This modular structure makes program debugging, testing and maintained easier.

11.1.2   C Menu

The C software is comprises of a main menu which is consist of several pads. These pads are used to create a new program, save a program or invoke an already existing program. The menu is also used to execute the program or compile the written program. The screen may appear slightly different for different versions of C.

The main menu which is presented horizontally on the top line is consist of Ten different pads. They are

File, Edit, search, run, Compile, Debug, Project, options, window, HELP. Each option of main menu has few more options associated with then. They are very easy to understand and use.

11.2 Structure of 'C' Program

A **C** program can be viewed as a group of functions. A function is a sub routine that may include one or more statement designed to perform a· particular task.

Usually following structure is followed to write a **C** program.
- Every C program is consisting of one or more functions, one of which must be main.

  The program will always begin by executing the main function.
- A function must contain
  - A function heading, which consist of the function name, followed by an optional list of argument enclosed in parenthesis.
  - A list of argument declaration.
  - A compound statement, which comprises the reminder of program.
- The program is to be typed in lower case.
- The first line of the program contains a reference to a special file (stdio.h) which contains information that must be included in the program when it is compiled.
- The second line generally contains a comment about the program. The comment generally expresses the purpose of the program and this may be in uppercase.
- The third line is a heading of the function main.

- Next line is a starting curly bracket (}) which indicates the starting of compound Statements.
- The first line of the compound program is a variable declaration.
- Next lines are the logic of the program.
- Each statement **I** of compound statement ends with a semi-colon except of compiler directives like define and include.

The program is terminated by a closing curly bracket (})

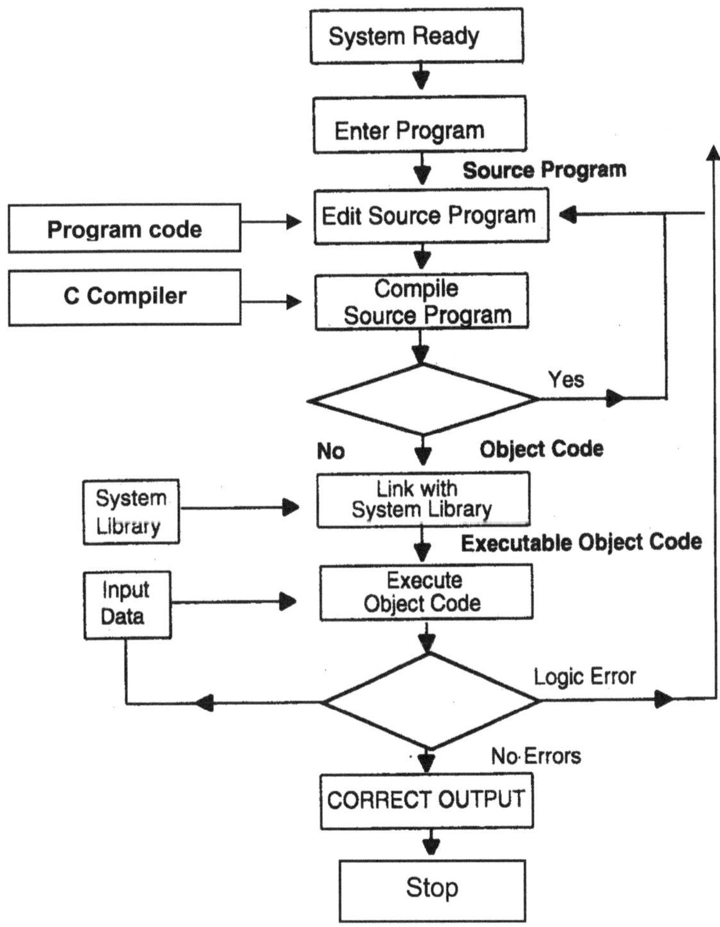

Fig. 11.1 Process of compiling and running a C Program

Main()   Function name

{   Start Program

----------------------   Program Statement

}   End Program

Format of Simple C Program

11.2.1 Execution of 'C' Program' .'

Executing a program written in C involves following steps.

1. Creating the program
2. Linking the program with functions.
3. Compiling the program.
4. Executing the program.

The program can be created with any word processing software in non-document mode with second name as C like area C or big C etc. The program can also be written with the inbuilt word processor of C compiler. The menu of C compiler contain many options to compile the program and then to run. We can save the program or reload a program using the option. Also we can debug a program by various ways if an error is occurred.

11.3 The C Character Set

Programmes are written to handle different types of values. The value may be a number or a character string or a combination of both. Further, the value may remain steady throughout the program or may be keeping changing at different stages.

Like any other language, C also used a fixed type of character set and provides several data types to handle these values. Data types are defined at a later stage of program and are used in the same way throughout the program.

C uses the uppercase litter's A to Z, the lower case letters a to **z,** the digits from 0 to 9, and certain special characters as building blocks to form words, numbers and expressions in a program. The characters in C are grouped into following categories.

- Letters   A - Z, a – z
- Digits   0 – 9
- Special characters
- White spaces

Special characters

,	Comma
.	Period
;	Semicolon
&	Ampersand
^	Caret
*	Asterisk
:	Colon
?	Question marks
"	Quotation
!	Exclamation
/	Slash
\	Backslash
-	Tilde
_	Under score
%	Percentage sign
#	Heber sign
!	Verticle bar

White spaces

- Blank space
- Horizontal tab
- Carriage return
- New line
- Form feed

C also uses certain combination of the character set like \b, \n and \t to represent special combinations such as back space, new line or horizontal tabs etc.

11.4 Data Types

C provides several data types. As it is very well known that a program has to handle several types of data. The data may be a number or character and the language should be strong enough to able to handle these data. C is sufficiently strong to deal with various types of data.

All C compilers support four fundamental data types. They are:

Integer (int)

Character (Char)

Floating point (Float)

Double precession (Double).

Integer types are used to store numeric data of integer nature. The value stored can be from – 32768 to 32767.

The character is used to store single character or string type of data. Float type is used to store numeric data of real numbers, while Double type of variable is used to provide more accuracy in float type of data.

Table 11.2 Size and Range of Basic Data Types

Data Type	Range of values
char	−128 to 127
int	−32,768 to 32,767
float	3.4e-38 to 3.4e+38
double	1.7e-308 to 1.7e+308

11.4.1   Constants

Constants are those value which remains stationary throughout the execution of the program. The value may be a digit or a character.

Classification & Constants

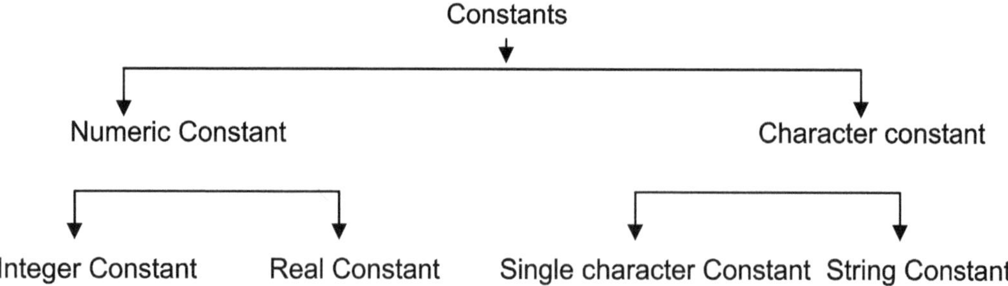

Integer Constant

An integer constant refers to an integer valued number. They are the sequence of digits. An integer constant may be written in decimal, Hexadecimal and Octal Number

Valid decimal integer constant is   101,   14675,   −12345

Embedded spaces, commas and non digit characters are not permitted.

Some invalid decimal integers are:-

15,750   -   Invalid character ',' used

15 750   -   Space not allowed

15.750   -   . is not allowed

Floating Point Constant

Floating point constants are those numeric values that may contain a decimal point or an exponential notation of the form (e^x), or both to accurately represent certain values that vary continuously like distance, weight, temperature, percentage, average etc.

Valid Floating Point Constants are:-

2.01, 0.2247, 22.467 2E+3,   0.45E-2

Invalid Floating Point Constants are:-

26   -   Decimal point or exponent must required

2,576,2.03 -   , is not allowed

Floating point constants have much greater range than integer constants. Typically the range from $3.4E − 38$ to $34E + 38$

String Constant

A string constant is a sequence of characters enclosed within single quotation marks. The characters may be letters, spaces, number, and special characters.

For example:

'Good bye', 'See you',   '2007'

Real Constants:

Real constants are those numeric values that may contain a decimal point or an exponential notation of the form (e^x), or both to accurately represent certain values that vary continuously like distance, weight, temperature etc. They are also called floating point constants.

Some valid real numeric constants are:

O. 1, 0.2827.625, 5000 2E+2, 0.6E-3

(Here E+2 represent E^2 and E-3 represent E^{-3}) Some invalid real constants are

50   - (either a decimal point or an exponent must present)

1,000.52 - (Invalid character',' used)

3E+ 10.2 - (Exponent must be an integer)

3E 10   (Blank spaces not allowed)

Floating point constants have a much greater range than integer constants. Typically the magnitude of, a floating point constant ranges from a minimum of 3.4E-38 to a maximum of 34E+38.

Floating point constants are normally represented as double precision quantity. However, the suffix f or F may be used to force single precision and I and L to extended double precision further.

Character Constants: Character constants are a single character or a string of characters enclosed in single quotation mark. Even if a number is written in the quotation mark, then it is treated as character constant.

Single Character Constant: A single character constant is a single character enclosed within single quotation mark. Some valid examples are' X', 'a', 's'.

String Constant: A string constant is a sequence of characters enclosed within the single quotation mark. The characters may be letters, number, spaces, and special characters. Some valid examples are

'Hello', 'Good Morning', '1999', 'X-Zone'

Backslash Character Constant: C supports several backslash character constants, also known as escape sequence characters that are used in output functions. These characters always begin with a backward slash (\) and are followed by one or more special characters.

11.4.2 Variables

A variable is a data name that may be use to store a data value. This variable may takes different values at different stages of execution. The data item must be assigned to the variable at some point in the program and it is then accessed or modified later in the program simply by referring to the variable name.

The data items stored this way may be of type like numeric, character or a combination of both. A variable name is chosen by the programmer in such a meaningful way so as to reflect its function or nature in the program.

A variable name may consist of letters, digits, underscores (-) or a combination of all these. Usually the maximum width of a variable name is eight characters. Lower case and upper case variables are treated separately (i.e. TOTAL and total are treated as two different variables). The standard keywords cannot be used as variable name.

Some valid variable names are.

Value

Amount

Grade

Some invalid variable names are

123   Area-of-square

Declaration of Variable

In a C program the variable has to be declared prior to use it. The declaration of the variable includes-

The Variable name

Its type.

The syntax for declaring the variable is

data type (Variable name (1,2,3).

Where variable name (1,2,3 ....) are one or more variable name used to store the data. If more than one type of data is to be defined in the program then they should be written in two different lines. A declaration statement must end with a semi colon. For example,

int avg;

float radius, area;

Char name ;

In order to provide more control over the maximum allowable length of variable, C provides three classes of integer storages namely short int, int and long int in both signed and unsigned form.

We declare long and unsigned to increase the range of the values.

The Variables can be grouped into four classes.

1.   Primary (or fundamental) data types.
2.   User-defined data types.
3.   Derived data types.
4.   Empty data set.

The four main data type, which we have discussed earlier (i.e. int, char float, double) comes under the primary data type group. The user defined types takes the general form **typedef** type identifier;

Table 11.3 Size and Range of Data Types on a 16-bit Machine

Type	Size (bits)	Range
Char or signed char	8	-128 to 127
unsigned char	8	0 to 255
omt+ pr sogmed omt	16	-32,768 to 32,767
unsigned int	16	0 to 65535
short int or signed short int	8	-128 to 127
unsigned short int	8	0 to 255
long int	8	-2147483648 to 2147483647
signed long int	32	
unsigned long int	32	0 to 4,294,967,295
float	32	3.4E-38 to 3.4E+38
double	64	1.7E-308 to 1.7E+308
long double	80	3.4E-4932 to 1.1 E+4932

Where type refers to an existing data type and identifier refers to the new name given to the data type.

For example.

    typedef int marks;

here marks is an integer variable. Later it can be used to declare variables as marks batch1, batch2;+ now batch1, and batch2 will also be of the same type as marks (i.e. integer)

Another user defined data type is enumerated data type. It is defined as follows:

    enum idenfier {value1, Value2, ... valuen};

The identifier is a user defined enumerated data type, which can be used to declare variable that can have one of the values enclosed within braces (known as·-enumeration constant). After this definition, we can declare variable to be this' new' type as below:

enum identifier V1, V2, ... Vn;

The enumerated variable V1, V2 .... Vn can have one of the values Value1, Value2 ..... Valuen.

For Example:

enum day {sunday, Tuesday, ... Monday}; enum day week_St, Week_end

Week_St = Sunday; +

Week_End = Monday;

The compiler automatically assigns integer digits begining with a to all the enumeration constant.

The definition and declaration of enumerated variables can be combined in one statement. As enum day {Sunday, Tuesday, Monday} week_St, Week_End};

Declaration of storage class: Variable in C has not only data types but also storage class that provides information about their location and visibility.

There are four storage class specifications in C. They are automatic, external, static and register and they are identified by keywords **auto, extern, static** and **register** respectively.

The storage class associated with a variable can sometimes be established simply by the location within the program.

Table 11.4 Storage Classes and its meaning

Storage Class	Meaning
auto	Local variable known to only to the function in which it is declared. Default is auto.
static	Local variable which exists and retains its value even after the control is transferred to the calling function.
extern	Global variable known to all functions in the file.
register	Local variable which is stored in the register.

Assigning Values to Variables: Values can be assigned to the variables using the assignment operator = as follows

Variable_name = Constant;

For Example;

Area = 234;

Sum = 1000;

Balance = 2832.64;

Result = 'First';

Multiples assignments can be made in single line also like

Start_val=O; Last_ Val=10 00;

It is also possible to assign a value to variable during the declaration of the variable. It takes the general form of - data type variable name = Constant;

For Example:

int count = 1;

char result = . PASS;

This process is called initialization. We can initialize more then one variable in a single statement.

For Example:

X=Y=Z =0;

This is equivolent to three statements x=0; y=0; z=0;

The following program shows typical declaration assignments and values stored in various types.

```
main()
/* Declaration of variables */
float x, P;
double y, q;
unsigned k:
/* Declaration and initialization */
int m = 54321;
long int n = 1234567890;
/* Assignments */
x = 1.23456789000
y = 9.876543210
```

k = 54321

p=q=1.0

We can define a variable in such a way that it will not change throughout the program. For this we can use the qualifier const at the time of initialization.

Const int class_size=40;

(This qualifier is used in ANSI C only)

Symbolic Constant: We often use some special value which is unique and fixed in all cases, for example, we use a symbol Pi whose value is 3.142 and it is fixed for all the programs. We can define such values at the start of the program. So that we do not have to change them separately in each statement. They can be defined in the following form.

#define symbolic name.

For Example:

#define PI 3.142

#define MAX_MARKS 100

#define SALARY 65289.00

Symbolic names are sometimes called constant identifiers. Following rules are applied to use the # define statement.

1. Symbolic names are written in capital letters.
2. No blank space is allowed in symbolic name. Also no space is allowed between # sign and the define command.
3. # define statement must not end with a semicolon.
4. The value of constant is not assigned with = operator as it is usually done. The value is assigned by putting the value one space apart from the symbolic name.
5. # define statement may appear any where in the program but the usual practice is to put then in the start of the program.

11.5 Operators

We know that data items are to be processed or joined by some operator to form an expression. An operator is a symbol that tells the computer to perform certain mathematical or logical operation on one or a group of data. They are used to manipulate the data and variables. 'C' includes a large number of operators which fall into several categories. The data items on which the operators acts are called operands. Some operator requires two operands while some other act upon only one operand.

C operators can be classified into the following categories.

- Arithmetical operators
- Relational operators
- Logical operators
- Assignment operators
- Increment and decrement operators
- Conditional operators.
- Special operators.

11.5.1   Arithmetic Operators

C provides all the basic arithmetic operations. There are five Arithmetic operators supported by C.

Table 11.5 Arithmetic Operators

Operator	Purpose
+	Addition
–	Subtraction
*	Multiplication
/	Division.
%	Reminder after integer division

The % is also referred as modules operator.

There is no exponential operator in C although there is a Library function (pow) to carryout this operation but you have to include a header file math. C at the top of the program.

Example of some arithmetic operations are a+b, a–b, a*b, a/b, a%b. The arithmetic operator may operate upon more than two values like.

a+b+c or a-b-c etc.

The operands must represent numeric constants or variables.

The remainder operator (%) requires that both the operands be integer and the second operand must be a non zero value. Similarly the division operator also requires that second operand must be a non zero value. The division always results in a truncated quotient (the decimal portion is dropped) if the values are integers while the result will be a floating point quotient, if one or both the values are floating point values.

For example 5/3 will result 1 and 4/3 and 3/3 will also results 1 while 5.0/3.0 will result 1.666 while 4.0/3.0 will result 1.33 and 3.0/3.0 will result 1.0.

If one number is negative and another is positive then division will always results in a negative value while if both the numbers are negative then the result will always be a positive number.

Multiplication (*) also obeys the same rules as division. In case of addition and subtraction, if one number is positive while another is negative then result will equal to their algebraic difference and the sign will be same as that of the higher numeric value.

If a and b are two integer variables and we have assigned the values 9 and 3 to these variables then following well be the result of several arithmetic operations.

Operation	Result
a+b	12
a–b	6
a*b	27
a/b	3
a%b	3.3

Now suppose a_1 and a_2 are two floating point variables whose values are 14.5 and 3.0 respectively then following will be the result of several arithmetic operations.

Operation	Result
a_1+b_1	17.5
a_1-b_1	11.5
a_1*b_1	43.5
a_1/b_1	4.89

The operands that differ in type may undergo type conversion before the expression takes on its final value.

If a is an integer variable whose value is 7, b is a floating point variables whose value is 5.5 and C is a character type variable whose values is w then several arithmetic expression show have following values.

Operation	Result	Type
a+b	12.5	double precision
a+b	126	integer
a+c+'Q'	78	Integer

Suppose A is an integer variable whose value is 7 and b is **a floating** point variable whose value is 8.5 then the expression (a+b) %4 is invalid because the return value of (a+b) is of floating point. However int (a+b)%4 will be worked perfectly.

Further suppose f is a floating point variable whose value is 5.5 then the expression

((int(f))%2

will first convert the variables into integer form and process it.

Among the arithmetic operators *; / and % fall into one precedence group and +, – falls into another group and first group has a higher precedence over the other. Within each of the precedence group, the execution takes place from left to right.

For example, the expression.

a-b/c*d

is algebraically equivalent to

a-(b/c)*d

and while execution b/c will executed first then the result is multiplied by d and then this result is subtracted from a.

Similarly the arithmetic equation

(a-b)/(c*d)

is equivalent to algebraic value of (a-b)/(c*d). Thus if a,b,c,d are 4 floating variables with the value 1., 2., 3., 4. respectively then the expression will be executed as,

(1. - 2.)/(3. * 4.)

= 0.083333...

Generally it is good idea to use parenthesis in expression that clearly distinguish the parts of the expression and this should be clearly noted that the execution within the parentheses proceeds over all other operators.

11.5.2   Relational and Logical Operator

Relational operators show the relation between two values. Any value must be equal to, less or greater than any other value, C supports following relational operators.

Table 11.6 Relational Operators

Operators	Meaning
<	less than
<=	less than or equal to
>	greater than
>=	greater than or equal to

Closely associated with the relational operators are two equality operators.

Operator	Meaning
= =	equal to
!=	not equal to

These six operators are used to form logical expressions representing conditions that are either true or false.

Example: Suppose A,B,C are three variables whose values are 5,10,15 then following relational expression with the resulting value are shown below.

Expression	Resulting Value
A>B	False
A>C	False
B>A	True
C>B	True
(A+B)== C	True

Arithmetic operators has a higher priority over the relational operators i.e. if arithmetic operators are used along with the relational operators then arithmetic expression will be evaluated first and then the relational operator is executed. For ex.

$(a+b-c) > K$

the expression $(a+b-c)$ is evaluated first and then the result is compared with the value of K.

The relational operators are used with decision making statements like IF-Else and looping statements like while or DO ..... while.

11.5.3   Logical Operators

We can use two or more relational operators in one expression using the logical operators. C supports following three logical operators.

Table 11.7 Logical Operators

Operators	Meaning
&&	AND
||	OR
!	NOT

The **AND** operator is used when we have to confirm that the entire conditional tested with relational operators are true. A single instruction or a group of instructions will be executed only if all the tested conditions are found to true. For example in the expression.

if a>b && p>q {

The group of statement will be executed only when a>b and p>q both the conditions are true.

The' OR' operator is used when a group of statements can be executed if anyone of the tested condition is found true. For example in the expression.

if a>b || p<q

{

The group of statements is executed if either a is greater than b or p is less than q.

The NOT operators causes an expression that is originally true to become false or vice versa.

The hierarchy of all the operators used so far is given below.

Operator category	Operator	Associatively
unary operator	-++--!	R->L
Arithmetic multiply, divide and reminder	*.1.%	L->R
Arithmetic add and subtract	+-	L->R
Relational operator	L <=> >= ==!=	L->R
Logical AND	&&	L->R
Logical OR	||	L->R

11.5.4   Assignment Operators

Assignment operators are used to assign values to variable. The most commanly used operator is =. It is written in the form of

variable = constant

where variable is any identifier and constant is a value or expression or a previously defined variable. For Ex. :

X=3

Avg=O.05, area=length X width, sum=a+b

The assignment operator = is different from the equality operator' ==. The assignment operator is used to assign a value to a variable while equality operator is used to check if two values are equal or not.

If two values used with an assignment operator are of two different data types then the value to the right of the operator is converted to the types of the left value. More than one assignment operators can also be used in a single statement. They take the form of

identifier ~ identifier2= ..... = expression, for Ex. : A=B=C=5

This statement will assign the value 5 to three variables A,B & C, If a, b are two integer variables and we write the statement

a = b = 5,9

then the value 5 will be assigned to the variable a and 9 to b. C also supports following additional assignment operators.

+=, --=, *=, /= and O/O=

The use of above operators can be understood by following example. If we give following command.

Expression 1 += expression2 then it is similar to

Expression1 = expression 1 +expression2

It means that above operators are used to add, subtract, divide, multiply or modules divide first expression with second expressions and store the result in the first variable.

Following are the examples and there equivalent expressions:

Example	Equivalent Expression
p+=5	p=p+5
P -=5	p=p-5
p*=5	p=p*5
p/=5	p=p/5
p%=5	p=p%5

11.5.5   The Increment/Decrement Operators

During a loop it is often required to increment or decrement the loop variable to reach to a particular point. Although this can be done by adding or subtracting 1 from the loop variable, C support two important operators.

Operator	Use
++	increment
– –	decrement

The ++ operator adds1 to the loop variable while – – operator subtracts 1 from the loop variable. Consider the following example.

C=C+1 ;

this could be written as C++;

Similarly   C=C-1 ;

could be written as C– –;

Under normal circumstances c++ and ++C are similar in use but they are different when they are used in expression on the right hand side of an assignment statement.

Consider the following example.

> b=120;

> C= ++b;

in this value of b and C will be 121. Now if we write this as -

> b=120; c=b++

then value of C will be 121.

11.5.6   The Conditional Operators

We generally use an if... else structure to evaluate a condition but a conditional operator (?:) can also be used to evaluate the condition. The standard form of this is-

> Expression 1? Expression2 : Expression3

Here expression1 is the condition evaluated. If the condition is found true the expression2 is evaluated otherwise expression3 is evaluated. Consider the following example:

> if (x>a)

> x=x+a; else x=x-a;

This could be written using the conditional statement (x>a)? x+a : x-a;

It means that if x>a then add the value of a with the value of x otherwise subtract the value of a from the value of x.

11.5.7   Special Operator

C supports two special operators the **comma** operator and the **size of** operator.

The comma operator is used to evaluate more then one expression in a single statement. Expression is written separated by commas and the expressions are evaluated from left to right and the rightmost result is the result of the expression. For Example-

> sgr = (x=10 0, y=5, x+y);

this statement will first assign the value 100 to x and then assign the value 5 to y and finally assign the value 105 (x+y) to the variable sgr.

The size of operator return the size of its operand in bytes. The operand may be an expression or a value.

These variables are seldom used by beginners but they are very useful for the professionals.

The following chart shows the order of execution of all the operators studied so for.

Table 11.8 Hierarchy of Operators

Operator Category	Operators	Associatively
unary operators	– ++ – – size of (type)	R – 7L
arithmetic multiply, divide and remainder	* / %	L –> R
arithmetic add and subtract	+ -	L –> R
relational operators	< <= > >=	L –> R
equality operators	==!=	L –> R
logical *AND*	&&	L –> R
logical *OR*	||	L –> R
conditional operator	?:	R –> L
assignment operators	= += _= *= /= 0/0=	R –> L

Now we will see a program which will illustrate some of the operators

```
main ()
int a, b, c, d;
a = 15;
b = 10;
c = ++a - b;
printf("a = %d b = %d c = %d\n" b, c);
printf("a/b = %d\n", a/b);
printf("a%%b = %d\n", a%b);
printf("a *= b = %d\n", a%b); printf("%d\n", (c>d) ? 1: 0); printf (" %d\n", (c<d) ?
1 : 0);
```

11.6 Arithmetic Expressions

We can use various type of data in a single expression but 'C' converts all of then in a single form before evaluating the expression. Here are some general rules for conversion of data from one type to another. Always converted into higher data types.

The 'lower' data types. In case of floating point operands the lower precision operand is converted into the higher precision operand and the result is the higher precision operands.

In case of float and double, the result will be a double, in case of float and long double the result will be a long double and in case of double and long double, the result will be a long double.

If one operand is a floating point and another is a character or integer then the char/int will be converted in to floating point type and the result will be a floating point value.

If one of the operand is longint and no operand is a floating point, then all the other operand will be converted into long int and the result will a long int.

We have just seen that C automatically converts the different data types of an expression to a higher precedence form. However, sometime we have to present the data in form, different from the usual form, for example, considers the example of finding the area of the circle. The formula for area of circle is

$$area = \pi r^2$$

where π is equal to 3.14. Now if we have define r as an integer variable, the formula will always give a result in the integer form which may not be correct all the time. So we have to modify the formula as

$$area = \pi float\ (r^2)$$

this will locally convert the value of r^2 into a floating point form and the result will be a floating point value. The original value of r and the data type of r will remain unchanged in the rest of the program.

The type conversion generally takes the form as

(type name) expression

where (type-name) is any valid C data type and expression is the value or expression whom we want to convert in another type locally.

Some changes must occur when we convert one type into another. The list below shows the response of some of the type-conversion activities.

Activity	Response
X=(int) 11.3	11.3 is converted to integer by Truncation.
z=(int) a+b	a is converted into integer and then is added into b.
a = (int) 9 .3/(int)4.5	will be executes as 9/4
Y = (int)(a+b)	the result of (a+b) is converted into integers

The first statement will define a variable **name'** and define its data type as character. The next statement will cause a single character to be input and after inputting the character, it will assign this value to the variable' name'.

It is to be noted that certain characters like white spaces and return key are also considered as a single character. We can use a numeric data also in response to the *putchar*() function but C will consider them as a character data. Also a character string can be entered against the getchar() function but C will accept only first character of the string.

More than one character can be entered using getchar() function with one character at a time but we have to use some looping structure.

11.7 Single Character Out Put: The Putchar() Function.

Single character can be output (printed) by using putchar () function. The return value of this function is a character type data.

The standard form is

|putchar (character variable) |

where character variable is any variable name which is previously defined as a character type and which has some predefined value.

For Ex.

char c; c=getchar(); putchar(c);

the last function will display the value of the variable C on the screen. The statement putchar ('\n'); will cause the cursor on the screen to move to the next line.

The putchar() function can also be used to display a string of the characters by using some looping statement.

ENTERING INPUT DATA: The Scanf() Function:

The scanf function is the most commanly used function used to input data from the keyboard. This can be used to enter any type of data including the numeric data, single character data or a character string. This takes the general form of

scanf ()control string," arg1 ,m arg2, arg3 ... argn);

where control string specifies the field format and type in which the data is to be entered and arg1, arg2, ... argn refer to various variables names for which the value is to be entered.

The control string comprises individual group of character with one character group for each input data. Each character group must starts with a percent (%) sign followed by the formatting group character.

Within the control string, more than one formatting character group can be written either continuously or separated by white spaces.

The arguments are written as variable started with an ampersand (&) sign. The variable or array must be previously defined and they must match with the type of formatting character group. However the array name should not begin with the ampersand. For Example:

        int mark1;

        scant ("%n", & mark1);

When we execute this, program will wait to get the value of variable mark1 and after getting the value of **mark1** it will assign it to the variable. Following table shows the more frequently used conversion characters.

Conversion character Meaning

    %c   data item is a single character

    %d   data item is a decimal integer

    %e   data item is a floating point value

    %f   data item is a floating point value

    %g   data item is a floating point value

    %h   data item is a short integer

    %i   data item is a decimal, hexadecimal or octal item

    %0   data item is a octal number

    %s data item is a string followed by a white space (the null character' 10')

    %y data item is a unsigned decimal integer

    %x data item is a hexa decimal integer

    [...J data item is a string which may include white space.

with the scanf function, data is accepted with its default width but we can locally change the width of the field to be read.

Formatted integer input: The formatted integer input values are given in the form of

        %wd

where w is the locally change the width of integer variable. For ex.

        scanf ("%4d", &mark1);

this command will read an integer variable (%d) mark1 and it will accept only a maximum of four digit value for this variable. We can read more than one variables in a single statement as stated earlier. For Ex :

        scanf ("%d %d", mark1, mark2);

this statement will read two variables mark1 and mark2 and wait to accept the values. Two values can be given either separated by white space or by a carriage return. If we given two values like 7255 5126, then first value 7255 will be assigned to the variable mark1 and second values 5126 will be assigned to the variable mark2. Input data item should not contain any punctuations mark.

An input field may be skipped by specifying * in place of field width. For example if we give command like.

scanf ("%d *%d%d", &a, &b)

and assign the data 212 222 344 then 212 will be assign to a and 222 will be skipped because of . *' and 344 will be assigned to b.

As stated earlier, the scanf function will read only the specified width of the variable. For example consider the following statement.

scanf ("%2d", &num)

and the input 4025 the variable num will be assigned the value 40 (first two digits of the variable as specified by scanf function). The remainder digits 25 will left unread by the scanf function.

Real number input: The real numbers (the floating point values) are specified by %f formatting code. For example.

scanf ("%1", & num) .

with the input data 536.54

will assign 536.54 to the variable num, More then one real number can be read in a single statement with multiple formatting codes and arguments like.

scanf("%f%f", &a1, &a2);

with input 58.55 36.62 will read two variables a_1 and a_2 and assign two values 58.55 and 36.62 respectively.

Like integer numbers, a real number can also be skipped using % *f specification.

If the data type is different than that of the formatting code then the scanf function will stop reading the function values. Consider some more examples of integer data input through scanf function. Suppose following is a part of some C program

#include <stdio.h>

main( )

int a,b,c,

scanf ("%3d %3d %3d", & a, &b, &c)

when we execute this program then C will wait for getting the values of variable a,b, &c.

If we provide the values as 1,2,3

then following assignments will automatically takes place a=1,b=2,c=3

If we provide the data like

212 222325

then assignments will be as a=212, b=222, c=325

but if we provide the data like 212 23334 then the assignments will be

a= 212 b=23 c=334

if the data is

2122334442

then the assignments will be

a=212, b=233,c=444

the last two digits42 will remain unused. So it is very clear that the scanf function will use only the specified number of digits (if specified) to assign the values to the variables. The same is also true for the floating point numbers. Also it should be noted that the actual data may be of lesser width than the width specified with the controlling code but it can not exceed to the specified width.

Inputting Character String : We know that single character can be inputted by getchar() function but there are situations when we have to enter more then one character (character string) as input data. Name of a person or address or city etc., are all character string. The scanf function can be used for this purpose. We can enter a single character or a character string with the help of scanf function. The inputting of character data with the scanf function takes the form of

%wcor %ws

where 'w' is the specified width of the character string. It is well known to us that the character type of data is defined with the type char, variable name and the width of the character variable, within the parenthesis. For Ex. the command

char sname[20);

will define a character variable with variable name as sname and the width as 20 character, an example of using scanf for character string can be char item [20];

scanf("%s", item)

this will wait for entering a character data of maximum 20 character and as we finish entering the data by pressing the enter key, the value will be assigned to the variable item.

like numeric values, more than one characters inputs can also be read with scanf() function. For ex. :

char sname[20]; char fname[20];

scanf(%20s%20s", &name, &fname);

These commands will define two character variables fname and sname with a width of 20 characters each. The value of these variables is read through scanf() function.

It should be noted that %s specification terminates as it encounters a blank space even if it is within the character limit. For example consider the following part of programmes.

char name [10];

scanf ("%s", name);

if we enter the value of variable' name' as Naresh Kumar

then scanf will read only Naresh and terminates when it encounters a blank space.

Reading Mixed data type

The scanf() function can be made to read different type of data in one statement using different control specifications. In such case, the care should be taken to ensure that the input data items must match with the control specification in order and type. The statement

scanf ("%d %f %s", & nm, &Avg, class)

will read the variable nm as integer, avg as floating point and class as the string data.

Printf() Function

The printf() function is the counter part of the scanf() function by which all the inputted data items or some calculated results can be printed on the screen. The printf() function can be used to print a single character or a character string or any numeric data. The general form of this functions is

printf("control string", arg1, arg2, arg3 .... argn).

where control string is some formatting string which will decide the type of data to be printed and is similar as used with scanf() function, and arg1, arg2 ..... argn are variables whose values are to be printed. For Ex.

printf(%d", cost);

in this example printf function will print the value of the variable cost which should be of integer type.

The arguments can, apart from the variables, may be some constants. In contrast to scanf function the variable name should not to be preceded with an ampersand (&) sign.

Output of integer number

The integer number are outputted in the form of

"%wd"

where w is the alloted width of the integer number. For Ex :

Printf ("%5d", num);

will print the values of the variable num with minimum width as 5 digits.

unlike scanf, if a number is greater than the specified field with, it will be printed in full, overriding the minimum specification. The numbers are printed in right justified order. Now we will see some examples of printf() function.

printf ("%d", 1234) will print 1234

but printf ("%6d, 1234) will print 1234 with two heading blank. printf ("% ~6d", 1234) will print 1234 with two trailing blanks. printf("%06d," 1234) will print the digit as 001234.

Like the constants, variables can also be printed in the same manner.

If the number is very long then it may be printed using ld inplace of d in the control format for ex. a digit 1234567 can be printed as

printf ("%ld", 1234567);

Output of real numbers: The real numbers (floating point numbers) can be outputted with printf using

"%w.pf"

where w is the minimum number of position that are to be used to display the entire number and p indicates the number of digits after decimal point. If the number of decimal places is not specified then it will displays 6 digits after decimal point. If the number after decimal point is longer than the specified decimal places, then it is rounded off to the specified decimal places.

The real numbers can also be displayed in the exponential form with the following format.

"%w.pe"

Here are some example of displaying the real numbers.

suppose avg is a floating point variable whose values is 1234.567 then printf ("%f", avg) will print 1234.567

printf(%7.2f", avg) will print 1234.57

printf("% 1 0.2e," avg) will print 1.2e03

printf("%-72f", avg) will print 1234.57

Printing of Strings: The strings can be printed by printf() function in the following format

%w.ps

where w is the specified field width and p indicates that only first p characters are to be displayed.

For Ex. :

prfntf ("%s", grade)

will print the value of character array grade which must be defined earlier.

The character constants can be printed with printf() function with putting the string with a quotation mark. Fox Ex : Printf ("welcome to C program");

will print the message inside the quotation mark as it is on the screen.

Now we will see a few examples of printf function used to print the character string "Madhya Pradesh". Note that the string has 15 characters. The array defined for this is of 20 characters

printf ("%s") will print the entire string as it is with left justified and 5 trailing blanks. Printf ("%20s") will print the text with 5 leading blanks because the string has only 15 characters and to fill 20 characters, it has to print 5 blank characters first.

printf ("20.10s") will print only the first 1 0 characters of the string with first 1 0 characters as blanks.

printf("%.5S"} will print only first five characters of the text with no leading blanks.

Now we will examine some complete programs to demonstrate various input/output functions read so for.

Prog1. Write a program to input two integer numbers and print them.

```
#include <stdio.h>
main( )
{
int a,b ;
printf("Enter two numbers\n");
scanf("%d%d",&a , &b);
printf("You have entered ");
printf("%d\ and %d" ,a,b);
getch () ;
}
```

After including the standard input/output file at the top of the program and calling the function main (), we have defined two integer variables a & b. Then to enhance the readability of the program, we have displayed a message to enter the number. This message is separated by the actual input by a new line character. Then the scanf () function is used to actually input the value of two integer a and b. The values can be entered in a single line with white space between them or they can be entered in two different lines by pressing enter after first input. Another message is again displayed and after this, the entered values are displayed on the screen.

Program: Write a programme to add, subtract, multiplies and divides two given numbers.

```
#include <stdio.h>
main()
{
float a,b ;
float tot,sub,mult,div
clrscr() ;
printf ("Enter two numbers\n");
scanf("%f%f",&a , &b);
tot = a+b
sub a-b
mult = a*b
div a/b ;
    printf("Addition is    %f\n",tot);
    printf ( "Substraction is                %f\n" , sub);
    printf ("Multiplication is %f\n" ,multl);
    printf("Division is                %f\n",div);
getch () ;
}
```

Since the result division may be of floating point type so we have defined the input numbers as **floating** point number. After inputting the numbers, we have performed all the calculations\and stored the results in four different variables. Then we have printed all the results with controlling specification as floating point. The output of the program will be as under.

Enter the number

41,20 Total=61.

subtraction=21. Multiplication=120. Division=2.05

Program: Write a program to find the area of a circle (Area=πr^2)

```
#include <stdio.h>
main( )
{
float r,area
clrs'cr () ;
printf("Enter radius of the circle \n");
scanf (" %f", &r) ;
area = (22*r*r)/7;
printf("Area of the circle is :%f",area);
getch();
}
```

Program: Write a program to find simple interest for specified sum, rate of interest and time period.

```
#include <stdio.h>
main()
{
float p,r,t,i
clrscr () ;
printf("Enter principle amount ");
scanf("%f",&p):
printf("Enter rate of interest ");
scanf ("%f", &r);
printf("Enter time period ");
scanf("%f",&t);
= (p*r*t) /100 printf("Simple Interest ;
getch () ;
}
```

THE GETS() AND PUTS() FUNCTION

We have seen that scanf() and printf() functions can be used to enter or print the numeric and character strings. Also we have studied about getchar() and putchar() functions, which are used to enter or print a single character. C function is provides two specialized functions to enter or print a character string. The gets() functions used to accept the strings while puts() is used to print the character string. Both these functions take the general form of-

```
gets (character variable);
```

or

Puts (character variable)

where character variable is an character array which is previously defined.

These two functions falls under the category of unformatted I/O functions. Although gets() is less powerful than scanf() but it is very advantageous because it reads strings that include blank space characters. For ex. with using scanf ("%s," name); we can only get the users first name because the scanf terminates as soon as it founds a blank space. To read the entire name, we have to use the gets() functions as.

gets (name);

The puts() is the counter part of gets() which is used to print the character string

11.8 Control Statement

The programs, seen so far are simple in their structure. The statements written in the programs are executed sequentially i.e. one statement is executed following by the next statement. So one statement is executed only once. We can not skip any statement nor can we repeat any statements. We cannot make the conditional execution of the statements, but the real life problems are not that easy. There are situations when we have to execute a particular statement or a group of statements based on certain conditions. The statements are executed only until a defined condition is found to be true.

This clearly indicates that two different set of statements are executed on the basis of the result of certain test condition. C, like many other languages, supports the traditional If else structure to test the condition and to follow the instruction. Apart from the if.. .. else structure, C also provides a switch statement and go to statement for this purpose.

11.8.1   Decision Making With If Statement

The if statement is the most commanly used statement to control the flow of execution of statement on the basis of the result of certain test conditions. A condition is checked with the If statement, If the condition is found true then a certain group of statements are executed otherwise the program executes the next statement written after the block. The if statement takes the general form.

If (test expression)

Block1 of statement

Block2 of statement.

The condition to be tested is written within the parenthesis. If the condition is found true then block1 of statement is executed otherwise block2 of statement is executed. However, block2 of statement is also executed after completing the execution of block1 of statement.

The following categories of the if statement are commonly used.

1. Simple if statement
2. If.. .. else statement
3. Nested if .... else statement
4. Else-if ladder

Simple if statements: This is the simplest form of if statement in which only one if statement is used in the program.

The program enters in the condition from a fixed point. Consider the following example

```
If (percent>45)
{
Pass=pass+1
}
Printf pass
```

In the above example a predefined variable 'percent' is checked against a fixed value 45. If the value of percent is greater than 45 then the value of another predefined integer value is increase by1 (pass=pass+ 1;) and then the current value of the variable pass will be printed otherwise the statement pass=pass+1; will be skipped and value of pass variable will be printed. Note that the if statement will not ends with a semicolon. Now we will see few examples which will illustrate the use of simple if statement in a C program.

Program: Write a C program to accept the number. If the number is 20, then it will print "well come Nishu!" otherwise it should terminate without doing any thing.

```
#include <stdio.h>
#include <conio.h>
main()
{
int no ;
printf ("Enter a number ");
scanf ("%d", &no) ;
if (no==20)
{
20 well come nishu
                    } getch (); }
```

A program must execute the statement block3 after executing either statement block1 or statement block2. It is very clear from the diagram that the program enters from one point but there are two possible exits.

Now we will consider one example which will illustrate the function of if .... else structure.

Program: Write a program to accept the age of a person and determine whether he is eligible for voting or not (A person is eligible to cast vote only if the age is greater then 18

```
#include <stdio.h>
main()
{
int age;
clrscr ()
printf ("Enter the age ") ;
scanf("%d",&age);
if(age > 18)
printf("Person is elligible ");
else
printf ("Not elligible"); }
```

This program will check a test condition. If the condition is found true then it will execute the statements marked as block1 otherwise it will execute the statement marked as block2.

A block of statement may contain a single statement or it many be a group of statements.

Now we will see one more example of if else structure.

Program : Write a program to get two numbers and print the bigger number out of them

```
#include <stdio.h>
main()
{
int a,b ;
printf("Enter two unequal numbers :\n");
scanf("%d%d".&a,&b) ;
if (a>b)
printf("First number is bigger ");
else
printf("Second number is bigger ");
getch () ;}
```

Nested if else structure: There are situations when one if conditions is nested within another if structure. It means that one test conditions is tested within another test condition. It takes the general form of

if (test condition I)

if (test condition2)

statement I;

else

statement2;

else

statement3

The above structure can be explained as: Test condition1 is tested first

If it is found true then test condition2 is checked

If test condition2 is found true then statement1 is executed, otherwise statement2 is executed.

If test condition1 is found false then statements3 is executed.

At the end, the statement marked *xxx* is executed.

Program: Write a program to accept the name, marks of a student in three subject. and then determine the result of the student. A student is declared as pass if the marks in all three subjects are greater then 40. If the student is pass then print the name, average, marks and grade.

```
#include <stdio.h>
main( )
char name [ 20] ;
float markl,mark2,mark3,tot,avg
clrscr() ;
printf("Enter the name :");
scanf ( "% [/, \n] " ,name) ;
printf("Enter marks in three subjects ");
scanf("%f%f%f",&markl,&mark2,&mark3) ;
```

```
if(markl>40)
if(mark2>40)
if(mark3>40)
tot = markl+mark2+mark3
avg = tot/3 ;
printf("Name :%s\n",name);
printf("Total marks = %f\n",tot);
printf("average marks = %f\n",avg);
printf("Grade pass);
getch () ;
```

11.8.2   The Switch Statement

The switch statement is a multilayer decision making statement which is used when if else structure becomes very complicated. The switch statement chooses a particular condition on the basis of the result of an expression. Various case statements are used to define various actions on basis of various values of the expression. If no value is matched with the expression then a default statements is executed. The general form of the switch statements is:

```
switch (expression)
case (value-l):
blockl of statements
Break;
case (value-2):
block2 statements

Break;
case (value-n):
blockn statements
Break;
default:
Default block of statements
Break;
statement-x;
```

This is obvious from above form that switch statement is associated with two other statements i.e. Break and Default. An expression, which may be an integer or character value, is compared with several labels. Each of such labels is unique within a switch statement. If the value of expression exactly matches with the case-lable, then the block of the statement associated with the case label is executed. After executing the statements, the break statement is executed which cause the program to come out of the switch statement and transfers the control to the statement-x. If no label value is matched with the expression value, then the Default part is executed and the statements associated with default statement are executed. However the statement-x must execute after executing the default statement. It should be noted that all the case statement must terminate with a colon (:) We will demonstrate the switch statement in the following program.

Program: Write a program to grade the students on the basis of their total marks as below

Marks	Grade
80-100	'Honors'
60-79	' First'
50-59	'Second'
40-49	'Third'
0-39	'Fail'

```
#include <stdio .h> !
#include <conio.h>
main( )
int marks ;
char grade ;
int index ;
clrscr () ;
printf ("Enter marks ");
scanf ( "%d" ,&marks) ;
index = marks!10
 switch(index)
{
Case10
Case 9
Case 8
Printf (Grade = Honours )
```

```
Break;
Case7
Case 6
Printf (Grade = First )
Break;
Case5
Printf (Grade = Second )
Break;
Case4
Printf (Grade = Third )
Break;
default
Printf (Grade = Fail )
}
Getch()
}
```

The above program has two special features. First the marks are converted in to expression

```
index = marks/1 0;
```

secondly it uses empty cases. The program will execute the same statement with first three case values.

```
Case 10; Case 9; Case 8;
grade = "Honors" break
```

The switch statement is mostly used with the menu programs where we have to select an option of menu to execute a particular program. After executing the program, the control again returns to main program.

11.8.3   The GoTo Statement

Like all or at least many other programming languages, C also uses a goto statement. It transfers the control of statement from one point to another. It will skip the statements between these two points. The goto statements transfer the control to a named paragraph which is defined some where in the program. The general form of GoTo statement is:

```
goto lable;
```

Where label is an identifier which indicates the place where the control is to be transferred

label:

}

Block of statement

The label may be above or below the goto statement. For Example:

goto calc;

The statement will transfers the control to some point which is labeled as calc. Consider an example which will accept a number and print it. The program will terminate when a negative number is entered.

11.8.4   The While Statement

```
#include <stdio.h>
main()
int sum, l;
sum=0;
i=1;
while (i<=lO)
sum=sum+i;
i=i+1
printf ("%d", sum);
getch() ;
```

This program will print the sum of first ten integer numbers. The value of the variable sum, in which the total is to be stored and the counter are initialized first. Then a while loop is established to execute till the value of counter is less than or equal to ten. The process within the while loop is executed ten times. The number of execution is counted by incrementing the counter variable i by 1. When the process is executed for ten times, then the control comes out of the loop and print the value of variable' sum'.

Now we will see one more example to accept one number and find the factorial of the number.

```
#include <stdio.h>
main()
int no,nol,fact=l
clrscr () ;
```

```
printf ("Enter a number ");

scanf ( " %d" , &no) ;

nol = no

while (no >=1)

fact =fact*no;

no = no-l ;

printf("Factorial of %d is %d',nol,fact);

getch () ;
```

We will see one more example to print the table of any given number.

```
#include <stdio.h>

main( )

int no, i=l;

clrscr() ;

printf ("Enter A Number ");

scanf ("%d", &no) ;

while (i<=10)

printf("%d\n",no*i) ;

i = i+l ;

getch () ;
```

11.8.5 THE DO.... WHILE LOOP

This loop is an exit controlled loop in which the control entered into the loop without testing any condition. The body of loop is executed once and then the test condition is evaluated. If the condition is found true then the body of loop is executed once again. The process is continuous till the condition is true. As soon as the condition becomes false, the control exits from the loop and executes the statement just below the while statement. This takes the general form of

```
do

body of the loop

while (test - condition);
```

Since the test-condition is evaluated at the bottom of the loop so the loop must executes once even if the condition is false from the start. This type of looping structures is used when it is known that the body of the loop should have to execute at least for one time.

Following is a part of simple do ....while loop.

```
do
scanf("%d", &no);
printf ("%d", no);
while (no>0);
```

It is assumed that the variable 'no' is already defined some where earlier in the program. As the program entered into the do loop, it will accept an integer number and then print that number. After printing the number, it will check whether the number is greater than zero or not. If the number is greater than zero then the loop will continue i.e. it will accept another number and print it otherwise the program will exit from the loop and executes the statement written just below the while statement.

Here is a program to demonstrate use of Do .... while loop.

```
#include <stdio.h> main( )
int no,nol
clrscr () ;
printf("Enter a number :");
scanf ("%d", &no);
                    printf ("Reverse is         : ") ;
do
nol = no % 10 ; no = no/lO printf ("%d" ,nol) ;
while (no>9)
printf{"%d",no);
getch () ;
```

It is very obvious from above program that although the program is checking for a number greater than zero but the first number entered will always be printed even if it is a zero or negative number.

Now we will see a program to print the numbers from 1 to 100 and print the sum of the numbers.

```
#include <stdio.h>
main( )
int i=l,sum=0
do
sum = sum+i
printf ("%d\n", i)
```

i = i+1 ;

while(i <= 100);

printf("Sum is : %d",sum);

getch () ;

More then one conditions can be checked with the do. ... While. This type of compound statement takes the form of

do

body of loop

while (conditionl relational operation) (condition2)

For example

do

while (code>IO 88 &&code< 100)

In the above example a do while loop will be executed second time only if both the conditions mentioned within while statements are found true.

More than one do .... while structures can also be used in a program. This is called the nested looping structure. It takes the general form as

do

body of loop

do

body of loop

while (condition

while (condition)

In such type of structures, the program enters into the loop through the outer do ..... while structure. Then for the first value of outer do----while loop, the inner loop Is completely executed. Then it checks the test condition of outer loop. If it is false then program comes out of the loop otherwise for the second value of outer loop the inner loop is again completely executed.

We will see an example to use two do ..... while loops in a program.

***Program:* Write a program to print the table of first 5 numbers.**

```
#include <stdio.h>

main( )

int i=1,k=1;

clrscr () ;
```

```
do

printf("'d\t ",i*k)

k = k+1 ;

while(k<=5)

k=l

i = i+1

printf("\n");

while(i <=10);

getch () ;
```

This program contains two nested do ..... while loops. The outer loop will control the numbers for which the table is to be written and the inner loop will control the actual table.

11.8.6 For Statement

For loop is the most effective and commonly used loop structure, used for repeating the execution of a group of statements. It is an entry controlled loop structure. The general form is

```
for (initialization; test condition; increment)

body of loop
```

The execution of a for loop consists of following steps.

1. Initialization of control variable
2. Comparing the value of test variable with the test condition.
3. If the test condition is true, then execute the loop once and increment the test variable as continued with the loop.
4. If the test condition is false then exit from the loop and execute the statement just below the for loop.

For example consider the following for statement:

```
for (i=0; i<=9; i=i+ 1)

{Body of loop
```

This statement will first initialize the test variable as O. Then it will compare the value of i with the value mentioned in the test condition (i<=9). Since the present value of i is less than 9 (condition is true) so· the loop is executed once. After executing the loop, the test variable is incremented by one and again the same process is repeated. The process will be repeated for ten times. After executing the loop for ten times, the value of test variable will become nine and the test condition becomes false. So the control comes out of the loop and the statement below the loop will be executed.

It is obvious from the above explanation that the test variable works as a counter which will control the number of times for which the loop is to be executed.

The value of control variable can also be decremented. For Example:

        for (i=9; i<=0; i=i-1)

In the above statement loop will start with initial value of control statement as 9 and after each pass of the loop the value will decreased by one, untill it will reach to the value zero.

We will consider a simple example using for loop.

Program:

```
#include <stdio.h> main( )
int i=l,sum=0
for(i=l; i <= 100; i++)
sum = sum+i
printf ("%d\n", i)
printf("Sum is %d",sum);
getch() ;
```

This program will display the integer numbers from 1 to 100 and then print the sum of the numbers.

More then one variable can be initialized at a time with for loop.

For example consider the following two statements.

        x=1 ;

        for (p=0; p<=10; p=p+ 1)

Both of these statements can be combined by a single statement.

        for (x=1; p=0; p<=17, p=p+1)

Note that the initialization part is separated by a comma (,) while other parameters are separated by semi colon (;)

More than one test conditions can also be made with for loop. For example for (p=1, q=1 ; p<=50, q<= 50; p=p+ 1, q=q+ 1) is a valid statement.

Also the compound test condition can be mentioned with the loop. For example: sum = 0;

        for (i=1; sum<20 && sum> 100; i=i+ 1)

One another important feature of the for loop is that any of the three expressions can be omitted provided that their values are supplied through some other source.

However the semicolons separating the sections must be shown. If the test condition is omitted then program will continue indefinitely unless it is to terminated by some other command.

Consider the example discussed just before once again. For statement of that program can be replaced with the following statement.

    for (; k=100;)

The initial value of the test variable must be specified some where in the program earlier for the use in the for loop. Although this form of loop reduces the parameters to be written but the readability also reduces and so it is less frequently used in the programs.

Where type is the data-type which the array is going to held, variable-name is the name of array and size is the maximum number of elements in the array. For ex. :

    int marks [10];

11.9 Recursion

We have seen in many previous examples that one function can call another function. But Recursion is a special process in which the function calls it self repeatedly until a specified condition is satisfied. This process is used in the case of repetitive computation where each further action can be defined in terms of a previous result.

The calculation of factorial is the most comman example of recursion. We have seen in the previous examples that factorial of a positive integer can be expressed as following expression.

    !n = nx(n-1)x(n-2)x(n-3) 1

However this can also be expressed as-

    n! = nx!(n-1)!

    (n-1)! = (n-1)x(n-2)! (n-2)x(n-3)!

    2! = 2x1!

This is a recursive approach to solve the problem. One stopping statement is used to terminate the program.

Calculation of Factorial with Recursion

```
#include <stdio.h>

main ()

int n;
```

```
int fact (int n) ;

clrscr(};

printf("Enter a number "}

scanf (" %d" ,&n) ;

printf("Factorial of %d = %d\n",n,fact(n) l;

getch{} ;

int fact(int n)

if (n<=l)

return(l) ;

else

return{n*fact{n-l»;
```

The program reads a positive integer number n and then calls the long iteger function factorial. The function 'factorial' calls it self recursively with an actual argument (n-1) that decreases by 1 after each successive call. The program continues until the value of actual argument is 1. The factorial of 1 is equal to 1 by definition.

Now we will see one more example in which a text is entered and then it is printed backward, using recursion method

```
#include <stdio.h>

 #define EOLN '\n'

main()

void reverse(void);

clrscr();

printf("Enter a line of text. Press enter when finished \n");

 reverse();

getch();

void reverse(void)

char c ;

il{(c = getchar(» l=EOLN) reverseO ; putchar( c);

return ;
```

THE TOWER OF HANOI

It is a very well know child game played with three poles and a number of different size disks. The disks arc stacked on left most pole in order of decreasing size. The object of the game is to transfer disks from leftmost pole to the right most pole without ever placing a larger disk on top of a smaller disk. Only one disk can be moved at a time and each disk must be stacked on any of the pole.

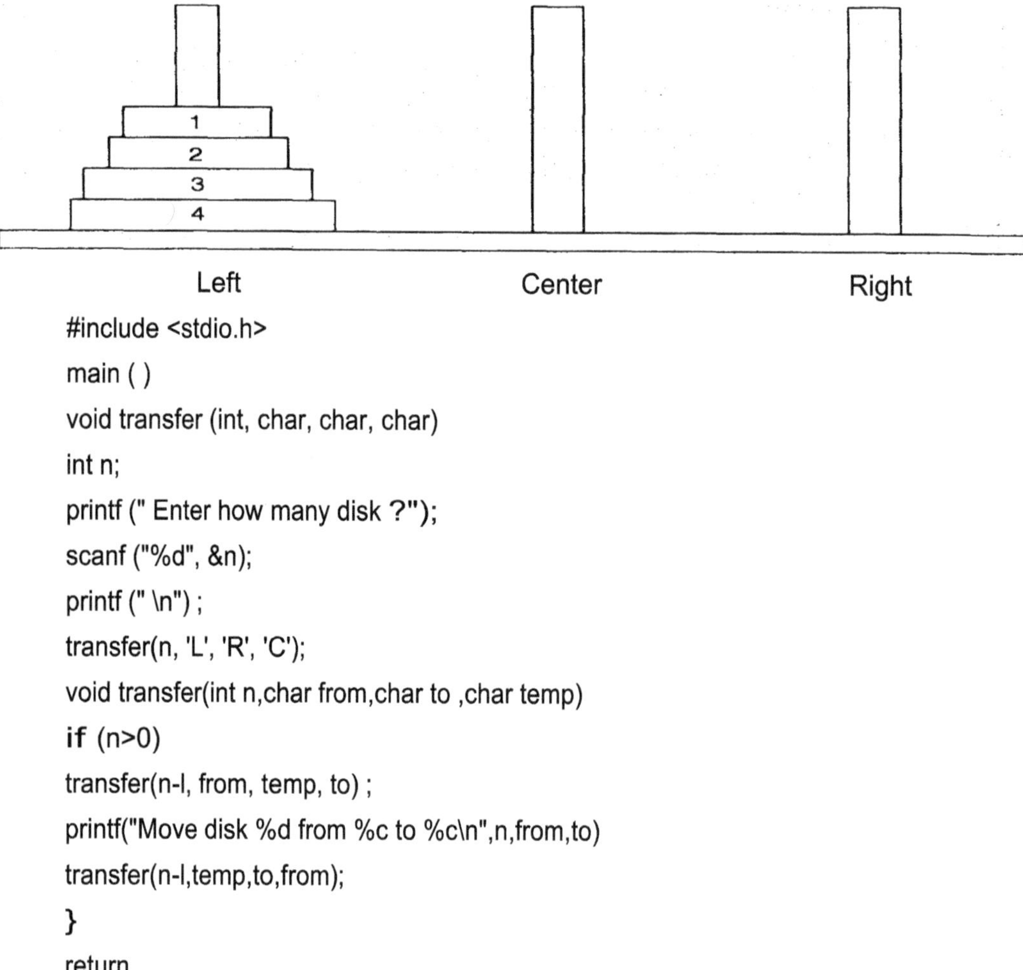


```
#include <stdio.h>
main ( )
void transfer (int, char, char, char)
int n;
printf (" Enter how many disk ?");
scanf ("%d", &n);
printf (" \n") ;
transfer(n, 'L', 'R', 'C');
void transfer(int n,char from,char to ,char temp)
if (n>0)
transfer(n-l, from, temp, to) ;
printf("Move disk %d from %c to %c\n",n,from,to)
transfer(n-l,temp,to,from);
}
return
```

The use of recursion is not the best possible approach to solve a problem. A non-recursive solution use less memory and executes fastly in comparison to a recursive program.

11.10 Array

It is often required to handle a number of data of same nature in a program. For example, in a program for mark sheet of students, we may have to use a thousand of names. We can not assign separate variables for each value nor can we retain all values within single variable name because the techniques we studied so far does not facilitate to do so because whenever we assign a value to a variable, the previous value of the variable automatically disappears. So we can use only the last value entered.

C, like much other programming languages provides an excellent way to store many variables under a single variable name. This is known as array. An array as a group of related data items that share a common variable name. The elements of the array are of the form of x1, x2, x3….. xn where x is the common variable name and n is the maximum number of element in that array.

Each array element is referred to by specifying the array name followed by one or more subscript with each subscript is enclosed within a square bracket. We can understand an array as a column which is divided into several parts.

X
1
2
3
--
--
n

Where x is the common variable name and 1,2,3....n are the elements of that array.

Defining an Array

Array is much similar to the ordinary variables except that the elements are subscripted within it. The general form of an array Is

Type variable-name (size);

where type is the data-type which the array is going to held, variable-name is the name of array and size is the maximum number of elements in the array. For ex. :

Int marks (10);

will define an array with its type as integer, name as marks and maximum number of elements as 10. The individual element of array will be defined as-

marks [0];

marks [1];

marks [2];

-

-

marks [9];

The subscripts of the variables i.e. 0,1 ,2, ... n can be controlled through some looping structure.

Whenever we define an array, the computer reserves the specified locations for the data to be entered.

If we have 10 values as 60, 65, 67, 68, 80, 79, 52, 59, 60,70 then computer will assign 60 to marks [0], 65 to marks [1], 67 to marks [2] and so on.

marks [0] = 60 marks [1] = 65 marks [2] = 67 .... marks [9] = 70

these elements i.e. marks [0], marks [1], marks [2] etc. can be used any where in the program as any other variable.

The subscript of an array can be a numeric constant or a predefined numeric variable those value is keep on changing.

The type of the array may be an integer, float or character. We have seen the example of an integer array earlier in this chapter.

float average [50];

define an array of 50 real numbers with the array name as average.

The C language treats all the character string in the form of arrays only.

char name [60];

declares the name as array name whose type is character and the string contains 60 character. The program will treat each character of the string as an element of the array. If we read following string constant into the string variable name

"INDIA"

then each character will become one element of the array and will be stored separately as below.

Name [0] = 'I' Name [1] = 'N' Name [2] = 'O' Name [3] = 'I' Name [4] = 'A' Name [5] = '\O'

When the compiler seas a character string it adds a null character at the end of the string which indicates the end of the string. So while declaring arrays of character type, we have to make provision for one extra character.

Data are most often read into an array through some looping structure and then each element of array is also processed through the looping structure. We can use any looping command to store and output the data into and from the array.

Now we will see one simple example that will accept 5 numbers and store them in an array and then print them.

```
#include <stdio.h>

main( )

int no[5];
```

int i =0 ;

clrscr ( ) ;

for{i =1 ; i <= 5 i++)

The general form of an array is

type variable-name [size]; |

The program defines the array of 5 integer number. Then through a for loop 5 digits are read using scanf command. The subscript of array is defined through the control variable i. when loop starts, then the value of **i** is zero. So the program reads the first value and store it as sum[O]. Then it will store another variable as sum [1]. Sum[2]. sum[3]. sum[4].

After reading the value it will print all the subscripts in the same way. Notice that reading and printing of the integer array is same as that of other integer variables.

Now here is an example that will accept a character string of 10 character and then print each character of that string.

#include <stdio.h>

main()

char name[10]

int i ;

clrscr() ;

printf("Enter string of 10 character \n"); for(i=I;i <=10 ;i++)

scanf (" %c", &name [i]) ;

for (i=1 ; i<=10 ; i++)

printf("%c\n",name[i]) ;

getch() ;

11.10.1 Initilization of Array

The array can be provided an initial value similar to that of other ordinary variables. The general form of an array initialization is

static type array name [size] = {list of values};

For example

static int code [5] = {101, 102, 103, 104, 105}

will define an array code with size five and will assign 101 to code [0], 102 to code [1], 103 to code [2], 104 to code [3], 105 to code [4].

If the number of values are less than the number of element, then only that many element will be initialized. The remaining element will be set to zero automatically. For Example:

Static int code [5] = {101, 102, 103}

will assign 101, 102 and 103 to code [0], code [1] and code [2]. The value of code [3] and code [4] will be zero.

The size of array can be omitted while initialization of array. This will allocate the same space as the number of elements. For Example:

Static int code [] = {101, 102, 103 104}

will define the array code which will contain four element (size is 3).

Character array can also be defined in a similar way.

For example:

char color [3] = ɾ R', "E", "D"};

This will assign "R" to color [0], "E" to color [1], "D" to color [2]. while the value of color [3] will '\0'

It is to be noted that the word 'static' is used before the type declaration. The automatic type of array cannot be initialized.

Now we will see some examples which use the feature of array.

Program: Write a program to enter 10 integers and then print the number, the biggest number among them. Also print the sum and average of the numbers.

printf ("Biggest Number is %f\n" ,big);

printf (" Smallest Number is %f\n" ,small) ;

printf("Total is   %f\n",tot);

printf("Average is %f\n",avg);

getch () ;

This is a typical use of array. An array is defined with its maximum size as 10 and then ten numbers are entered which are assigned to various subscript of array. After this, the first element is assigned to avariable big and then subsequent value is campaired with this variable. If the value is less than the value of variable then it is skipped and next element is read, otherwise the value of variable big is replaced with the value of element and then the next element is read. The process of adding continuous simultaneously with each step.

Now we will see an example which will deal with the character array. Recall that each character including the blank character of the string are considered as the element of the array.

Program write a program to accept a string of five characters and then print it in reverse order.

```c
#include <stdio.h>
main()
char str[5];
int i ;
clrscr() ;
printf("Enter the string of 5 characters ");
for (i=0;i<=5;i++)
scanf("%c".&str[i]);
i - 5;
printf("Reverse is :" );
for (i=5;i<=1;i--)
printf("%c",str[i]) ;
getch();
```

11.10.2 Two Dimensional Array

All the arrays soen so for are single dimension arrays in which there is only a single colum. C allows the elements to arrange in double dimension also in which the array has more then one row and column. This takes the general form as.

Type array-name [i],[j];

where type is type of array, array-name is the name of array and i is the number of rows and j is the number of column in that array Note that no. of rowl[i] and columns are indicated in two different brackets. The total number of element in the array is equal to the multiplication of the number of rows and columns.

when we issue data to a double dimension array, it is accepted there row-wise. The first data is placed at first row first columns, 2nd data is placed at first row second column. 3rd data at first-row third column. When first row is completed then it starts to occupy the second row in the same manner (second row first column, second row second column, second row third column etc.)

For example if we have defined an array of 2 rows and 3 columns and data provided is 5,6,8,10,2,20 then the position of data in the array will we

first row-first column	5
first row - second column	6
first row - third column	8
second row - first column	10
second row - second column -	2
second row - third column	20

This can be represented as

$$\begin{bmatrix} 5 & 6 & 8 \\ 10 & 2 & 20 \end{bmatrix}$$

Initializing a two dimensional array : The two dimensional arrays are initialized in the same way as the single dimension array. The initialization starts with the static command.

For Ex. :

Static int count [2] [3] = {1, 1,1 ,2,2,3}

This command will initialize all the element of first row as 1 and second row as 2. It is obvious that initialization done row by row. The above statement can also be written as

static int count [2] [3] = {{1 ,1,1}, {2,2,2}};

Two dimensional arrays can be initialized in a form of matrix.

static

int count [2] [3] ={

{1,1,1},

{2,2,2}

};

As stated earlier that total number of elements in an array is equal to the multiplication of number of rows and columns. If the values are less in the initialize then they are automatically set to zero.

For Example:

static int count [2] [3] = {1, 1 ,2,2};

This will assign following values to the elements. count [1] [1] = 1

count [1] [2] = 1

count [1] [3] = 2

count [2] [1] = 2

count [2] [2] = 0

count [2] [3] = 0

It is obvious from the above discussion that the two dimension arrays are of the form of a matrix. We can perform several matrix operations by using a double dimension array.

Now we will see a program which will accept integers for two 2x2 matrix and then add the elements of array and print it in a form of third matrix.

```
#include <stdio.h>

main( )

in t a [2] [2] , b [2] [2], c [2] [2]

int i, j;

clrscr ()

prin~t ("Enter numbers for first array \n")

for(i = 1 ; i<=2 ; i++)

for(j=1;j<=2 ;j++)

scanf("%d",&a[i] [j]l

printf("\n") ;

printf("Enter numbers for second array\n")

for (i=1 ; i<=2 ; i++)

for(j=1 ;j<=2 ;j++)

scanf ( "%d" ,&b [i] [j ]) ;

e[i] [j] = a[i] [j] + b[i] [j] printf ("\n")

printf("Additionof array is \n");

for(i=1 ; i <=2 ; i++)

                        for(j=1; j<=2; j++)

printf("%d\t",e[i] [j] );

printf (" \n") ;

geteh ()
```

If first matrix is A and second maxtrix is B then their sum can be shown in the third matrix C as-

C [i] [j] = A [I] [j] + B[i] [j]

The element of first row-first column of first matrix is added with the element at first row-first column of second matrix and placed at first row first column of the resultant matrix. Similarly the other elements are also added. Note that two matrix can be added only if they are of same order.

Here is one more example of using a double dimension array.

Write a program to transpose the elements of a two dimensional array. Transpose means interchange the elements of rows and columns.

```
#include<stdio.h>
#include<conio.h>
main( )
int x[3] [3j,i,j;
clrscr () ;
printf("ENTER THE ELEMENTS OF MATRIX \n");
for(i=0;i<3;i++)
for(j=0;j<3;j++)
scanf ( "%d" , &x [i] [j] ) ;
printf ("MATRIX IS \n");
for(i=0;i<3;i++)
for(j=0;j<3;j++)
printf ( "%d\ t" ,x [i] [j ] ) ;
printf (" \n");
printf("THE TRANSPOSE OF MATRIX IS \n"); for(i=0;i<3;i++)
for(j=0;j<3;j++)
printf( "%d\t" ,x[j] [i]);
printf (" \n");
getch () ;
```

We will be seeing one more Example of double dimensional array.

Program: Write a program to determine

(a) Total marks obtained by each students

```
#include <stdio.h>
main( )
int roll,marks;
int class[2] [3]
int tot
int i,j
clrscr () ; for(i=1;i<=2;i++)
printf("Enter marks for student %d\n",i)
for(j=1;j<=3;j++)
scanf("%d",&marks)
class[i] [j] =marks
for(i=0 ;i<=I ;i++)
for(j=0;j<=2 ; j++)
tot = tot + class[i] [j]
printf("Total marks of student %d = %d\n ",i,tot);
tot = 0
getch ()
```

11.10.3 Multidimensional Arrays

Three or more dimensional arrays can be defined and used in the same way as a double dimensional array. The general form is

type array-name [81] [82] [83] ..... [8n]

where type is the data type, array-name is a valid array-name and 81, 82,83 .... 8n are positive valued integer expressions that indicates the number of array elements associated with each subscript.

For Example:

int score [3] [5] [10]; float marks [5] [3] [2] [5]

The score array is a three dimensional array with 150 integer elements while marks is a four dimensional array with 150 float elements.

Remember that a three-dimensional array can be represented as a series of two-dimensional array as shown below.

Year 1

Year 2

month city	1	2	....	12
1				
5				

month city	1	2	....	12
1				
5				

The initialization of multidimensional array can be made as any other array. For Example:

```
int p[l0] [20] [30]
{l,2,3,4} {5,6,7,8} {9,10,1l,12}
},
{21,22,23,24}
{25,26,27,28}
{29,30,31,32}
} ;
```

this table can be understand as 10 tables each having 20 rows and 30 columns.

Prog. Now here is one example which uses single dimension array and do the: following.

1. Read 10 number into an array.

2. Sort the item in increasing order

3. Find the median of the number.

we will explain each aspect of this program in detail.

```
#include <stdio.h>
#include <conio.h>
main( )
```

```
int i,j ;
float median, a[10],t
clrscr() ;
printf("Enter 10 numbers \n");
for(i=1;i<=10;i++)
scanf ("%f\h", &a [i]) ;
for(i=1 ; i<=9 ;i++) for(j=1
j<=9-i ;j++)

if(a[j] <= a[j+1))
t = a [j] ;
a[j] = a[j+1];
a[j+l] = t
else
continue
median = (a[5]+a[6])/2
for(i=0 ;i<=10 ;i++)
printf("%f \n",a[i]);

printf ("Median getch () ;
%f" ,median)
```

Prog. A test consisting of 25 multiple choice items is held from 5 students. Correct answers and the responses are tabulated in array. Write a program to:

- Read correct answer into an array
- Read the response of a student and count the correct ones.
- Repeat the above step for each statement

Print the results.

```
/*PROGRAM TO CHECK THE ANSWERS OF FIVE STUDENTS DISPLAY
THE NUMBER OF CORRECT AND WRONG ANSWERS*/
#include<stdio.h>
#include<conio.h>
main( )
int i,a=0,b=0,k=0;
```

```
char x[25] ,y[25];

clrscr () ;

printf("ENTER THE ANSWER OF 25 MULTIPLE CHOICE QUESITION ");

for(i=0;i<25;i++)

scanf ( "%s" , &x [i] ) ;

while (k<5)

printf ( "\nENTER THE ANSWER GIVEN BY STUDENT ");

for(i=0;i<25;i++)

scanf("%s",&y[i)); if(x[i]==y[i]}

        a++i

else

        b++;

printf("\nNUMBER OF CORRECT ANSWERS ARE ");

printf ("%d", a) ;

printf("\nNUMBER OF WRONG ANSWERS ARE "); printf("%d",b);

k++;

a=0;

b=0;

getch () ;
```

Three arrays are defined at the beginning of the program.

Array1 to store correct answers. Array2 to store responses of the student. Array3 to store correct results to prepare the result. Then the correct answers are stored in first array through a for loop. After storing correct answers the evolution starts. A for loop is executed to count the number of students and within this loop one more loop is executed to accept the answer of each student. After keying the answer, each answer is compared with the correct answer in the form of subscripted values and at the end, the result for first student is printed. The process is continued for all the students.

11.10.4 Handling of Character String

It is stated earlier that the character strings are processed in the form of array. All the reading and processing of character string can be done only by defining them as an array. After defining a character string we can perform several operations on that character string. Some of them are:

Reading/writing string

Combining two or more string

Extracting a portion of string from any other string.

Copying one string into another.

Comparing two strings for equity.

Reading String from Terminal

We can use the scanf function to input character string we may use %s format specification for this purpose.

    scanf ("%s", address);

where address is a character type of variable and is defined earlier in the program in the form of character array.

The only problem with scanf function is that it terminates the input as soon as a white space is apper in the input. For Example:

11.11   User Defined Functions

Functions are the basic strength of C language. Although C does not provide in built command for most of the works but it has got several strong inbuilt functions. We have read several of such function in the previous chapters. Main() is the most important one. Scanf(), printf(), putchar(), getchar(), etc. are other com manly used functions. All these functions come under the category of library functions because they are the part of a C library. Apart from the usual library function, C also allows user to write their own functions and use them anywhere in the program. These user defined function are very useful in the programming and they determine the modular nature of C language.

Before going deep into defining and using of functions, let's first see what a function is and why it is so useful in the program. A function is self contained segment of a program that is used or written to perform a particular task. They are written within the program or tney may be in a form of separate program which could be called by any other program.

11.11.1   Need for user Defined Function

There are situations where a particular operation or calculation is repeated from many points of the program. These repeated instructions can be placed at a single place with one function name and can be called from any part of the program. The function also enables the logical clearity in the program. It makes the testing and debugging procedures easy. A program with functions is easy to understand and modify. Several functions can be stored within a user defined library and can be accessed by any programmer in his program. So it reduces the job of writing similar program segments for different applications. The advantages of using function in a program can be summarised in following points.

It determines the modular approach of C language in which the program logic is solved at different levels from higher to lower (Top-down approach).

Since the function can be kept outside the main program and can be called when required so the length of source program is very less.

A function can be used by many other programs. This reduces the spaces and the time effectively.

It is easy to modify small segments (functions) in comparison to the large programs.

11.11.2 The form of a C Function

The general form of C function is function-name (argument list) argument declaration;

```
{
local variable declaration
statement1
statement2
 statement n
return (expression)
```

All functions do not follow this standard format. Many of the objects of this standard form can be skipped on the basis of the requirement and nature of the function. Many programs does not have any argument associated with them like main() does not have any argument. Argument list can also be skipped in this case. Declaration of local variable is also not necessary if no local variable is to use within the function. A function is terminated by using the return command. As soon as a return is occurred, the control returns to the calling function. The return function can also be used to return a particular value. So we can conclude that only the function name and the executable statements are the necessary part of a function. All other objects mentioned in the standard form are optional and can be omitted if not actually required.

If used, the argument list is a list of variables separated by comma and surrounded by parenthesis. Some valid examples are

sqr(a, b) tot(a,b,c)

fact (x) exp (x, n)

Note that the functions name is not end with a semi-colon.

The variables used with the argument list must be declared after the function header and before the opening braces of the function.

Now we will see a program that will define and use a function within the program.

```
#include <stdio.h>
main( )
int ax, sum = 0;
ax=add (sum) ;
printf("Total is %d ",ax);
getch ()
add (tot)
int i;
for(i=1 i <=10 i++)
tot tot+i
return (tot) ;
```

11.11.3 Return Values and Their types

We have seen that a function is called through a program. When the execution of the function is completed, the control returns to the main program. While returning to the calling program, the function may or may not return some value of the function through the return function.

This return function passes aJ'1Y desired value from the function to the calling program. If the function is terminated with just the return, then it will not pass any value to the calling program. It acts just like the closing braces of the function. When the return is occurred, the control is immediately transferred to the calling program. An example of such return is.

```
if( error)
return:
```

The second form of return is one which passes some value to calling program. An expression is used along with the return and the value of that expression is transferred to the calling program. For example

```
add (a, b)
int a, b;
int p;
p = a +b;
return(p):
```

This program will return the value of p to the main program.

The function may have more than one return statement and they may return same or separate values to main function. These are used when different values are to be returned on the basis of some test conclusion. For example

if (a>b) return(a);

else

return(b);

All functions by default return an int type of data. If the return value is of some other type, then it must be specified while defining the function. For example

float mul(a, b);

long int(prod);

11.11.4 Accessing a Function

A function can be called by using the function name in the statement. The function name is followed by a list of arguments enclosed in parenthesis and separated by comma. If no argument is required then an empty pair of parenthesis must follow the function name.

Now here is a complete program in which a function is defined and used within the program.

```
#include <stdio.h>
Main()
int a,b,c,d
clrscr () ;
printf("Enter2 integer values \n");
scanf("%d%d%d",&a,&b,&c)
d = max (a , b) ;
printf("Maximum is %d",max(c,d));
getch ()
max(x,y)
int x,y
int z
z = (x >= y) ? x: y
return(z)
```

In this program the same function maximum is called at two places. At first call, the actual arguments are a, b and in the second call, the arguments are c, d. The two statements can be replaced by a single statement.

```
printf("maximum=%d", maximum (c, maximum(a, b));
```

11.11.5 Types of Functions

We have seen that many functions are used with an argument list but some does not have any argument associated with them. Similarly some functions passes values to the calling function while other does not pass any value. On the basis of presence or absence of argument list and return value, the functions are catogorised into following classes.

No argument and return value

In this type of function, there is no data transfer between the calling function and called function. Only the control of the program is transferred to the called program and returns back to the calling program.

```
calling function

called function
```

Here is an an example of such program where there is no data communication between the functions.

```
#include <stdic.h> stdio

main( )

clrscr() ;

printline ()

area() ;

printline () ;

getch () ;

printline ()

int i

for(i=1 ;i <=35 ;i++)

printf("%c", '-');

printf (" \n") ;

area( )

int radius

float area
```

```
printf("Enter radius of circle ");
scanf("%d",&radius) ;
area = 3.l4l*radius*radius
printf("Area of circle = %f",area)
printf ( "\n" ) ;
```

Following is the calling program which calls two other functions. Both the called functions do not have any argument with them. It means that they do not receive any data from the main function. Similarly there is no return statement in the program indicating that the called functions does not returns any thing to the calling functions.

Arguments but no Returns Value

In this type of functions the called function has some argument but it does not return any value to the calling function. We will modify the above program to depict this.

```
#include <stdio.h>
main( )
int radius ;
printfl"Enter radius of circle "); scanf("%d",&radius) ;
print line ( , * , ) ;
value (radius) ;
print line ( , * , ) ;
getch () ;
print f (line ch)
char ch ;
int i

forli
for (i = 1;i<=30;i++)
printf("%c",ch);
printf (" \n") ;
value (radius)
int radius ;
float area ;
area = 3.141 * radius*radius
printf("Area = %f",area);
```

Argument with Return Value

It is required many times not to just display the result but also to return them to the main program for some other calculation.

We will modify our currently used program to show this two way data communication.

```
#include <stdio.h>
#include <conio.h>
main( )
int radius
float area
printf("Enter radius of circle ");
scanf("%d",radius)
pline('*',40);
area = value (radius)

printf ("Area
pline('*',40);
pline(ch,len)
int len
char ch
int i

for(i=1;i<=40 ;i++)
printf("%c",ch) ;
printf("\n") ;
value(r)
int r;
float area;
areal = 3.l4l*r*r
return (areal) ;
```

11.11.6 Function with Arrays

By using the array name as the argument of function, the entire array can also be passed to the function. The size of the array is not specified with the argument. The argument must be declared as an array within the formal argument declaration.

For example

```
main( )
Int n;
float list[l0]; j* array definition
float avearge(); j*function definition
avg=average (n, list)
float average (a, x) j*function definition
int a; (*formal argument declaration
float xl]; j*formal argument (array) declaration.
```

A function. average is called within the function main. In the first line of function declaration we see two formal arguments called a & x. The formal argument declarations establish as an integer variable and x as a floating point one dimensional array. There are two actual arguments also shown in the example. One is the integer variable n and another is a one dimensional floating point array list.

Now we will see a **program to reorder a list of n integer.**

```
#include <stdio.h>
 #define SIZE 100
main( )
int i,n,x[SIZE] ;
void reorder(int n,int xl]) clrscr () ;
printf ("How many numbers ?");
scanf ("%d", &n);
for(i=0;i<=n ; ++i)
printf("i=%d x = ",i+1)
scanf("%d",&x[i])
reorder(n,x)
printf  ("Reordered list is ,,);
for(i=0;i<n ; ++i)
printf("i=%d x = %d\n",i+1,x[i]);
```

```
void reorder(int n ,int xl])
int i,item,temp ;
        for (item = 0;item<n-1;++item)


        for(i=item+1 ; i<n ;++i)
        if(x[i] <x[item])
temp = x[item] x[item] xli] xli] = temp;
return
getch ()
```

The re-arrangement will begin by scanning the entire array for the smallest number. This is done by comparing first number with the entire arrays. This number will then be interchanged with the first number in the array. Now the next (n-1) integers are again scanned for the smallest value and the smallest value will be placed at the second position. Then remaining (n-2) integers are again utilizing the same process to find the smallest number which is placed at the third place. The complete rearrangement will require a complete (n-1) pass through the array.

The declaration for reorder that appear in main is written as a function prototype.

It should be mentioned that return' statement can not be used to return an array. Therefore, if the element of an array is to be passed back to the calling portion of the program, the array must either be defined as an external array whose scope includes both the function and the calling portion of the program, or it must be passed to the function as a formal argument.

Every variable used in C, comes under any one of the following category.

1. Automatic variable

2. External variables

3. Static variables

4. Register variables.

Each type of variables behaves differently when used within the functions. Automatic variables are declared within each function. They are private to the function in which they are used. It means that the variable is applicable only within the function. All the variables, which are defined without any storage class are considered as automatic.

Now we will see a program which will demonstrate the working of automatic variable.

```
#include <stdio.h>
maln( )
```

```
int m = 1000
function2 () ;
printf ("%d\n" ,m);
functionl ()
int m=10 ;
printf ("%d\n" ,m);
function2 ()
int m=100 ;
functionl();
printf("%d\n",m) ;
getch () ;
```

The function main has two sub functions function1 and function2. An automatic variable m is declared at start of each function. During the executions the main function calls function2 which in turns called function1. Since last active function is function1, so the active value of variable m is 10. As soon as the function1 is finished, function2 will be active (m = 100) and after this main (m = 10000) will become the active function.

The external variables are declared outside a function and can be accessed by any function in the program. Because of this nature, they are also called as global variable. If a variable of same name as global variable is defined inside a function, then this local variable has the higher precedence over the global variable. Now here is an example of working of global variable.

```
#include <stdio.h>
#include<conio.h>
int x;
main()
.{
printf("Enter value of x:");
scanf ("%d", &x);
printf("x = %d\n" ,x);
printf("x = %d\n",funl()) ;
printf("x = %d\n",fun2());
printf("x = %d\n",fun3());
getch () ;
```

```
funl ()
x = x+10 ;
return (x)
fun2 ()
x= x*10 ;
return (x) ;
fun3 ()
x = x/10 ;
return (x)
```

A value of x is defined outside the function which is used in all the function except in function2 where a local variable of same name is also defined. A variable can be defined with the storage class **extern** for use by the function above the variable also. The static variables persist until the end of the program. A variable can be defined static by using the key word **static.**

For Ex.

static int x; static float y;

The program given below shows the working of a static variable. The static variable is initializes only once and during first call to state, x is incremented to 1. These value pasts and therefore, the next call adds 1 to x giving the value to 2.

```
#include <stdio.h>
main ( )
int i;
for(l=l i<=3 i++)
stat () ;
stat ()
static int x=0;
x = x+l ;
printf( "x=%d\n" ,x);
getch() ;
```

The Register variables are kept in machine's register rather than in memory for faster execution of the program.

For example register int score; only a limited number of variables can be defined as register variable.

11.12   Pointers

Pointers are the most important feature of 'C' language. A pointer is a variable which contains the address of some other variable. The pointers are used within the programs with arrays or structures. They are used for following reasons:

1. The use of pointer reduces the complexity of the program and increases the execution speed of the program.
2. Pointers provide a way to return multiple data items from a function via function arguments.
3. They can be used to handle single or multidimensional arrays more effectively in comparison to simple array.
4. The pointers enable to represent a collection of string of different length within single array.

11.12.1 Pointer Fundamentals

All the programs and the values of variables are stored in some storage cell. Each cell has a unique address associated with it. It means that every information is stored at a particular address. These addresses are numbered sequentially starting from zero. Consider the following statement.

int x = 100;

This statement will define an integer variable x, and assign the value 100 to it. These values will be stored on a particular address. Suppose this address is 2000. This can be shown in the following figure.

x --1 variable 100 --1 value 2000 --1 address

During execution of the program we can access this value of variable either by using the variable name or by using the address number. Since memory addresses are simple numbers so they can be stored under some other variable name. Such variables that hold the address are called the pointers. The link between the variable, its values, its location and the pointer is shown in the following diagram

Variable	Value	Address
X	100	2,000
Y	2000	2,500

In the above diagram a value 100 is stored under a variable name X which is located at address 2000. This address is stored at another location (2500). With the variable name Y. It means that the variable Y indicates the location of X. So Y is the pointer of X.

11.12.2 Accessing the Address of a Variable

As a simple user of 'C' language, we can not determine the exact address of storage. We have to use the address operator & for this. The operator immediately preceding the variable name provides the address of that variable. For Example

      P= &x

will assign the value 2000 to the variable P because 2000 is the address of variable X. The & variable is applicable only to a simple variable or an element of the array. A constant or entire array name can not be used with the & variable. Following are some invalid uses of & variable.

      &200   - Points a constant

      int P[10]; - Points to an array name &P

      &(P+V)   - Points to an expression.

11.12.3 Declaring and Initilizing Pointers

Like any other variable, the pointer must also be defined before using. To differentiate an ordinary variable from a pointer variable an astrix(*) is used. The declaration takes the general form as

   For Ex.

   Here,

      Idata-type *pointer variable name. **I int * balance;**

      *** represents that the variable 'balance' is a pointer variable.**

The data type int indicates the type of value which the variable 'balance' is going to point. It should be noted that the type int is not the type of the variable 'balance' but it is the type of that variable to which the pointer variable is pointing.

P is a pointer variable to a floating point variable. It should be noted that the pointer variable always points to the corresponding type of data. If we define the type of pointer variable not similar to that of original value then the program will produce some result

   int x;

   float a, b;

   int *p;

   p = &x; p= &a;

Here the pointer variable p, points towards an integer value. So p = &x;

will work properly because x is also an integer value, but

p= &a;

gives some improper result because a is of floating type variable while the pointer variable points towards an integer value.

In the statement p = &x, the pointer variable takes the value of the location of the variable x. This is called the pointer initialization. The initialization can also be done in the following manner.

int x, *p = &x;

Here x is defined as an integer variable and then its location (&x) is stored under the pointer variable p.

Accessing a Variable through its Pointer

After assigning the address of an ordinary variable to a pointer variable, we can get the value of that ordinary variable by using the indirection operator . *. Consider the following example.

int rollno, * roll, n; rollno = 20010; roll = &rollno;

n = *roll;

11.12.4 Pointers and Arrays

We have seen in arrays that every array has two parts. The name of the array and number of elements in that array. Consider the following array.

int x[5];

This array has got five elements of integer type.

x[0], x[1], x[2], x[3] and x[4]

Every element occupy some location in the storage. If the first element is located at address 1000 and every integer occupies two bytes then the location of five elements will be:

x[0]   x[1]   x[2]   x[3]   x[4]
1000   1002   1004   1006   1008

Now if we define p as a pointer variable then it is clear that

p = &x[0];

we can access the location of every element by using increment operator to move from one element to other.

P = &x[0] = 1000

P+1 = &x[1] = 1002, P+2 = &x[2] = 1004, P+3 = &x[3] = 1006, P+4 = &x[4] = 1008

It is obvious from the above that the address of ith element of an array can be defined by the either &x[i] or as (x + i). That means that we can write the actual array element which preceded by ampersand (&) or by adding the subscript with the base address.

Similar to address of an element, the content of the address can be expressed either by x[i] or by *(x + i).

Now we will see a program which will use both type of expressions for array element and their address.

The first line defines two integer variables roll no and n and a pointer variable *roll pointing towards an integer value. The second line assigns a value to the variable roll no. The third lines assigns the location of the value of variable 'roll no' to the pointer variable roll. In the last, the indirection operator is used. When the operator is placed before the pointer variable in an expression, the pointer returns the value of the variable of which the pointer value is the address. Here *roll returns the the values of the variable roll no.

The use of indirection operator is shown in the following program.

```
#include <stdio.h>
main( )
int x,y ;
int *ptr;
x = 10
ptr = &x
```

11.12.5 Pointers and Functions

A method called "call by reference" can be used to pass the address of a variable as an argument of the function. Also a pointer can be defined to point towards a function. When we pass address to a function, the parameters receiving the address should be a pointer while it is possible to declare a pointer to a function which can then be used as an argument in another function. A pointer to a function is defined as-

```
data-type (*function-name) 0;
```

where data type refers to type of the value returned by the function. The function can be accessed by the indirectional operator(*). The indirectional operator and the function name should be placed within single parenthesis. A blank parenthesis is also used after the function name.

```
Int(*group)0;
```

This indicates that group is a pointer to a function which will return an integer value. Now we will see an example that will use a function pointer as a function argument

```
#include <math.h>
#define pi 3.1415926
main( )
double y(), COS(), table();
prinft("Table of y(x) = 2*x*x-x+1\n\n' ');
table(y, 0.0, 2.0, 0.5);
printf("\nTable of cos(x)\n\n' ');
table (cos, 0.0, pi, 0.5);
double table(f, min, max, step) double min, max, step;
double a, value;
for(a = min; a <= max; a += step)
value = (*f) (a);
printf(' '%5.2f % 10.4f\n", a, value);
double y(x) double x;
return(2*x*x-x+l) ;
```

11.13   Structures and Unions

We have seen in the previous chapters that various data of similar nature can be stored under one variable name using arrays. The limitation of using an array is that all the element of an array should be of same type. Consider an example of the data of employees of an organization which comprises of name, section and basic salary of the employee. The name and section are of character type while the basic salary is of numeric type. We cannot use this data within a single array. The C language provides an excellent way to store these type of data called **structures.** The structure is a special data structure whose individual element can be of different type. It can be used to represent different attributes like employee-name, section or basic salary.

Another related concept is unions which also contains multiple elements but the number of a union share the same storage area.

11.13.1 Defining a Structure

The keyword **struct** is used to define a structure. The general form of a structure definition is:

```
Struct tag;
data type member1;
```

data type member2;

data type member n;

} ;

where tag is a name that identifies the structure and member1, member2 ..... etc. are individual member declaration. The individual member can be any ordinary variable, array, pointer or other structures.

Consider an example of employee data base consisting of Account name, card no. type and basic salary of an employee. We can define a structure to hold this information as below.

Struct employee;

Char name[30];

char cardno[10];

char section[10];

Here employee is the tag name and name, cardno, section and salary are the element of that structure. This can be illustrated as

employee (structure)

name member 1

cardno member2

section member3

salary member4

It should be noted very carefully that member of the structure are not the variable. They donot occupy any memory until they are associated with some structure variable.

After defining the structure, the actual structure variables can be defined as

Struct employee emp1, emp2, emp3. Each are of these variable has four members as specified by the template. The complete declaration may look like:

Struct employee

char name[30];

char cardno[10];

char section[10];

struct employee Empl, Emp2, Emp3;

The structure composition can be combined with the structure variables as shown below

Struct Employee;

char name[20];

char cardno [10] ;

char section[10];

float salary;

Empl; Emp2; Emp3;

In this example Emp1, Emp2, Emp3 are three variables of type employee.

As it is stated earlier that a structure can contain another structure as one of its member. Consider the following Example :.

Struct name;

Char First name[20];

Char mid_name [20] ;

char last_name[20];

} ;

struct Employee;

Char cardno [10] ;

char section[10];

struct name;

int pf;

} ;

static struct pay_roll.Empl = {2500, 500, 100};

static struct pay_roll. Emp2 = {3000, 250, 100};

In this example basic will be initilized as 2500, hra will be initialized as 500 and pf will be initialized as 100 for Emp1 while for Emp2 basic will be initialized as 3000, hra will be initialized as 250 and P.F. will be initialized as 100.

11.13.2 Arrays of Structures

We can define a structure in the form of an array. For example, in a structure of Employee, we can declare Employee name and basic salary, and then declare all the Employee as structure variable. In such case we may declare an array of structures, each element of array representing a structure variable. For example

Struct plant Employee [10] ;

will define an array of 10 Employee. Each element will be of type struct plant. This structure 'plant' must be defined some where in the program. Consider the following Example.

```
Struct date
int math;
int day;
int year;
};
static struct date student[3] =
{{5,20,1968}, {6,25,1978}, {10,12,1982}};
```

This will define an array, student, with three elements in it. The elements are of type struct date. The values will be initialized as

```
printf("Input data");
scanf("%s%d%d%d%d" student. stu_name, &student.day&student,
math, & student.year, & student.tot_marks);
print ("%s%d%d%d%d", student.stu_name, student.day,
student.math, student.year, getch(); student.tot-marks);
```

11.13.3 Structure Initilization

The members of a structure variable can be assigned initial values similar to that of any other variable. However, the structures must be declared as static if it is to be initilized Inside a function. Consider the following example:

```
main ()
static struct
int roll;
int marks;
student
```

```
{l045, BO};
```

This will assign 1045 to student roll and 80 to student. marks. The values can be initilized in many other ways. For example-

```
main ()
struct pay_roll;
```

```
int basic;
int hra;.
for(j=0; j<=2 j++)
student[i] .total += student[i] .sub[j];
total.sub[j]+= student[j] .sub[j]
total. total += student[i] .total
printf ("STUDENT TOTAL\n")
for(i=0;i<=2;i++)
printf("student[%d] %d\n",i+1,student[i] .total)
printf("\nSUBJECT TOTAL\n");
for(j=0;j<=2 ;j++)
printf("Subject%d %d\n",j+l,total.sub[j]) ;
printf("\nGrand total = %d\n",total.total);
getch();
```

11.13.4 Structures within Structures

A structure can also be a member of another structure. Following example shows the structure of a result database

```
structure result
char name [50] ; char f_name[50];
int mark1;
int mark2; int mark3;
int day;
```

initial value, we can just define an array of structure and can provide the values at some later stage.

For Example

```
Struct account
int AC_no;
char name [80] ;
int balance;
static struct account customer[10];
```

Instead of giving

This will define following type of structure variable

    customer [0] . AC_no

    customer [0] .name[8D]

    customer[O]cbalance

    customer[I] . AC_no

    customer[9] . balance

    student [1] .month = 6

    student [2] .year = 1982

It is very obvious from the above that the array of the structure is stored as a two dimensional array.

Now we will see a program to define an array of structures for student data base and then calculate the subject wise and student wise totals and store them as a part of structure.

STRUCTURES AND UNIONS

    student[0] .month = 5

    student [0] .day = 20

    student[0] .day = 1978

    struct pf

    char mp_name[30]

    float basic

    int pfp;

    } ;

    main( )

    struct pf update() int p_pfp;

    float p_in;

    static struct pf rec = {"Parag",2525.25,10}; printf("\nInput increment pf% by\n");

    scanf ("%d", &p-pfp);

    p_in = 2525.25;

    rec = update(rec,p_in,p-pfp); printf("Updated values of -\n\n"); printf ("Name
    printf ("Basic \n", rec. emp_name) ;

%f\n",rec.basic) ;

printf("P.F. perc.: %d\n",rec.pfp); getch () ;

struct pf update(name,bas,pff) struct pf name;

float bas;

int pff;

name.basic=bas; name.pfp+=pff; return (name) ;

puts(s) rewind(f) scanf(...)

<stdlib.h> abs(i) atof(s) atoi(s) atol(s) callic(u1,u2)

exit(u)

free(p)

malloc(u)

rand(void) realloc(p,u)

srand(u) system(s)

Send string s to the standard output device. Move the pointer to the beginning of file f.

Enter data items from the standard input device.

Return the absolute value of i.

Convert string s to a double-precision quantity. Convert string s to an integer

Convert string s to a long integer.

Allocate memory for an array having u1 elements, each of length u2 bytes. Return a pointer to the beginning of the allocated space.

Close all files and buffers, and terminate the program. (Value of u is assigned by the function, to indicate termination status.)

Free a block of allocated memory whose beginning is indicated by p.

Allocate u bytes of memory. Return a pointer to the beginning of the allocated space.

Return a random positive integer.

Allocate u bytes of new memory to the pointer variable p. Return a pointer to the beginning of the new memory space.

Initialize the random number generator.

Pass command string s to the operating system. Return 0 if the command is successfully executed; otherwise, return a nonzero value typically-1

11.13.5 Arrays within Structures

It has been stated earlier that arrays can be used as a member of structure. Single or multidimensional array can be used as the member. Integer, floating point or character array may be use in this place. For Example

```
Struct marks
int number;
float subject[3];
} student [2] ;
```

In the example the member subject contains three elements subject [0], subject [1], subject [2].

Each element can be accessed with suitable subscripts.

Now here is an example of demartialy array within a structure

```
#include <stdio.h>
main ()
struct marks
int sub[3] ;
int total ;
} ;
static struct marks student[3]
= {{ 88, 52, 54,0}, {45, 59,79,0} , {82, 79, 58, 0} }
static struct marks total ;
int i , j;
clrscr ()
for(i=0 ; i<=2 ;i++)
```

In the above structure we can group the marks into another structure.

```
struct result
char name [50] ;
char f_name [ 50 J ;
struct
int mark1;
int mark2;
int mark3;
marks
student;
```

The result structure contain marks as a member of it which itself is a structure. The member contained in the inner structure can be referred in the form of

variable.member.submember

student.marks.mark1

11.13.6 Structure & Functions

Function can be used within structures to pass entire structure or a single member of structure to a function. Individual structure member can be passed to a function as actual argument of function call and a single structure member can be returned via return statement. The complete structure can be transferred to a function by passing a structure-type pointer an argument.

The second process i.e. transferring of entire structure is more commonly used. We will see a program which will illustrate the method of sending entire structure as a parameter of function program.

CHAPTER 12

BASIC Programming Language

12.1 Introduction

The word BASIC stands for Beginners All-purpose Symbolic Instruction Code. This language was developed in Dartmouth College, USA, under the directions of professors John G. Kameny and Thomes E. Kertz in 1964. Though it was developed as a beginner language, it has become very popular due to its simplicity, among beginners and learners.

BASIC is available on all types of computers – from micro to mainframe. There is very little difference between the several version of the BASIC language.

BASIC language is provided with both interpreter and compiler. The interpreter is more suitable for the learner because editing a program is more convenient to an interpreter than a compiler. The different version of BASIC is available as BASIC, GW BASIC etc.

12.2 Format of Basic Statements

Statement is the fundamental unit of BASIC program. Each command or instruction in BASIC is called a statement. It you want to store a value in the computer memory, compare any two values or display the result on the screen, you have to write separate statement. The statement or instructions should be given according to the rules of the layers in which the program is written.

For Example :

A statement for storing a value in the memory may be given in different formats in different languages as below:

BASIC   10 LET A = 90

FORTAN   A = 90

C   A = 90

PASCAL   a: 90

BASIC statement consists of three parts:

Line or statement number, i.e. 10

An optical command A = 90

Remark statement - [Good].

12.3 Line Number or Statement Number

The line number or statement number consists of one to five depending on the size of program. The program will be executed in the order of the line numbers. The BASIC compiler/interpreter will automatically insert any given line according to the sequence before executing the program or before printing the complete program. Zero and negative numbers should not be used as statement numbers.

Let us assume that we have entered a program with five statement with line number as 1, 2, 3, 4, 5.

1. -----------------------------------

2. -----------------------------------

3. -----------------------------------

4. -----------------------------------

5. -----------------------------------

In case, you want to insert a statement between 3 and 4, then you are required to remember all the statement from 4 as 5 and 5 as 7. The new statement has to be entered with line number as 4. It will be very difficult to do such renumbering of the number of statements if the programs are large. Hence, to avoid this difficulty it is always better to give the statement number in steps of 10. If we type the auto command and press the entry key, line number 10 will appear on the screen. Now if we type the statement against it and press the entry key, we will automatically get line number 20.

After typing all the statements, press the entry key. Then press the ctrl and break key together. This will stop the execution of the auto command.

12.4 Elements of the BASIC Language

The elements of any programming language consist of the character set, operators, data types, variables, and statements, which are recognized by its compilers.

Character set:

(a)   Digital   :   0 -9

(b)   Letters   :   A-Z

Constants / Data

Constants / data are the values stated in a program. Based on the type of value, they are classified as string or numeric constants.

String constants : The computer also processes, non-numeric information such as names, address etc. These data do not involve any mathematical calculation but can be used for comparison and references. Such types of data are called alphanumeric or string data. Strings consist of a set of alphanumeric or special characters enclosed within quotation marks. Blank space is also allowed in a string.

Valid string constants :

"Gold"

"28/8/1964"

"Come in"

The maximum number of characters that can be included in a string varies from computer to computer and has between 255 to 4095 characters. Strings are used in print headings, expander remarks etc.

Invalid string

"Record	-	Quotation mark missing at the end.
"I am "Seven" year old"	-	Quotation mark inside the string not allowed.
187	-	Not enclosed inside quotes.

Numeric Constant : At any numeric value on which mathematical operations can be performed is called numeric constant. It is made up of a string of digits, positive or negative, with or without a decimal point. Numbers may consist of an exponent part, the letter E followed by an optical sign and one or two digits. This form of representing the numbers is called exponent or scientific format. These are used in scientific or engineering applications to represent very high or low values.

Valid Numeric Constant

246	5	2.5 E + 04
256.75	- 626.0	2.5 E – 10

Invalid Numeric Constant		Reasons
24/6/1964	-	It is an arithmetic expression
"1265"	-	It is enclosed inside quotes.
193/B	-	Alpha numeric are not allowed.

Variables

A variable is an area of computer's memory within a program and can be referred to by name. Any reference to that name mode by the program is the current value at the storage area. BASIC has numeric variable: - The numeric variable always represents a numeric constant.

Alphabets and digits may form the string variable. In subtraction the first character must be on alphabet then combination of alphabets and digits.

The maximum number of character to be used is a numeric variable, which varies from version to version of BASIC. In IBMPC version of BASIC up to 32 characters are allowed.

Valid numeric variable

C44   X DII

Invalid numeric variables

2 x   -   The first character is must be alphabet

M#   -   # is not permissible

Numeric variable can be classified into flooting and real variables. It we want to store only whole number, % symbol must be given at end of the variable number.

For example,

A % = 12.4

Computer will store only 12

It we give A = 12.4

Then computer will store value as 12.4.

Real variables may be followed by special characters $ or #. If a numeric value is followed by $ then it is called a single precision variable (which is the default). This means that it can store up to 7 digits at accuracy (in decimals). If a numeric value is followed by # symbol, then it is called a double precision variable. This will take more memory storage and will provide 14 digits of accuracy.

Examples:

Calculate %	Integer variable
Interest	Single precision variable
Interest /1	Single precision variable
Principle #	Double precision variable.

String variable : A string variable represents a string of characters or alphanumeric constants. This variable start with alphabet that may have further characters of alphabets and digits. The last character must be a $ symbol.

Example :

X $ LOCATION $ LESSION $

Invalid string variables   Reason

4 $ [First character must be a letter]

$ 5   [Letter must precede $]

XY $$ [To many $ parameters]

Operators:

In BASIC we used three types of operations i.e. arithmetic, relational and logical.

Arithmetic Operators : The operator with numeric constants and variables is called an arithmetic operator. It will always give numeric output. The arithmetic operators used in BASIC are as follows:

Exponentiation   ** or ^

Multiplication   *

Division   /

Addition   +

Subtraction   –

More then one arithmetic operator may be present in an arithmetic expression i.e. $(A * B) / 4 * C - D \wedge 2$.

The hierarchical order of operators for evaluating the expression is follows :

- Breaket   - Small ( )   Middle { }   big [ ]

- ^

- * and /

- + and -

Relational operators

The relational operators are used to compare two values. The comparison may be done with the following operators.

=   Equal

<   Less than

>   Grater than

< =   less or equal

> =   grater or equal

< >   not equal

Logical operators. The following logical operators are used in BASIC :

AND

OR

NOT

These operators are used to combine two or more relational expressions to evaluate single logical values that are true or false.

12.5 Basic Statement

Basic has following statements:

Assignment Statement	-	LET
Input Statement	-	READ AND INPUT
Output Statement	-	PRINT
Transfer Statement	-	GOTO GOSUB-RETURN
Conditional Statement	-	IF-THEN-ELSE,-GOTO
Loop Statement	-	FOR-NEXT, WHILE-END

LET Statement

The LET statement is used to assign a value or data to a variable. This statement will store the data into the variable.

The general format of this statement is,

Statement number LET Vrb = Vrb / Data / Expression

Where Vrb is a variable name of numeric or string type. On the right hand side, data, variable or expression can be given. If data is given, it will be stored into the variable on the left side of the statement. If variable is given, then the value of the variable will be stored into the variable on the left side of the statement. If expression is given, it will be evaluated and the result will be stored into variable on the left side of the statement.

The data, variable or expression should be of the same type on either side of the statement, i.e., if the variable is numeric, the data assigned to it should also be numeric. You cannot mix numeric and string type in the using an assignment statement.

Some examples of LET statement are given below:

10 LET X = 20

20 LET RATE = 25.04

30 LET COST = 22.35

40 LET X = X + 4

You can see from the above examples that string variables with string expressions and numeric variables are used with numeric expressions. In the last example, the variable X appears on both sides of the "equal" sign. Thus, this line asks the computer to add the value of X and store it as the current value of X. Thus, the LET statement is easier to understand if the "=" sign is considered as "is replaced by".

Strings can also be assigned values from complex expressions but only the plus operator may be used. In this case, the plus is used to mean combination rather than addition. String variables can be combined together or can be combined with string constants as in the following examples.

250 LET A$ = "COMP" + "UTER"

The resultant value of A$ in the above example will be "COMPUTER".

240 LET B$ = "Type" + "Writer"

In the above example, the string data "Typewriter" and the value of the string variable B$ are joined together and stored in another string variable B$.

In most BASIC compilers or interpreters, the word LET may be omitted.

Thus, we can write the statement as:

245 A$ = B$

275 A = (B + C)/2

Print Statement

The PRINT statement is used to display the output on the screen. This statement will print constants, variables or expressions. The general format or syntax of this statement is,

Sr. No. PRINT list of variables/ constant / expression.

If more than one value is printed, they may be separated by either a comma or a semicolon (;) leaving a space in between.

If an arithmetic expression is directly given in the PRINT statement, it will be evaluated and the result will be printed. If any constant has be to printed, either numeric or string, it must be enclosed within quotes.

Example

20 PRINT X

30 PRINT X, Y

40 PRINT "The value of X is" , X

80 PRINT A = B

50 PRINT X = B

60 PRINT "The sum is" , X + Y

Formatting Output

The PRINT statement has a lot of options to format the output on the screen.

If you print any value using the PRINT statement, the output will be given in a fresh line, i.e, the display will begin from the very next line. If more than one data has to be displayed on a line, the PRINT statement must be given with the variable separated by a comma or a semicolon.

Effect of Comma in PRINT

A line is separated into 5 zones, each with 14 spaces. For the following statement,

100 PRINT X, Y

the value of X will be printed from the first column, i.e., at the first zone. Then the control will be moved to the second zone, at the 15th column. Here the value of Y will be printed.

100 PRINT P,Q,R,S,T

will print all the five values in the same line each in one zone. If you give one more variable, then it will be printed in the first zone of the next line.

100 PRINT P,Q,R,S,T,U

Here, the values of P,Q,R,S and T will be printed in one line, and the sixth value, U, cannot be accommodated in the same line. Hence it will be printed in the next line.

If any one of the values exceeds the length of the zone, it will be printed in the next zone. For example, you see the following statement.

100 PRINT "MARKS IN SCIENCE" , M

You will get the result as

MARKS IN SCIENCE 85

Here the length of the string constants exceeds 14 characters. It is extended into the second zone and hence the value of M (85) is printed in the third zone.

If you give comma at the end of any PRINT statement, then the next statement of your program will be printed from the same line and not from a new line.

Execute the following statements and note the difference.

1. 10 PRINT "BASIC", "PROGRAMMING"
2. 10 PRINT "BASIC"
   20 PRINT "PROGRAMMING"
3. 10 PRINT "BASIC"
   11 PRINT "PROGRAMMING"

Instead of using comma as the separator, if you use the semicolon, the values will be printed much closer to each other with only one space in between.

Hence, if you want to accommodate more data in one line, use the semicolon to separate the variables.

1. 20 LET X = 10
   40 LET Y = 20
   60 LET Z = X + Y
   80 PRINT X,Y,Z
   100 PRINT X;Y;Z

Using TAB

The data can be printed at a specific column on the line using one of the library functions called TAB. You know that each line has 80 columns. You can shift or move the cursor to a specific column – using TAB.

Example :

50 PRINT TAB (10); "HELLO"

This statement will move the cursor to column 10 and print HELLO. If TAB (10) is not given, then HELLO will be printed from the first column.

The TAB function, should have the column reference in ascending order, i.e.,

100 PRINT TAB (5); "COMPUTER", TAB (15); "PROGRAMMING"

Column 5 is referred first and then column 15. You cannot give column 15 first and then 5, because once the column is crossed, the cursor cannot go backwards. If the crossed position is referred again in the PRINT statement, the value will be printed in the next line. For example,

200 PRINT TAB (20); "COMPUTER"; TAB (5) ; "PROGRAMMING"

Will print as   COMPUTER   PROGRAMMING

Note : If you use TAB function in PRINT statement, use semicolon in place of comma. This is because comma may print the data at different zones. Thus the effect of TAB function may not be realized.

Leaving Blank Lines :

To leave blank lines in between printing an output, you can give the PRINT statement without any data or variable.

    100 PRINT "BASIC"

    200 PRINTS

    300 PRINT "PROGRAMMING"

Will print as

BASIC

PROGRAMMING

1. Write a program to print the following:

    ONE

    TWO   THREE

    FOUR   FIVE   SIX

    SEVEN   EIGHT   NINE   TEN

    ELEVEN   TWELVE   THRTEEN FOURTEEN   FIFTEEN

2. Type the following program and execute.

    10 LET N = 10

    20 LET X = N*2

    30 LET Y = N*5

    40 LET Z = N*2

    50 PRINT N; "*2 = ": Y

    60 PRINT N; "*3 = "; Y

    70 PRINT N; "*3 ="; Z

3. Find errors, if any, in the following PRINT statement

    (a)   10 PRINT A, B, C, D,

    (b)   20 PRINT A, B,

    (c)   30 PRINT "QUESTION" =

    (d)   40 PRINT: X, Y

    (e)   50 PRINT R * S1

4. Show how the output will appear in the following:

   (a)   10 PRINT "AVERAGE OF"; X:

           TAB (20); "AND";

           20 PRINT TAB (30) ; Y; TAB (40);

           "IS"; TAB (50); (X+Y)/2

           (Where X = 10, Y=20)

   (b)   10 PRINT "SUM OF" ; TAB (4) ;

           20 PRINT "A + B"; TAB (30);

           30 PRINT "IS EQUAL TO" A+B

           (Where A =25, B=55)

INPUTTING DATA

The data for the variables can be either from the program itself using the LET and READ statements or it can be read from the user terminal device using the INPUT statements.

INPUT Statement

This is used to request data items from the user terminal. As each value is typed in, it is assigned to the appropriate variable. Thus if the statement

    10 INPUT X

is executed, the terminal will print ? And then awaits user's response (Note : The program execution is suspended until the user enters the value and presses the Enter Key). The data typed by the user must be in the INPUT statement.

If the user enters more or insufficient data, BASIC will respond by prompting the error message as "Redo from start".

If the data type does not match with the variable type, then BASIC will display Redo from start, and allow you to type the data again.

To make the user clear about the input, this statement may be provided with an optional message. This message will be displayed when BASIC awaits the user's input. This will make you understand what the program expects as INPUT general format or syntax of the INPUT statement is,

Statement No. INPUT "say"; variables

For example,

    10 INPUT "YOUR NAME"; N$

    20 INPUT "YOUR AGE"; AGE

    30 INPUT "YOUR MARKS" TM

If more than one variable is used in the INPUT statement, the variable must be separated by a comma. While entering data from the keyboard, the data must also be separated by a comma.

Try Yourself

1. Input your name and print the same in two lines.

2. Input your age, your brother's age and print the difference between them.

3. Write the LET statement for the following:

   (a) $a = \dfrac{Y_2 - Y_1}{X_2 - X_1}$ (b) $d = y_1 - mx_1$

   (c) $p = ut + \dfrac{1}{2} at^2$ (d) $a = \dfrac{x + i}{z}$

4. Find the error in the following statements.

   (a)   10 LET X = Y = 5

   (b)   20 INPUT "ENTER NUMBER"

   (c)   30 PRINT X, Y:Z

   (d)   40 END AMOUNT

   (e)   50 RENUM

5. Write a program to input two values and find the addition, subtraction, multiplication and division involving them.

6. Write a program to input your name and marks in Hindi, Maths and Computers. Find the total and average.

7. Write a program to input three sides of a triangle and find the perimeter. (perimeter of triangle = x+y+z, and x,y and z are the three sides of the triangle).

8. Write a program to input the side of a square and find the perimeter and area.
   Perimeter of a square = 4* x

   Area = x * x

   (Where x is the side)

9. Write a program to input the salary of an employee and calculate the DA, which is 25% of the salary.

10. Guess the output for the following :

    (a)   10 LET X = Y

           20 LET Z = X + Y

           30 PRINT Z

           40 END

(b)   05 LET N $ = 1
        10 LET A = 10
        15 LET C = A + 2
        20 PRINT C
        25 END

(c)   10 LET N$ = "COMPUTER"
        20 LET X = N$*2
        30 PRINT
        40 END

(d)   10 INPUT "WHAT IS YOUR NAME" , A
        20 PRINT "WELCOME TO BASIC" , A
        30 END

(e)   10 INPUT "ENTER A VALUE"
        20 LET X = A * A
        30 PRINT "THE SQUARE OF" , A, "IS" , X
        40 END

Lab Exercise

1. Write a program to input five number and find the sum of all number
2. Write a program to print the fillowing :

   P
   PR
   PRO
   PROG
   PROGR
   PROGRA
   PROGRAM

3. Write a program to print the following using TAB function.

   C
   CO
   COM
   COMP
   COMPU
   COMPUT
   COMPUTE
   COMPUTER

4. Input the value of A and print the result of the following equations :
   (a)   A + A2
   (b)   2A + 10
   (c)   20 – A/2
   (d)   A
   (e)   3A2 + 4A
5. Write a BASIC program inputting the values of A and B and print the result.
6. Write a program to input the size of your study room i.e. the length, width, and the height of the walls and find out the area of wall paper required.
7. Write a program to input the radius of inner and outer diameter of a circle and find the area of the circle.

   Hint : Area of the circle = Area of the outer circle – Area of the inner circle.
8. Find the errors, if any, from the following programs.
   (a)   10 LET A = 5
         20 LET A = B
         30 LET C = 5/A
         40 PRINT C
         50 END
   (b)   10 INPUT "NAME" , n
         20 INPUT "MARK" , m
         30 PRINT N$; "HAS GOT GOOD MARKS"
         40 END
   (c)   10 INPUT "YOUR HEIGHT" , h
         20 LET w = HEIGHT * 5
         30 PRINT "YOUR WEIGHT SHOULD BE AROUND" ,w
         40 END
   (d)   10 LET X = 21/x
         20 INPUT X
         30 PRINT X
         40 END
   (e)   10 LET RADIUS = 5.5
         20 LET PI = 22/7
         30 LET AREA = PI * S *S
         40 PRINT "AREA = " , AREA
         50 END

12.6 Library Functions in Basic

Library functions are readymade program codes available in the standard library of a language. These functions can be invoked from any program written in those languages to perform specific task.

1. ASC Function

It is also known as ASCII function. This functions is used to find out the ASCII value of a character or ASCII value of the first character of a given string.

Syntax :

Line No. ASC (Alphanumeric Variable String or Constant)

Example 1 :

```
100 CLS
110 Let A$ = "A"
120 LET B = ASC (A$)
130 Print "Character is – " , A$
140 Print" ASCII equivalent of this characters is " , B
150 End
```

Example 2 :

```
10 CLS
20 Input " A String of Characters – " , A$
30 Let B = ASC (A$)
40 Print "String" , ASCII"
50 Print A$, B
60 End
```

2. STR Functions

It is also known as String function. This function is used to convert a numeric value into an alphanumeric value.

Example:

```
10 Let x = 50
20 Let y = 100
30 Let z = x + y
40 Let x $ = STR $ (x)
50 Let y $ = STR (y)
60 Let z$ = x$ + y$
```

```
70 Print "First Value = " , x
80 Print "Second Value = " , y
90 Print " Third Value = " , z
100 Print " First String = " , x $
110 Print " Second String = ; y $
130 End
```

Output of the above program will be :

```
First value = 50
Second Value = 100
Third Value 150
First String = 50
Second String = 100
Third String = 50100
```

3. VAL Function

It is also known as Value function. This is used to find out digit value as numeric value of a string. This digit value should be written at left most column of a string.

Example 1 :

```
100 Let A$ = "100 Chandni Chowk"
110 Let V = VAL (A $)
120 Let B = 200 + V
130 Print "A$ = "; A$
140 Print "Value = " ; V
150 Print B
160 End
```

Output of the above program :

```
A$ = 100 Chandni Chowk
V = 100
B = 300
```

Example 2 :

```
100 Let X$ = "1000"
110 Let Y$ = "500"
120 Let Z$ = X$ + Y$
130 Let X = VAL (X$)
140 Let Y = VAL (Y$)
150 Let P = X + Y
```

160 PRINT "X$ = " ; X$, "Y$ = " ; Y$

170 Print "X$ = " ; Y$, = "Y$ =" ; Z$

180 Print "X = "; X, "Y = "Y = " ; Y, "P = " ; P

190 End

Output of the above program is :

X$ = 1000 Y$ = 500

X$ + Y$ = 1000 500

X = 1000 Y = 500 P = 1500

4. Left Function

This function is used to find out the number of characters from the side of a string.
Syntax : Line No. Left $ (String, Number)

Example :

100 Let X$ = "Computers"

110 Let Y$ = Left $ (X$,5)

120 Print "X$ = " ; X $

130 Print "Y $ = "; Y$

140 End

Output of the above program is :

X $ = Computer

X $ = Compu

5. Right Function

Just like the above function this Right function works vice versa. This function is
used to find out the number of characters from the right side of a string.

Syntax : line No. Right $ (String, Number)

10 Let A$ = "Friends"

20 Let B$ = Right $ (A$, 5)

30 Print "A$ = " ; A$

40 Print "B$ = " ; B$

50 End

Output of the above program is

A$ = Friends

B $ = iends

6. MID Function

MID function is used to find out the number of characters presents from the middle of a given string.

Syntax:

MID $ (String, Starting Character Number, Number of Characters to be searched)

Example :

100 CLS

110 Let X$ = "Computers"

120 Let Y$ = MID$ (X$, 4,6)

Output of the above program is :

PUTERS

i.e. It Starts from the fourth Character i.e. 'P' and extracts six characters after it.

7. CHR Function

It is known as character function. This function is used to convert the ASCII value into its character equivalent.

Syntax : line No. CHR$ (Numeric Value or variable)

Example :

100 Let X = 65

110 Let Y$ = CHR $ (X)

120 Print "ASCII Code", "Character"

130 Print X, Y$

140 For X = 0 TO 100

150 Let Z$ = CHR $ (X)

160 Print X' "ASCII Code value in characters" ; Z$

170 Next X

180 End

The above program will print the character equivalent of number 0 to 1, as A,B,C,D……. so on.

8. LEN Function

The len function is used to find out the length of a string to know the total number of characters present in that string.

Syntax : LEN (String)

Example :

    100 CLS
    110 Let X$ = "Computer"
    120 Let Y$ = LEN (X$)
    130 Print X$, Y
    140B End

Output of the above program is

computers 7

12.7   User Defined Functions and Subroutines in Basic

User defined functions

Basic allows its users to define their own function and write formula for those functions. The define statement in BASIC is used to define the user defined functions.

Syntax : Define A (X) = Expression,

where A is a one-letter name of the function and X is the argument of the function defined. This argument appears as a variable in the expression on the right hand side.

$$A (X) = ax^2 + bx + c$$

The above formula can be defined as a user defined function in Basic by the following:

    100 Define A (X) = (A * X + B) * X + C

As only on single letter is allowed to name a function, a maximum of only 26 functions can be defined in a program.

Subroutines

In large program, usually the main problem is broken into small units or sub problems. This breaks a large program into small program modules or codes. In such situation, a particular calculations or a set of calculation appears more than once in a program. If these calculations can be included in a single statement, then we can define a function and use this function wherever required. But if more than one

Statement is required then the better way of doing this task is a subprogram, which is also known as subroutine.

A subroutine is a set of program Statement that may be used repeatedly at different places throughout the main program. This subroutine is normally placed at the end of the main program. The structure of the subroutine is as under :

```
100 REM 'Subroutine ABC'
110 :
120 :
130 :
140 :
150 RETURN
```

These line numbers should be in a sequence and must not appear elsewhere in the program. The control from the main program can be transferred to a subroutine at any point by using the GOSUB Statement. This statement is :

```
GO SUB n
```

Where n is the number of first line of the subroutine. When the GO SUB n statement encounters, it transfers the program control to the statement number n. The execution of program now continues from n statement until a RETURN statement is encountered. The RETURN statement returns the program control to the statement immediately following the GO SUB n statement.

GOSUB RETURN

Syntax : line No. GOSUB (Line No.)

< Statements>

Line No. RETURN

Example 1 :

```
100 CLS
110 GOSUB 140
120 Print A$
130 End
140 Input "Your Name : " ; A$
150 RETURN
```

Example 2 :

```
10 CLS
20 GOSUB 80
30 Let A = X + Y
40 Print "Value of X : " ; X
50 Print "Value of Y : " ; Y
60 Print "Value of X and Y" ; A
70 End
80 CLS
90 Input "First Number : " ; X
100 Input "Second Number : ' : Y
110 Return
```

Example 3 :

Write a program to input name, address, city & state of a person assign GOSUB statement. Print them in mailing label format.

```
10 REM "Program to Print Mailing Labels"
20 CLS
30 GOSUB 100
40 Print Tab (2) : "TO"
50 Print Tab (5) ; "Ms/Mr" ; N$
60 Print Tab (5) ; Permanent Address " ; Add $
70 Print Tab (5) ; "City" ; City $
80 Print Tab (5) "State" ; State $
90 End
100 Input "Name : " ; n$
110 Input Permanent Address : " ; Add $
120 Input "City : " ; City $
130 Input "State : " ; State $
140 Return
```

The Output of the above program will be

Name	-	Robin Hood
Address	-	240, Jungle Woods
City	-	Royal Castle
State	-	Green Nature

To

Shri Ms/Mr Robin Hood

Permanent Address 240, Jungle Woods

City Royal Castle

State Green-Nature

The same program can be modified further to print as many mailing labels as the user wishes and stop printing by accepting user's choice.

CHAPTER 13

Application Software

13.1 Word Processing

Word processing is software package for processing of words as is suggested by the name. Letters project reports etc. are some common results of Word processing. In computer terminology Word Processing refers to typing, editing and formatting any kind document that has already been keyed into the computer.

Earlier means of communication was by way of handwritten letters, with the invention of the typewriter, method of communication changed to some extent. But the typewriter had some disadvantages like typed letters can't be stored and errors have to be retyped. Inspection of the electronic typewriter solved the drawbacks to some extent but could not store large reports or data.

Invention of the computer and computerized Word processing solved many of the problems faced in typewriting. WORD STAR is the earliest Word Processor which is DOS based. With this software one could create long documents, spell check, mail merge etc. Its limitations were that only one document can be opened at a time and charts and graphics could not be inserted into it. Advent of Windows changed the entire scene.

Advantages of Word Processing

Word processing is different from conventional typing in many ways. Here the document is not printed while being keyed in. However its image is displayed on the computer screen and the information is also stored in computer memory. The computer operator can verify the document which is displayed on the computer screen and can correct the mistakes before printing i.e. it helps to print relatively error free documents in desired format. Any number of copies can be printed without retyping and all print outs look as the first copy.

Word processing helps prepared such documents with special features like bold face, underline, and strikeout.

Microsoft Words (MS-word) uses the standard Windows procedure for starting programs, saving and printing files. Word utilities the Windows graphical user interface (GUI), a mouse can be used to complete many Word Procedures. It combines a Word processor, desktop and spread sheds.

13.2 Installing Word in Computer

Microsoft Word (MS-Word) can be installed in your computer, if you have the M-S Office CD or installer floppy. The CD/Floppy is to be inserted into the concerned drive and its contents displayed. There will be a setup of install icon. Double clicking on it will start the installation procedure, which can then be completed by following the step by step instructions given on screen.

Steps to Load Word

Before starting Word, make sure that the computer can run Windows based software and that Windows and Word are properly installed. Word can be loaded in the following steps.

Step 1 : Switch on the computer. If Windows is already loaded, skip to step 3.

Step 2 : To start Windows from DOS prompt (C :\>), type of windows please enter, type win and press enter.

Step 3 : Locate the MS-Word icon in the group windows displayed within the program Manger Window.

Step 4 : Point to the MS-Word icon and double click the mouse to start Word.

Exiting Word

This is done in any of the following ways:

1. Open the file menu and click on Exit command
2. Double click on the word window control menu box
3. Press the [Alt] key and press [F4] ([Alt]+[F4]).

Inserting Text into Existing Paragraphs

This is done in the following manner

1. Place the pointer at the point where the text is to be inserted and click to anchor the insertion point at that location.
2. Type in the text to be inserted.

It can be seen that the existing text moves to the right and down to the next line in the document.

Deleting Text with the Backspace and Delete Key

Deleting text is easily done using the back space or Delete keys. Pressing the backspace key removes character to the left of the insertion point, while that at the right is removed by the Delete key.

Selecting and Replacing Text

Changing a string of text involves a two way process of identifying the text, selecting it and replacing it. Selection of and replacement of text is normally done in the following manner.

Move the beam pointer (cursor) first in front of the text string to be replaced. Click the mouse button to position the cursor and then selected the text by dragging the pointer across the word until they appear in reverse video followed by release of the mouse button.

When the selected the matter which has to replace it shall have to be keyed in.

Other ways of selecting text are as following

One Word can be selected by double clicking on it.

An entire sentence is selected by double clicking on it.

An entire sentence is selected by placing the cursor anywhere on the sentence press the [ctrl] key and clicks the mouse button.

Undo and Redo

Some time after changing a text, it is seen that original text has to be brought back. Clicking on undo button in the standard toolbar helps to resort changed text to previous condition. In case the text that has changed needs the originally edited matter, this can be done by just clicking on the redo button.

Saving a Document

Any information keyed into a document is temporarily stored in the computers memory and will be erased unless the document is saved as a file.

Documents can be saved after giving them a name and specifying the location (Drive and Directory) where the file is to be stored. Document are saved by clicking on the SAVE button on the left side of the standard toolbar to display the SAVE AS dialog box (Fig 12.1). Fill in the blank space to complete the procedure to save the document.

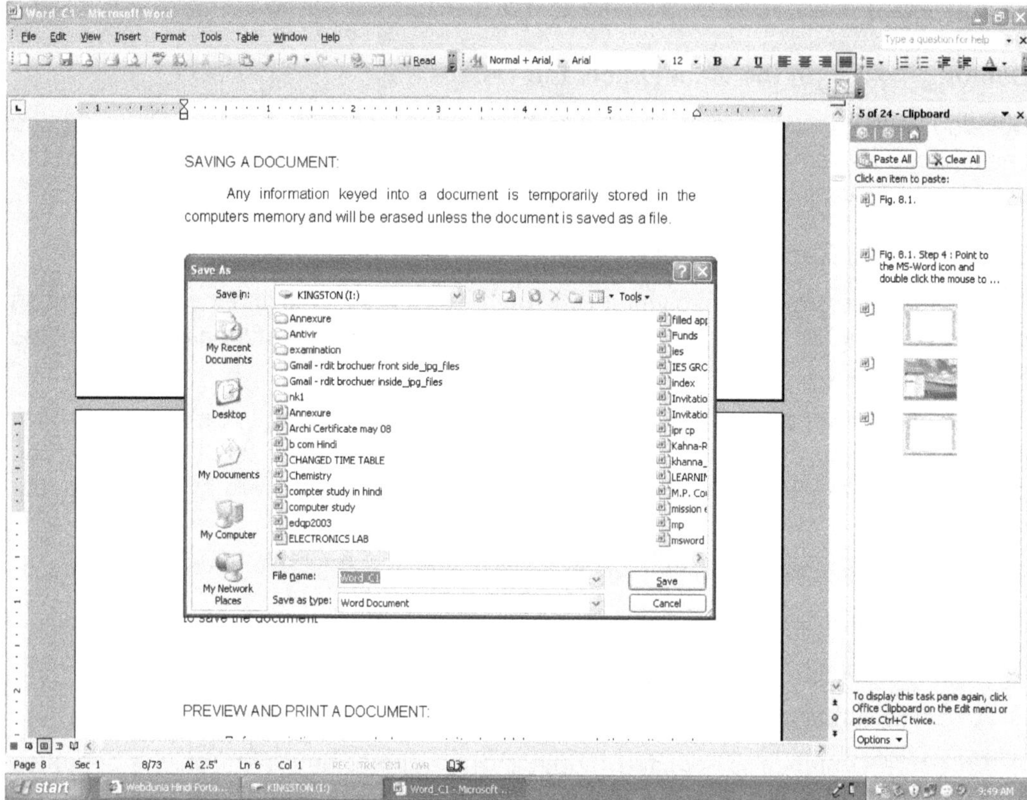

Fig. 13.1

Preview and Print a Document

Before printing a word document it should be ensured that attached printer is properly attached and installed. Previewing a document helps in that one gets an idea of how the printed output would look.

The print preview window has many options to view and improve a document. Some of the basic functions are enumerated below:

1. When a document is seen on the screen and we click the PRINT PREVIEW button the window displayed will be similar to the one in Fig. 12.2. This window will have its own toolbar and the pointer appears as a magnifying glass when placed inside the document.

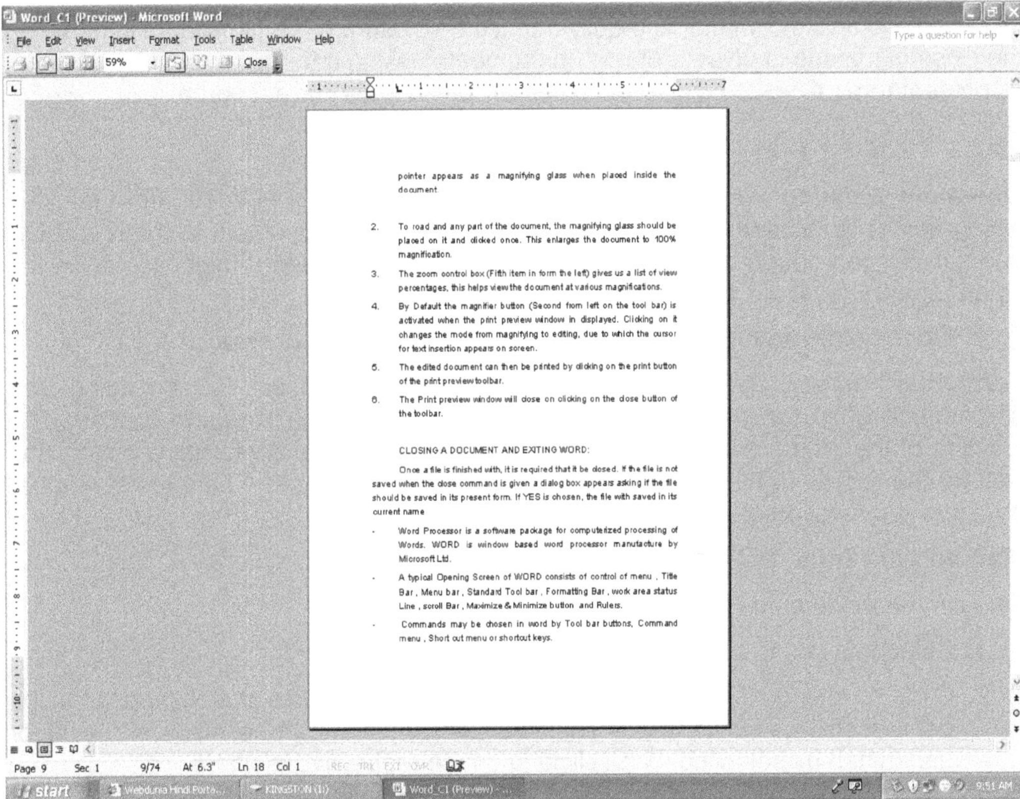

Fig. 13.2

2. To read and any part of the document, the magnifying glass should be placed on it and clicked once. This enlarges the document to 100% magnification.

3. The zoom control box (Fifth item in from the left) gives us a list of view percentages, this helps view the document at various magnifications.

4. By Default the magnifier button (Second from left on the tool bar) is activated when the print preview window in displayed. Clicking on it changes the mode from magnifying to editing, due to which the cursor for text insertion appears on screen.

5. The edited document can then be printed by clicking on the print button of the print preview toolbar.

6. The Print preview window will close on clicking on the close button of the toolbar.

Closing a Document and Exiting Word

Once a file is finished with, it is required that it be closed. If the file is not saved when the close command is given a dialog box appears asking if the file should be saved in its present form. If YES is chosen, the file will saved in its current name

13.2.1   Editing Text

Operating Existing Files: A previously saved document is opened with the open dialog box. it is initiated in the following manner. Go to 'file' option in the menu bar and select open option or click the open button on the standard toolbar to open the Open Dialog Box. A file can be opened in the following steps.

1. Move pointer to the file name textbox and double click to select the file

Formating Toolbar: This contains the common tool used for changing the appearance of a document. Its button work like that of the standard toolbar. The function of the button can be known by positioning the tip of cursor on a button and wait for the tool tip to display the name of the button at the same time the status bar will show the function of the button.

Making Text Bold, Italic or Underlined

Text can be made bold in the following steps

1. Select the text to be made bold as explained in chapter1.

2. Click on the bold button on the formatting toolbar. The button appear to be depressed when bold text is selected Similarly text can be made into italic or underlined by selecting it and clicking on the respective toolbars .

Changing Font

Font is the general shape and size and design of characters display on the screen. The size is generally measured in points (where 1 point = 1/72 of an inch). Word's default font and point size is Times New Roman and 10 respectively. Fonts may be printer fonts, screen fonts and True Type Fonts. To ensure that what is displayed on screen is the same in the printed output, it is suggested that True Type fonts be used. These fonts are display with a double T icon. Fonts can be change in the following step.

1. Select the text whose font is to be changed.

2. Click on the drop-down box next to the font box on the formatting toolbar that will show the list of available fonts.

3. Click on the fonts you want to use.

4. Similarly select point size from the font size box next to the font box on the formatting toolbar.

The Help System

Word comes with help, a complete online reference tool that includes step by step procedures that you can follow as you work examples, demos and reference information about using word commands.

You can view word help contents window by choosing contents from the help menu or by choosing Microsoft Word help menu.

You can also use Help button on the standard toolbar to search for a specific topic or to get context sensitive help about item on the screen and commands.

Index: Word includes an on-line index. To look up a topic in the help index choose index from the help menu and click the first letter of the topic you want to read about.

Contents: To get an overview of the help, choose contents from the help menu and click the topic you want to read about in windows you can display step by step procedures while you are working in a document. To do so choose Contents from the help and click.

Context Sensitive Help: To find about an item on the screen click the help button on the standard toolbar and when the pointer changes to a question mark choose the command or click the window item on which you want help. World display the help topic for the selected commands or window item in Help window.

Moving and Copying Text

There are a number of ways in which text can be moved or copied, the commonest being the Drag-and-Drop editing. This method can be used to drag text from one location to another. Text can be dragged in the following steps.

1   Click on the tools menu and select the OPTION' option. This opens the option dialog box, which is a tabbed dialog box.
2. Click on the Edit tab to display the dialog box.
3. Check to see if Drag and Drop text editing option is on it, if the check box in front of the option has an X in it.
4. After this double click on the text to be dragged
5. Place the tip of the pointer on the selected text. This changes the pointer to a left pointing arrow.
6. Hold the left mouse button. This places the selected text in a dotted box at the bottom of the arrow. Drag the mouse so that the insertion point is located at the new location.
7. Click the mouse out side the selected text to remove the highlighting.

This method can also be used to copy text.

1. Select the text to be copied.

2. Point to the selected text, holding down the [Ctrl.] key, then presses the mouse button (Keep both depressed). The pointer looks similar to that in the earlier procedure the pointer includes a plus sing near the tip.

3. The dotted insertion point is then dragged to the location where the text is to be copied and then the mouse button is released followed by the release of the [Ctrl.] key.

4. Click outside the selected text to remove highlighting.

Text can also be moved and copied through the clipboard. This is useful to carry and copy text from one page to another page of the same document or for that matter of the document, since this places the text on a temporary storage location. The edit menu can be used for the 'Cut and Paste' or Copy and paste. Procedures in the following steps.

1. Select the desired text

2. Open the edit menu and click on the cut or copy command to place text on the clipboard.

3. Move the insertion point to the desired location.

4. Again open the edit menu and click on the paste command to insert the text into the new location.

Changing Case

To change the case of selected text does the following:

1. Click on the format menu

2. Click on change case command to display the change case dialog box.

3. Select the case option.

4. Click OK.

Spell Check

Word helps to catch and correct typographical and spelling errors. The spelling program is started by clicking on the spelling button on the standard toolbar. The spell check will begin at the cursor point and process downwards comparing each word to the standard dictionary the Not in dictionary textbook at the top of the dialog box will appear.

The second text box then display suggest replacement from which the desired word is Deleted and then the change button is clicked to apply it. To change a word spelt incorrectly in the entire document click on the change all button. If an unrecognized word is used throughout the text click on the ignore all button each time the word is encountered. When the spelling program reached the end of the document. a dialog box informs you for the same. Click on OK to close the box.

Formatting Paragraphs

Aligning Paragraphs

To make a document attractive and presentable it is necessary that text be aligned in a definite manner. To align a paragraph we use the concerned buttons on the formatting toolbar. For aligning text we can do so with the button on the formatting. Toolbar or through the keyboard.

Button	Keys	Paragraph Containing Cursor is
Align Right	[Ctrl] + [R]	Right Aligned
Center	[Ctrl] + [E]	Centered
Justify	[Ctrl] + [J]	Justify
Align Left	[Ctrl] + [L]	Left Aligned

Setting Tabs

By default tabs are set at a distance of half inch apart across the document. Alignment of text depends upon the type of tab set. There are four types of major tab sets shown in Fig. 13.3.

Type of tab	Ruler Symbol	Function
Align Right	L	Characters shift to the left on the tab stop
Center	⊥	Characters are centered on the tab stop
Align Left	⌐	Characters shift to the right on the tab stop
Decimal	⊥.	Numbers and Characters are aligned on the Decimal point.

Fig. 13.3

Line Spacing

The paragraph indents and spacing dialog box helps to sent paragraph indention spacing and alignment at the same time. This is done as follows.

1. Open Format menu and click on the paragraph to display paragraph dialog box. Select indents and spelling tab.

2. Select the values of both left and right textboxes in the indentation section by moving the adjacent scroll buttons.

3. Set the spacing of the paragraphs by selecting the option form the line spacing down list.

4. Alignment can be changed by clicking an option from the alignment dropdown list box (at the lower right portion of the dialog box).

5. After making the necessary selections, click on the OK button.

Line spacing can also be changed from the keyboard by placing the cursor in the paragraph to change line spacing and doing any one of the following.

Single Spacing   :   [Ctrl] + [1]

Double Spacing   :   [Ctrl] + [2]

Spacing at 1.5   :   [Ctrl] + [5]

Bullet and Numbering

Whenever a list is presented with bullets or is numbered, if marked it easier for the reader to understand the key points. Word can present lists with bullets, numbers or multi level formats in the following manner.

1. Type out a list without any change in indentation, pressing Enter after each item.

2. Select the entire list.

3. Click on bullets button of the formatting toolbar to place a bullet in front of each item.

4. Numbering is also done in a similar way by clicking on the numbering button of the formatting toolbar.

Appearance of bullets and numbers can be controlled by the Bullets and Numbering dialog box which can be evoked from the format menu and styles selected by clicking on it.

13.3 Page Layout

Document Views: When working in Word we have the choice of working with four basic views.

1. Normal

2. Page Layout

3. Outline

4. Master Document

The views or modes can be accessed from the view menu. The normal, page layer and outline modes can be directly activated by clicking on their corresponding buttons located above the status bar to the left of the horizontal scroll bar.

- *The normal view* is the default view used when word is started. This mode allows viewing of regular text, text enhancements and graphic. Graphic displayed in normal view may not appear in the same location in the pointed document, certain page layout elements like Headers; footers etc. are left out in the normal mode to speedup editing.

- *The page layout* mode shown the document as it will appear when it is printed. This mode is useful in finalizing the page element will appear will be display on screen since all details are displayed, this view will take longer time to display changes made in complex documents.

- *The outline page* view display the topical outline of a document, when heading styles are assigned to the section titles of long documents. Working from this view also helps to quickly rearrange topics or promote or demote document headings.

- *The master document* view is commonly used when creating long documents. Working from within this view allows the creation of sub document for a master document. This view also provides an outline of the document and makes it easy to add manipulated or remove subdocuments.

Paper Size and Orientation

It is vary to set the paper size; page orientation (portrait or Landscape) editing of headers and footers and other option before beginning of the document.

When you start a new document word uses the default setting for the pages size, orientation, margins and other options.

if you want to vary the pages layout within a page or between pages you can divide the document into sections.

Pages can be oriented vertically or horizontally.

Option that effect the document are as follows:

- Paper size
- Page orientation
- Margins
- Headers and footers
- Page numbers
- Line numbers
- Number of Newspaper style columns

To select the paper size and page orientation:

- Select the text which needs a different paper size or page orientation, or place the cursor at the point where you want to change.
- From the file menu choose page setup. Now, select paper size tab.
- Select the paper size you want to print and page orientation.
- In the apply To box, select how much of the document you want to print on the selected paper size or the selected orientation.
- Then choose OK button.

Margine

Word provides you with different margins for different section of the document.

To adjust the margins in a document, you can use rulers or the page setup command or Document Layout command on the File menu. By using the rulers in either print preview or page Layout view you can drag the margin boundaries to change the margins.

If the document doesn't contain section, the margin setting affect the entire document. if the document is divided into section you can specify the margin setting that effect the whole document or only the section that contains the insertion point.

To set margin with the ruler:

1. In page Layout view or print preview, place the insertion point in that section where you want to change the margin. If the document does not contain multiple sections it make changes of margin applicable to the whole document.
2. With rulers drag the margin boundaries on the horizontal and vertical rulers, the mouse pointer becomes a double headed arrow when it is over a margin boundary. Word updates the page setup or document Layout dialog box.

You can also use the margin tabs in the page setup or Document Layout dialog box.

Margine and Indentes

A margin specifies the distance from the edge of the paper while an indent specifies additional distance usually measured in from the margin.

When you indent a paragraph word adds the indent measurement to the margin measurement. For e.g. if the document has the 1" left margin and you specify a 5" left indent for a paragraph being with 1.5" from the left edge of the paper.

To specify the Exact measurement and other margin setting :

- Select the Exact the margin you want to change, or place the insertion point in the section whose margin you want to change.
- From the file menu choose page setup or document layout.
- Select the margin tab, and dialog box appears.

Dialog Box Option

Top	:	Distance between the Top of the page and the Top of the first line on the page.
Bottom	:	Distance between the bottom of the page and the bottom of the last line on the page.
Left	:	Distance between the left edge of the page and the left end of the each line with no left indent.
Right	:	Distance between the right edge of the page and right end of each line with no right indent.
Gutter	:	Amount of extra space you want to add to the margin to allow for binding. The extra spaces are added to the left margins of all pages, if you clear the mirror margin.
Mouse Margin	:	If you want to print on both side of the page, select the mirror margin option. This makes the margin of the falling pages, minor images of one another.
Selected section	:	Applies the setting to a selected section.
Preview	:	Display the result of the margin setting before applying to the document.

In apply to box, select, how much of the document you want to apply the new margins and choose OK.

Headers and Footers

A header or footer is text or graphic that is usually printed at the top or bottom of every page in document. A header is printed in the top margin and footer is printed in the bottom margin.

To Create a Header or Footer:

1. From the View menu choose Header and footer.

2. When word display the Header and footer tool bar click the switch between Header and footer button to move to the header or footer area.

   The header and footer area are enclosed by a nonprinting dashed line. Text and graphics in the document are visible but dimmed. To type the next, Type with in the dashed line that surround the header and foot area.

3. To return to the document choose the close button on the header footer toolbar or double click in the main text area.

To delete Header or footer:

1. Position the insertion point in the section with the header or footer you want to delete.
2. From the view menu choose Header and Footer.
3 Select the Header or footer you want to delete and press the backspace or delete key.
4. If you have different Header and Footer in the other section of the document click on show Next/Show Previous button on the Header or Footer toolbar to find the next header or footer you want to delete.
5. To return to main document choose the Close button in header and footer toolbar or double click on the main text area.

Word prints Headers and Footers in the top and bottom margin and if the Header and Footer is too large to fit in the margin, word adjust the top and bottom margin to accommodate the Header and the Footer.

To create different Header and Footer for the first page of the document or section:

1. From the view menu choose Header and Footer.
2. On the Header and Footer toolbar click on page setup option or document Layout button.
3. Select the layout tab.
4. Under headers and footers select the different First page check box, and then choose the OK button.
5. Select show next or show Previous or switch between to move to the page header or footer area in the document and then create the header or footer you want to apply in the rest of the document.

To create header or footer for odd and even pages:

1. Choose the View and select Header or footer.
2. On the Header and footer toolbar click on pages setup option or document layout button.
3. Select lay out tab.
4. Under Header and footer, select the different check box, then choose the OK button.
5. Select show next or show previous or Switch between to move to the pages header or footer area in the document and then create the header or footer you want apply in the rest of the document.

To return to main document, choose the close button to the header and footer toolbar.

Page Numbers

There are two primary ways to add page numbers to your document.

Choose the page Number command from the insert menu. Use this command to add a page number to each page of the document.

Choose the Header and Footer command from the view menu and use this to include additional text with a page number.

When you add page numbers, word insert a page number in every page which can be seen in the document in the print purview. Word updates the page number automatically.

When you inert a page number word put it in the header or footer in the top and bottom margin and aligns it as specified.

To Insert Page Numbers

1. Place the insertion point where you want to add numbers, and then choose page number from the insert menu.

2. To specify where you want to print page numbers, select location in the position box, and an alignment box.

To remove page number

- Position the insertion point in the section from which you want to remove page number and then choose Header and Footers from the view menu.

- Select a page number and the press back space or delete. Word removes the page number in the document.

- After you finish removing the page number choose the close button on the header and Footer toolbar.

To Format Page Numbers

1. Place the insertion point in the section whose page number format you want change.

2. From the insert menu, chose Page numbers.

3. Choose the format menu.

4. In the Number format box select the format you want and choose the OK button.

After you finish changing the page number format choose the close button.

Dialog Box Option

Left	:	At the left margin
Center	:	Centered between left and right margin

Right	:	At the right margin
Show number of first page	:	Display a page number of the first page. To hide the page number on the first page clear this check box.
Format	:	Select formatting option for page numbering.
Preview	:	Show the result of the option you specify before you apply them to the document.

To Insert a Section Break

1. Place the cursor where you want to start a new section.
2. From the insert menu choose break.
3. Under Section breaks select the option that describes where you want the next section to begin.
4. Choose OK button.

Do Delete a Section Break

- In normal view select the section break you want to delete and press backspace or delete.
- When you delete a section break you also delete the section formatting for the text above it. That text becomes part of the section that follows.

Footnotes and Endnotes

Footnotes and Endnotes explain comments on or provide references for the text in a document. You can include footnotes and endnotes in the same document.

To Insert Footnotes and Endnotes:

1. In normal view, position the insertion point, where you want to insert the note reference mark.
2. From the file menu choose print preview.
3. Word the document so that the page numbers are correct and it displays one or more pages including the pages that contain the insertion point.
   - To display one page at a time click the one page button on the preview button.
   - To display two or more pages at a time: click the multiple pages button and select the number and configuration of pages.
   - View a magnified area of the document: Move the mouse pointer to the location you want to view.
   - To hide all screen elements expect the display pages and the print preview toolbar: Click the full screen button on the print preview toolbar. To return the hidden elements to the screen click the full screen button again.

To Print a Document

1. Open the document to print.

2. On the standard toolbar choose the print button.

If the document contains an envelope or a section with a page size that envelop or a section with a page size that is different from the default page size word display the print dialog box again for that envelope or section.

Word displays the print dialog box so that different options of print setting are available.

Through the key board you can print by selecting print command from the file menu.

Dialog Box Options

Printer	:	Display the name of the printer.
Print what	:	Select the information to print.
Copies	:	Type the no. of copies print.
Document	:	Prints the whole document.
Summary info	:	Print the summary information of the document.
Styles	:	Prints only the description for any style in the document.
Page range	:	Specify the page you want to print.
Current Page	:	Prints the selected page containing the insertion
Pages	:	Print the pages you specify.
Print to file	:	Print a document to a new file on the drive you specify instead of routing it directory to a printer.

To print the multiple copies of the entire document: in the copies box type given in the number or selected the number of copes.

To print only odd or even pages: In window select odd pages or Even pages from the print box.

To print selected text: In window under page range select the selection option button.

Choose OK.

When you print a document word formatting is translated into a set of instructions describing each page. The code is then sent to the printer which interprets the instruction to produce the printed document.

Creating and Printing Envelops and Labels

You can use Envelop and Label option under Tools menu to print an address on envelop.

Delivery address: Word locates the mailing address in the document.

If the document contains several addresses select the one you want before choosing the Envelopes and Label command.

Return Address: To print a return address on an Envelop or a mailing label, word uses the address specified in the Mailing Address box on the user info tab of the Option dialog box.

To create and print envelop:

1. If the document contains more than one address, select the delivery address you want to use.
2. From the Tools menu choose Envelop and Labels.
3. Select the Envelops tab.
4. Delivery address.

   In the delivery address box, accepts the proposed delivery address or type the address to which you want send the letter.

5. Return Address.

   To print a return address, accepts the proposed return address in the Return Address box or type the address.

   - *Omit:* This options does not print the return address on the envelope. It is useful when envelop already contains the return address.
   - *Print:* Prints envelop directly to printer
   - If you don't want to print return address select the omit Check Box.
   - *Print preview:* Show the preview of envelops to be printed.
   - *Feed:* Show where to place the envelop in the printer before printing.
   - *Option:* Set option for the size position of the envelop.

6. To select the envelop size, type of Paper feed and other option provide Choose the Option button.

Chang Document

To change an existing envelop that is already attached to a document as a separate section.

The Envelope and Labels commands formats and position address on envelopes.

To print a single Label or same address on an entire sheet of labels

1. From the Tools menu choose Envelopes and Labels.

2. Select the labels tab.

Address	:	Accept the proposed address.
Return Address	:	Prints a return address label that contains
Print	:	Prints a single mailing labels that on an entire sheet.
Label	:	Show the current setting in the label option dialog box.
Option	:	Provides information about the printer and label product and you are using and to specify height and width of each label.

3. To print the deliver address, accept the proposed address in the address box or type the address.

4. To print the return address select the use return address check box and then in the address box either accept the proposed address or type the return address.

5. Under print in the lower left corner of the Labels tab.

   1. To print a single label select the single label option. in the Row and column number or the label sheet type the row and column number for the label you want to print.

   2. To print the same address on an entire sheet of labels select the full page of the same label option button.

   3. To select the label type choose the option button, select the option you want and choose OK.

13.3.1 Column and Table

Coloumn

Many document are formatted into columns like newspaper, brochures etc. For such case word provides not only predefined column layout also provides for customized layouts.

Creating Columns

Columns are created in the following steps:

   1. If the Show /hide option is not already found on, activate it

   2. Place insertion point at the beginning of the document and then press the enter

   3. To create a 2 column layout, drag the pointer across the first two columns that appear in the group column box.

   4. Normal view will show only one column at time. Changing to the page layout mode enables viewing and editing the columns on screen.

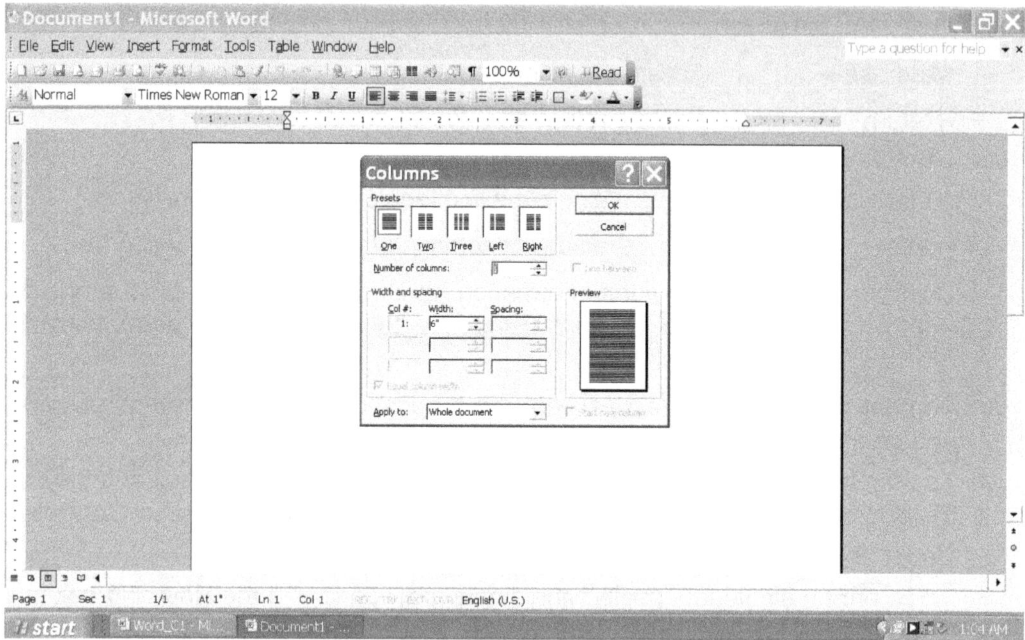

Fig. 13.4

The columns dialog box has 5 present column buttons, along with a width and spacing section width of each column (Fig. 13.4.)

- open the format menu and click the column option to open the column dialog box. it is seen that one present button is already selected by default, having a width of that one present button is already selected by default, having a width of the single column of 6 inches.

- Click on present button two to see the changes in the dialog box.

- Click OK to change the document into two columns.

- Other present option can be chosen in a similar manner.

Change Column Width, and Inserting A Line between Columns

When column are uneven in width, the width of a column can be adjusted by dragging one of its margin marker to a new location. When all the columns are equal in width changing one margin marker affects the dialog box

- display the column dialog box and turn off the equal column width option

  - Select the desired column number in the width and spacing section.

  - Enter desired width and space

  - Repeat above two steps as needed

  - Click OK.

Creating Manul Column Breaks

Word automatically breaks each column at the bottom of the page and sends the remaining information to the top of the next column. A manual column break is created in the following steps.

- bring the screen to page layout view and place the insertion point at the top of the document
- Place the insertion point at the top of the document. point at the point from where you want the text to appear in the next column i.e. the where the manual column break is to be inserted.
- The manual break is created by pressing [Ctrl]+[Shift]+[Enter].

Inserting Section Breaks

Section breaks are inserted to vary the number of columns displays within a document. Insertion of a section break followed by selection of the continuous option word starts the next section on the same page as the section preceding the section break marker.

Section breaks are inserted in the following manner:

- Open format menu and click on column to display columns dialog box.
- Open the insert menu and click the break command to display the break dialog box.
- Click the continuous option, in the section breaks section. This allows for the second section to be printed on the same page as the first section.
- Click OK
- To start a section on the next page, under the section breaks option of the break dialog box and click Next page to start this section at the top of the next page Click OK.

13.4 Electronic Worksheet or Spreadsheet

An electronic spreadsheet or worksheet is used to store information in the memory of a computer, ask the computer to calculate results, and display the information and results on the computer screen in a desired manner. In other words, it replaces the normal paper sheet or ledger, pencil, eraser and calculator. In such a worksheet, information is entered through the keyboard and displayed on the computer screen. The information thus entered can be easily changed or modified. The worksheet calculates results for example it can calculate the total sales by multiplying the quantity sold with the unit cost. If any of the original information is changed, the worksheet automatically recalculates all results. The worksheet displays results in the graphical form, and the output thus obtained can also be printed.

The applications of worksheets are varied and all kinds of information can be stored in them. Some common applications of a spreadsheet are in the following areas.

1. Annual reports of business firms.

2. Income statement and income tax calculations.

   - Payrolls.
   - Billings
   - Accounts payable and receivable.
   - Production and marketing analysis.
   - Investment and loan analysis
   - Banking and other financial services.
   - Inventory control
   - Tender Evaluation
   - Scientific calculations
   - Cost-effective Analysis

13.4.1   Advantages of Electronics Spreadsheet

The Major advantages of Electronic spreadsheets are as follows:

- The results are accurate.
- Excel has the facility of automatically recalculating all formulas that are used, even if a small change is made in any of the figures. This saves lot of time in manual recalculating and changing of figures.
- The worksheet can be quite big in size and any part of it can be viewed and edited.
- Data entered can be formatted in several ways to give a professional look.
- Several mathematical, trigonometric, financial and statistical functions are built in and all types of complicated calculations can be performed using these built in functions, facilitating rapid operation.
- Data can be viewed graphically and these graphs are of different types and can also be printed.
- Worksheet is saved as electronic files that can be retrieved and modified later.
- Existing worksheets can be merged with any existing or new worksheet.
- The information entered in a worksheet can be sorted in any desired format.
- With the electronic worksheet, one can easily and quickly produce reports and get answers to what-if questions.
- The information stored in a worksheet can be transformed to other software programmed like Word, WordStar, Fox Pro, dBase etc.

13.4.2   Excel

Excel is an integrated electronic worksheet developed by Microsoft Corporation, USA. It has three basic components of Worksheet, Graph and Database management. It lets you create a worksheet and enter information. It performs all types of calculations and displays results on the screen in the form of figures and graphs. Various database management functions on the data entered in the worksheet can be performed. Excel has all the advantages mentioned in. Besides it has other important features like:

- Date and time related functions
- Manipulation of character data (strings)
- Database management
- Keyboard macros.
- Drawing toolbar to create Graphics.
- A worksheet can have several multiple sheets.

Creating a New Workbook

Excel makes it easy to design a new workbook to suit your purpose. It is done in the following steps:

1. Open a new worksheet.
2. On the File menu, click Save As.
3. Type Technology as the file name.
4. Click the Save button.

Enter and Format Titles

Using titles on the worksheets makes it easier to read and understand the information shown. You can retain the existing styles, create your own styles or customize your own workbook template. The next exercise illustrates how easy it is to enter and modify font styles and sizes in your worksheet.

Entering and Formating a Title on the Worksheet

1. With the Technology worksheet open, move the pointer to cell E3, type Technology, Challenge and then press enter.
2. Click cell E3
3. On the formatting toolbar, click the Font box, and click Arial. (You may have to use the down arrow next to the Font box to find Arial)
4. On the formatting toolbar, click the arrow next to the Font size box, click 14 and then click the bold button.

   You can add other formatting characteristics to your titles. To make the text bold, click the text cell, and click the bold button on the formatting toolbar.

Entering Column Headings and Adjusting Column Widths

Column headings help you and others understand the data or information you have entered on your worksheet. Sometimes the column heading is too large to fit into a column. Even though it does not show the entire title or formula, the cell still contains every thing you entered into it. This exercise show you how to increase or decrease the column width to fit the information you are entering.

Entering column heading and adjusting its widths:

(i)   Using the Technology worksheet, click cell B5, and type Dates in cell B5.

(ii)   Press tab to go to cell C5, and then type Elementary schools.

(iii)   Press tab to go to cell D5, and then type Secondary schools. One cell will overlap the other.

(iv)   Press enter.

Arranging Text with the Copy, Paste, and Cut Commands

With Excel it is easy to modify data. When the features in Excel are used to create a table you may decide on a different order of column heads or you may want to revise them. It is important to make changes before you build a formula for the chart in order to maintain correct calculations.

Usually Cut is used to remove the contents of a cell or cell to a different location. Copy is used to duplicate the contents of a cell in another location

Using the Cut, paste, and copy commands to arrange text

1.   Using the Technology worksheet, right –click cell C3, and click Cut.
2.   Right- click cell C1, and click Paste.
3.   Right- click cell D5, and click Cut.
4.   Right- click cell D10, and click Paste.
5.   Right- click cell C5, and click Cut.
6.   Right- click cell D5, and click Paste.
7.   Right- click cell D10, and click Cut.
8.   Right- click cell C5, and click Paste.
9.   Try dragging cell C5 and cell C5 to new location as you did in the previous exercise.
10. Close the file without saving.

Entering Data

Using Excel is a powerful way to enter and display data or text. For example, you can have Excel display a date showing the month, day, and year with the time, or showing only the first letter of the month, followed by a two –digit year. Numbers can be display as whole numbers, numbers with decimals, or numbers written in scientific notation.

Doing Simple Calculations

Using Excel, You can perform a wide range of mathematical calculation and function according to what you need from your data. To calculate sums (total) and percentage, use the mathematical operation of adding number to get a total, and then divide each number that was just added by that total.

Note:Office Assistant has information on different ways to enter a formula so that you can perform a variety of mathematical calculations.

In the Technology workbook, click E5, type Total Sites, and press enter.

Click cell E5 again, and on the formatting the toolbar, click the Bold button.

Click cell E6, and on the formula toolbar click the Edit Formula button (the =sing).

Click the Function arrow, and choose Sum.(C6:D6 appears in the window.

Click OK.

To sum each pair of numbers, click E6 and drag the fill handle from E.

Calculating the percentage of school
1. Click cell F5, type % of RDIST schools, and then press enter.
2. Click cell F5 again, and then click the Bold button on the formatting toolbar.
3. Click cell G5, type% of Sec. Schools and then press enter.
4. Click cell G5 again, and on the formatting toolbar click the bold button.
5. Click F6, and click the Edit Formula button (the = sign)
6. Type C6/E6 and click OK.
7. On the formatting menu, click cells. On the Number and tab, choose percentage, and the type 2 in the decimal places.
8. Click F6 and drag the fill handle to F12 to calculate the percentage for each pair of number click OK.
9. Repeat step3 through 8 for Secondary Schools using the formula D6/E6 to calculate the percentage.
10. Save the worksheet and close it.

Customizing the Enter Key

You can change the direction in which the pointer moves when you press enter. If the default direction is to the right, and you are entering data in a column, you can change the default to down. You can change the direction of the pointer to support your movements.

Changing the direction of the enter key:

1. Open a new workbook.
2. On the Tools menu, click Option.
3. Click the Edit tab.
4. Click move selection after Enter, and in the Direction box, click Right, and click OK.
5. Repeat step 1 through 4 to change the direction back to Down.
6. Close the workbook without saving it.

Creating a One-Input Data Table

Using Excel, you and your student can learn the cost associated with making payments on purchases. You can easily calculate monthly payments based on interest and balance due on purchases. In the next exercise, you can calculate monthly payments based on interest and total cost of a car, showing how the loan term and interest rates affect monthly payments.

Note

All formula start with the =sing in a cell.

Calculating car payments:

1. Open a new workbook.
2. Click Sheet2 at the bottom of the window.
3. In cell 2, type car payment Schedule.
4. Type the text and formulas in the cells shown in the chart:

    Note: When you enter a formula and press enter, the result appears in the cell, and the formula is displayed in the formula box.
5. Click cell C11, and on the formula toolbar, Click Edit Formula button (the=sing).
6. Click the Function arrow, and click PMT, if visible.

    -or-

Click more Functions.

7. In the Function category, click Financial.
8. In the Function name, click PMT, and then click OK.
9. Click the Shrink button at the right of the input area, click D5 on the worksheet, and then press enter.
10. In the Rate box, click after D5, and type /12.
11. Click the Nper window, and click the Shrink Button.
12. Click D6 on the worksheet, and press enter.
13. Click the Pv window, and click the Shrink Button.
14. Click D7 on the worksheet, and press enter.

15. Click OK.

16. To change the months of the loan to 24, type 24 in cell D5.

17. To change the interest rate to 12.5 percent to demonstrate how the payment changes, type 12.5 in cell D4. Try several combination on your own, and see how it works.

18. Close the workbook without saving.

Order of Calculation in Excel

You have just discovered one easy formula in Excel. There are many other that help you calculate or analyze everything from finance to statistical sampling plans. When you combine several mathematical steps in a formula, they are performed in a specific order. Excel will start calculating from the left to the right according to the following order of operations:

- - ()   Parentheses
- - -   Negative number if used with one operand
- - %   Percentage
- - ^   Exponentiation
- - *and/   Multiplication and division
- - +and-   Addition and subtraction
- - &   connects two text values to produce one continuous text value
- - =,<,<=,>,>=,<> Comparison operator for reference, the Comparison operator.
- - =   Equal to
- - <   Less then
- - <=   Equal to or less than
- - >   Greater then
- - >=   Equal to or greater than
- - <>   not equal to

Note: for example and meanings of calculation operator in formulas, click office Assistant, and type Operators.

Copying Formulas

Once you have created a formula, you can quickly and easily copy it into adjacent cells to calculate student records that contain the same type of data.

1. Using the worksheet from the previous lesson, click the L4 cell to select it.

2. Click and drag the file handle at the lower-right corner of the cell to the bottom of the column, and release the pointer.

3. Save your file with the name student List.

Note: Refer to Office Assistant for more information on conditional Formatting.

Applying a Formula to Equally Weighted Tests

Now that you have recorded test scores and calculated averages, you can easily figure letter grades from numbered scores using Excel.

For this type of formula, Excel Computers data with a formula that evaluates the data to a logical value of true (1) or false (0). Using Excel to calculate grades is quick and easy. The formula interprets a range of data such as>89 (Which means 90or more) and assigns a letter grade if the data meets the criteria (score is >89-true or false). Therefore, you have a conditional commonly known as an If- Then statement for equally weight tests.

Creating letter grades from number scores

- Open the file named Student list that was saved from the previous exercise.
- Position the pointer in cell M3, type grade, and then re click M3.
- On the formatting toolbar, click the bold button to make the heading bold.
- Click cell m4, and enter the following, very carefully: =IF (L3>89,"A".IF(L3>79,"B".IF(L3>69,"C".IF(L3>59."D","F"))))
- Click and drag the fill handle in cell M4 to cell M10
- Save the workbook.

Analyzing Scores

Sometimes the test and assignments you give are not equal in importance, making the grading process more complex. Excel can help you analyze these types of test scores.

Calculating mean, median, and standard deviation for each test

1. Continuing in your student list workbook, click cell B12, and type Average.
2. Click cell B13, and type Median.
3. Click cell B14, and type Standard Deviation.
4. Click cell D12, and on the Standard toolbar click Paste Function.
5. In the Function category, make sure Statistic is selected, and in the Function type, click Average, and then click OK.
6. if D4:D10 is not in number 1, type it in.
7. Click OK.

8. Click cell D13.

9. On the insert menu, click Function.

10. In the Function category, click Statistics, and in the Function   type, click Median, and then click OK.

11. If D4:D10 is not in number 1, type it in.

12. Click OK.

13. Click cell D14, and type = STDEVP(D4:D10)

14. Select cell D12, D13, and D14.

15. Click and drag the fill handle to column L.

16. Right-click the row header 12,and click Format Cells.

17. In Decimal place, type 1.

18. Adjust the decimal to 2 places for the standard Deviation.

19. In Decimal places, type 2.

20. Save the workbook.

13.4.3 Calculation by Using Formulas

In MS-Excel a formula always begins with an equal to Sign C=S. In a simplest formula of Excel the Excel to Sign is followed by a set of values separated by +, -, *, or / for example :

   = 20+6 + 5

The above said formula when entered in any blank cell of Excel worksheet gives the result 31.

	A	B	C	D	E	F	G
	NAME	MATHS	HINDI	SCIENCE	ENGLISH	SUM	%
1	RAM	89	68	95	92	=B2+C2+D2+E2	=F2/4
2	NAIVEDYA	92	70	92	88	=B3+C3+D3+E3	= F3/4
3	NEETA	86	90	91	66	=B4+C4+D4+E4	=F4/4
4	NISHTHA	72	89	86	72	=B5+C5+D5+E5	E5/4

The above worksheet is a sample worksheet to calculate the total mark obtained by the four students of a class. The marks of four subjects Math, Hindi, Science, English are given. Formulas are used in column E and Column F to calculate the total marks obtained by each student and their percentage.

Calculation by Using Functions

The spreadsheet software provides built in functions to perform the simple mathematical functions. Functions provide by MS-Excel are as shown in the Table :

S.No.	Function Name	Operation
1.	Average	Find Average
2.	Max	Find the maximum Value
3.	Min	Find the Minimum Value
4.	Round	Convert the integer with decimal places into whole number
5.	Sum	Find the sum of given numbers
6.	IF	Check for given condition
7.	Count	Counts the number
8.	Lookup	Look up the value in vertical coloumn

Although there are a lot of functions besides the above listed functions.

SUM

The function SUM is used to find the sum of given numbers. In this function entered the ranged of cells specified with the function.

Syntax:

= SUM (First cell, Last cell)

e.g. (In Table 1)

= SUM (B2,E2) = 334

13.4.4   Graphs Creation

In MS-Excel, charts and graphs are made to represent the data in pictorial methods. These graphs are plotted very easily using the chart wizard available as a button on the tool bar. A varity of charts or graphs can be plotted by using the data stored in the worksheet. The various types of charts are : Line, Pie, Bar, Area, Doughnut, 3-D etc.

Steps for plotting Graphs :

- Select the range of cells
- Click the next button to confirm your selection
- Select the type of chart and click next.
- Tables of the chart, chart title and other information to be added to your chart.
- Finally the preview comes in front of you.
- Click the finish button.

13.4.5 Databases in a Worksheet

Databases are an organised collection of related information. All information Pertaining to a single individual are present in one line and called a Record. In a record information may be broken up into different categories like name, locality, city, pin etc. each of these categories are called fields. The column headings are called fieldnames. The row containing the field name is the header row.

Database can be located any where in the worksheet, and may contain labels, numbers etc. All worksheet commands and functions; number of database related commands and functions are available. Information in a database can be arranged in any manner as desired.

Essential of Database

Database can be entered into any area in the worksheet and is based on the following rules

- The first row of the database not necessarily the row 1, must contain fieldnames.

- Fieldnames are not case sensitive.

- Each fieldname must be unique and indicative of the information it contains.

- Rows below the fieldnames contain records and one set of information must fit into one row. If this dose not happens, either the column width must be increased or the field must be broken into two or more fields.

- There should be no blank rows or divider lines between fieldnames or records.

- One has to make sure that correct information is fed into the correct field; else wrong output will be obtained when information is to be retrieved from the database.

- Space should not be typed before numbers while entering them into the database.

- No extra space should be typed after typing entries in the database.

Creating a Database

This is done in the following steps:

- Press ^N to create a new worksheet

- Change the width of column A, B, and C11 and enter data

- Save the worksheet as STAFF1.

Sorting a Database

With excel one can arrange stored information in any desired order. For example the above created database can be arranged in an alphabetical order or one can even sort on multiple fields at the same time.

Using the Sort Buttons

Database can be quickly sorted in an ascending or descending order using the SORT buttons provided on the standard toolbar. This is the following steps

- Move the cell pointer to anywhere in column A which has to be sorted.
- Click the button to sort in ascending order or the button to sort in a Descending Order. The change takes place immediately.

The SORT button can sort out only on a single field, to sort on multiple fields the Data, sort command has to be used.

Using the Data, Sort Command

Position the cell pointer anywhere in the database. If the cell pointer is Position in the column on which you want to sort, Excel automatically picks up that column as the Sort order.

To sort the database on the Name field, move anywhere in Column A in the database range.

- Open the data menu and then choose the sort Command from the Data menu. Excel automatically select the database range and opens the Sort dialog not provided.
- This dialog box allows you to sort the selected database on up to 3 fields. The 'my list has' box at the bottom is to ensure that the header row is not including in the sorting process.
- When we want to sort on multiple fields, Excel sort on the first field called the primary key and then sorts all records within the primary key on second field.

Maintaining a Database

Efficient maintenance of information in a database is possible by using data form. This allows one to view and edit one record at a time and also allow adding or deleting records. We use the data form on the employees' database in STAFF1 worksheet created above.

The cell pointer is moved to any where in the database range

Use the data, from the menu and Excel display a data form on the worksheet.

- Move the cell pointer to F5 and enter department
- In cell F6 enter Personal (so space should be typed before or after the word)

- Move the cell pointer any anywhere in the database range A5:D13. This will enable Excel to automatically pick the database range for the advanced filter.
- Use the Data, Filter, Advanced Filter command from the menu. Excel display the Advanced Filter dialog box.
- Specify the criteria range by clicking against it in the advanced filter dialog box, and enter the criteria range.
- After the list and criteria ranges in the Advance dialog box has been specified, ask Excel to apply the criteria to the data base. All the records not meeting the criteria are hidden.
- Selecting the data, Filter, Show All command from the menu, and excel display all records in the employee database.

Values as well as formulas can be used as criteria to search records in a database. Formula can be used as criteria when the corresponding field contains numeric data.

Sometimes we may have to search for records that satisfy a particular formula. When this done excel evaluates the formula for each record in the database. If the result of the formula is true for a record, it is included when the Data filter and advanced filter command is used. The records that do not satisfy the criteria are excluded from the result.

Copying Records

When records satisfying particular criteria need to be copied to another location, we use the copy to location option in the Advance filter dialog box. This is done in the following steps:

- Place the cell particular anywhere in the range
- Choose Data, Filter, Advanced filter command from the menu
- Click to another location option
- Specify an output range where the data is to be copied say we are to start from A15, place cell pointer at A15
- Click OK

Using Subtotals and Grand Totals

In excel calculate grand totals for a database. For example in the above example, we can calculate how much the salary for the employees is working in various departments and the total salary for all employees. This is done in the following steps:

- Move the cell pointer to anywhere in the database range.
- Use Data, Sort command, Excel displays the Sort dialog box.

- If the sort by field contains Department, click OK else use the drop-down arrow for the Sort by field box and choose Department and click the OK.
- Choose Data, subtotals command from the menu and Excel displays the subtotal.
- Click the OK button and Excel calculate the subtotal and grand total for the department field.
- Excel automatically inserts the required number of rows to enter the subtotal for each department and the grand total at the end of the list.

To remove the subtotals and grand totals

- Choose data, subtotals command from the menu
- Click the remove all button.

13.4.6   Printing the Worksheet

The print button on the standard toolbar or the print command on the file menu enables you to print the entire or a specified part of the worksheet. We a work sheet id printed, the page setup and margins can be changed. This facilitates printing of reports in any desired format.

Printing a Worksheet

To open a file the following is done

- Open the worksheet file.
- Open the file menu and choose the print command
- Excel display the print dialog box
- The print dialog box helps in selecting the matter to be printed and also helps in setting up option like number of copies, page range etc. The top left corner of the dialog box is the name of current printer and printer port.
- Choose the option in the dialog box and click OK.

Removing Gridlines from the Printout

To remove the gridlines from the printout change option in the page setup dialog box in the following way:

- Open the file menu
- Select page setup command
- A page setup dialog box is displayed, select sheet from it
- Click the gridline checkbox and ensure that it is not selected (shown by a cross if selected)
- Click OK button to close the page setup dialog box

Other Ways to Start to Print a Worksheet

Press ^P or click the print button. On clicking the print button Excel start   printing the worksheet. On pressing ^P, Excel display the print dialog box, in which case click ok to print the worksheet.

Using Print Preview

Sometimes after printing the worksheet, we realize that worksheet need some modification then we modify it and print again. If we missed some change and we want to make that change and print the worksheet again, instead of it, the print preview can be used, which allows us to view the printout on the screen. The print preview command can be chosen either from the print preview button or from the file menu.

In the preview mode the complete page including header, footer and actual margins along with a new toolbar are displayed. The standard and formatting toolbar will not be displayed. The print preview toolbar also contains the print button through which we can directly go to the print dialog box. The setup and margins buttons can be used to adjust page setup and margin respectively, while the close button closes the preview mode.

Page Setup and Margins

To select page size

- Open File menu
- Choose Page setup command
- In the page setup dialog box displayed select page tab
- Here selected from the option of paper size, Orientation and other options
- The print quality box at the bottom of the page setup dialog box helps select print quality
- The margin option helps in defining the height and width of the page and actual print space
- The headers and footers can also be defined from the page setup option.

Defining Header and Footer

The header and footers are defined in the following manner:
- Open the page setup dialog box through the page setup command.
- Select the header/Footer page in the page setup command.
- Select the custom header button to display the Header dialog box.
- Select the option to create a customized header

Print Option

It is also possible to select what is to be printed from the print dialog box. In the print what box are three option of Selection, Selected sheet(s) and entire workbook. By default, the selected sheet (sheets) button is selected. The selection option is used to print a specified range and in case there are multiple pages, the entire workbook option is chosen. By default one copy of all pages is printed, however multiple copies can also be printed by entering the desired number.

13.5   Powerpoint

13.5.1   Starting power point

- Click the start button in the lower-left corner.
- On the Start menu, click the insertion point on programs.
- Click Micro power point.

13.5.2   Exploring the power point dialog box

When you first open the program, the power point dialog box present four way to create a presentation

- Auto Content wizard creates a slide set within theme you select presentations
- Template create slides from pre-designed slide sets for standard presentations
- Blank presentation creates slide that you design from scratch
- Open an existing presentation allows you to modify a presentation that you someone else has already created.

Starting a presentation from the power point:

Start-up window

Click Blank Presentation and click OK.

On new slide click OK.

Here is the dialog box you see when you first open power point.

13.5.3   Creating a new presentation

You can create a new presentation at any time even if you others are open. You can use a wizard or template when you create a new presentation to save time. Wizards help you design meeting planners, project updates, personal home pages, and other presentation. You can also select from more than 25 presentation styles.

Designing the first slide

Creating a title slide

- On the file menu, click new.
- On the General tab, click Blank presentation, and click OK.

o In the new slide dialog box, click the upper-left page layout that show

o Close the presentation.

   ▪ Creating a document using a template

o On the file menu, click New

o Click each tab to view presentation design templates and presentation wizards.

o On the presentation design tab, click high voltage-pot, and view the presentation template in the preview window.

o Click OK.

o On the new slide tab, click the Bulleted list Auto Layout (top, row, second column), and click OK.

o Close the presentation.

Using template to create presentation in power point saves time. You can create a series of slide or presentation with a common look, or you can create different design to distinguish one set of concept from another

Using the Auto Content wizard

The Auto content wizard is an easy-to-use wizard that help you create a presentation by leading you through some basic question. From your answers to the questions, power point selects the best style and built-in out line to suit your presentation. The wizard asks you to respond to question and then uses your answer to automatically lay out and format your presentation.

Using the Auto Content wizard to create a presentation

- On the file menu, click New

- On the presentation tab, click Auto Content Wizard. pwz, and click OK.

- Click the next button to move to presentation type on the flowchart.

- In the select the type of presentation you're going to give list, click Generic.

- Click next to move to out put option on the flowchart.

- To move the How will this presentation be used? Question, click presentation, informal meetings, handouts, and then click next to move to presentation style flowchart.

- To the what type of out put will you use? question, click On-screen presentation.

- To the will you print handouts? question, click No, and then click next to move to presentation option on the flowchart.

- In the presentation title box, type welcome to fall open House.

- In the name box, type Pat Kirkland.

- In the Additional information box, type music class, click next, and then click Finish.

- Your presentation is now in out line view.
- If you exit the wizard before you finished creating your presentation, you will not be able to save your work.

Closing a new presentation without saving it

- On file menu, click Close.
- Click No to the question 'Do you want to save the change you made to presentation'?
- Each presentation is numbered consecutively until it is saved with a specific name. The x used at right is a placeholder because the number will vary from user to user.

Creating and editing slides

Editing and creating slides in power point is easy. Power point identifies the slide area that you can fill by placing sample text in them

Creating a Slide

- On the File menu, click New.
- On the presentation Design tab, click high voltage pot, and then click OK.
- Click to add title, and type this is the title.
- Click to add text, and type this is text. Then Press enter to add the next bullet.
- Type this is next, tool to match the screen shot.
  You can edit slides at any time by clicking the text you want to change. Then you can delete text, add text, or change text.

To edit a slide

- Suppose you have typed the word "The" and want to edit
- Click in front of h in the title you just typed
- Press back space until you see the word "The".
- Press the right arrow key to move the insertion point to the end of the line in front of the period.
- Add one space and type is "good".
- Position the insertion point in front of "good", press delete to remove the word "good", and then type short, to create The title is "short".
- Press backspace to delete text in front of the insertion point.
- Press delete to delete text after the insertion point

13.5.4   Viewing Presentations

There are five different ways to view your presentation in power point. As you become familiar with the power point view, you can customize the menu and add buttons to the tool bar to make it even easier and quicker to create presentations. The view are accessed by button (shown below) which are located in the lower-left corner of your screen.

- Slide view is the easiest to use when you are designing your presentation slide by slide.
- Outline view helps you organize your presentation in out line format.
- Slide Sorter view show your entire set of slide on-screen, so that you can check the order and completeness of your presentation.
- Notes page view presents the slide in miniature so you can add notes to each one for your presentation.
- Slide show view puts your presentation together so you can view it complete with sound and animation.

Creating and viewing slide in different formats

Power point provides several ways to create and view slides within your presentation. You can create master slide style or default slide formats. The formats include bullets, two column, tables, charts, clipart, and blank slides. These formats make it easy to quickly make slides that support your classroom instruction.

To create a view slide from the menu bar

1. On the insert menu, click New slide.
2. Double-click the 2Column Text Auto layout.
3. Repeat step 1, and then double –click the Text & Chart Auto Layout.

Creating and viewing slides in different formats

Use the vertical scroll bar to move from slide to your presentation:

- Click once above or below the shade portion (i.e., the scroll box) of the scroll box.-or-
- Drag the scroll box up and down.-or-
- Click the up or down arrow on the scroll bar.

13.5.5   Saving your work

When you create a presentation, you must save your work in a logical place on the computer. Just like filing a document in a file drawer, storing a computer document requires some attention to how you name it and where you place it, in order for you to be able to find it again, once you have saved the presentation. Be sure to save to a location that makes sense and is easy to find. Saving files can be accomplished in many ways. If you forget to save, don't worry : Office Assistant will remind you.

Saving for the first time

When you save the file for the first time, you should name the file as descriptively, but a briefly, as possible. Sometimes, you will want to name it as a particular version or as a type of presentation (i.e., fall Open House or Technology Grant). The steps involved in saving a document:

- On the file menu, click Save.
- In the file name box, enter a relevant and specific name, to make it easy to identify the memo again.
- Click Save.-or-press enter to save the file.

Saving to a different location

To save a different name or to a different folder or disc drive

- On the file menu, click Save As to save the document with a new name
- In the save in box, select a folder or drive.
- Enter a different name in the fill name box.
- Unless you specify otherwise, the program saves all files to a default folder on your computer called my documents.

Saving your document as another file type

If you are saving your document to share with other who may have a version of power point that is different from yours or other kinds of presentation software or files, you may need to select a different file type. By saving your file as a specific type, you make it possible for others to read and download your presentation on their computer system and software.

Saving to other Power point file types

You may want to save your presentation in a different file type. Using power point you can create a slide show presentation and present it on a computer that dose not have power point installed. With the pack and go wizard, you can take the presentation on a disc and run the slide show using only the power point viewer (instead of the entire software program) that the wizard copies on your disk or laptop computer.

Saving to earlier versions of power point

- On the file menu, click saves as.
- Click the Save as type down arrow to see format types.
- Click Power point show (*.ppt) to save as another power point program file type.
- Click Save.

Saving to other presentation programs

If you want to share a file with someone who has different presentation software or transfer the file to another computer that has different software, you can save your presentation in the file format used by another program.

- On the File menu Click save as.
- Click the save as type down arrow to see format types
- Click outline/RTF (*.rtf) to select a generic file format.
- Click Cancel.

13.5.6 Printing your presentation

Power Point offers several print option to help you. Prepare your presentation. Using Power point you can print to transparencies, slides, handouts and notes to support your lessons. When you print transparencies, make sure that film appropriate to your printer type is in the paper tray. Always quit the program before you turn off your computer.

Printing presentation slides involves the following :

- On the File menu, click print –or – press ctrl + p.
- In the print what drop-down list box at the bottom, click slides (without animations).
- Click OK

Printing other outputs

You can print other types of presentation output using the Print what list.

- Handouts print two, three or six slides per page. You may use Handout to provide an outline of your presentation to your class.
- Notes pages print one slide per page and have room for your presentation notes.
- Outline view allows you to print the outline you used to develop your presentation.

Quitting Power Point

There are several ways to quit power point97. Always follow proper procedure. All office applications prompt you to save changes.

Quitting Power Point with the Standard toolbar

- On the File menu, click OK.
- Click yes to save your document and you want to quit word now.
- Click No, If you do not want to save the document for future use and you want to quit power point now.

Using power point templates you can quickly and easily create presentations for many purposes, including meeting handouts and agendas, speaker introductions, academic content and information or invitational flyers.

Using a template to create a flyer.

Creating a school activity flyer.

1. Open Power point -   Click Templates and click OK

2. Click the presentation tab, and then double-click Flyer (standard)

3. On slide 1, click to add title, and type French club meeting.

4. Click to add sub-title, and type Tuesday

5. Position the insertion point before the T and Tuesday, and press enter.

6. Click the double-down arrow on the vertical scroll bar to move to the -next slide.

7. After you cerate the title on one slide of your hand out, you need to include all of the necessary information about the meeting on the other slide. The power point wizard helps you cover all the important items.

Adding key information to a flyer wizard.

1. Click in front of the E in Event name, and press delete until Event Name is erased.

2. Type French Club.

3. Click in front of the T in time of Day, and press delete until time of the day is erased.

4. Repeat step 3 to delete the template text and add the rest of the information about the meeting, as shown in the screenshot which follows.

5. After you have entered all the information, you can print the flyer.

6. Close the file without saving it, and quit power point.

7. For extra effect, you can copy the flyers onto colored paper to attract more attention.

Presentation Printing

- On the file menu, click print.

- In the print what box, click Slides.

- Select scale to fit paper, and click OK.

13.5.7   Developing a Presentation Style with Power Point

Selecting a presentation style

Power point has many different presentation styles from which to choose. Depending on what you are creating, different presentation styles may fit your needs. First you have to select an overall look for your presentation.

Creating a presentation style with power point

- On the format menu, click and preview several designs.
- Under presentation Design, click and preview several designs.
- Click Notebook pot, and click Apply.

Changing the presentation style

Using power point it is easy to change presentation styles. Depending on the material and audience you are addressing, you may want to select specific style or keep a consistent style for a topic or series of lesson.

Changing an existing presentation style

- On the view menu, click slide sorter.
- A shortcut to a different view is to use the buttons on the view toolbar
- Double click Contemporary. Pot.

If at any time you select a style that you do not want to use for your presentation, you can easily and quickly change to another style. Or you can try several different styles to find one that fits your presentation.

Undoing or redoing a design choice

- On the Edit menu, click undoes Apply Design.
- On the Format menu, click Apply design.
- Double-click zesty. Pot.
- On the edit menu, Click Undo Apply Design, click Redo Apply Design, and then click Undo Apply Design.

Customizing the background

Depending on how you presentation, a change in the background may make it easier to see and read your information. Customize the background allow you to change the color behind every side.

Changing the background color for each slide

- On the format menu, click Background.
- In the Background dialog box, click the down arrow, and the click the red square.
- Click Preview to see how the color change will look in your slide.
- Click Apply to all to make the change to your entire presentation.

Selecting color and fonts

Changing the color scheme is more dramatic than changing the background color. Completing your color selection is the next step in customizing your presentation.

There are two make change to almost all parts of a presentation including notes and handouts.

Changing the color scheme for all slides

- On the Format menu, click Slide color scheme.
- Click the standard color scheme in the second row.
- Click Apply to all to make the change to your entire presentation.
- Customize the color scheme.
- On the format menu, click Slide color scheme.
- Click the custom tab, and then click the Background color scheme box.
- Click change color, click a blue spot at the top of the hexagon, and then click OK.
- Click preview to see how the color will look.
- Chang the rest of the option under scheme colors as desired.
- Click Apply to all to make the color changes to the entire document.

Replacing fonts in a presentation

The second step in customize your presentation to choose appropriate fonts. Whether you have completed a presentation or are working on one, you can easily change some or all of fonts. With power point, it is easy to make comprehensive replacing fonts in your presentation.

- On the Format menu, click replaces Fonts.
- In the with drop-down box, click Arial Black.
- Click Replace.
- Repeat steps 1-3 until you have selected the most effective fonts for your presentation.
- Click close when you have finished.

Creating headers and footers in your presentation

As you create presentation, you may go through several drafts or of several people working on a presentation. Using the headers and footers is an easy way to ensure that version and author do not get mixed up.

Adding page numbers, author and creation dates to presentation

- On the view menu, click Header and footer
- On the Slide tab, under including on slide select Date and time and Update automatically.
- Select slide number to print a number on each slide.
- Select Footer, and type How a Bill Become a Law in the Footer text box.
- Select don't show on title slide.
- Click Apply to all to make these changes throughout the presentation.

Power point gives you two choices of dates:

- Update automatically
- Fixed.

The Update automatically option insert the current date and then updates the date every time presentation is opened. The Fixed option freezes it. Date to whatever date you type. Use Update automatically as you create and modify your presentation to keep track of most current version. Add the time if you are printing more than one copy of your presentation in a day.

13.5.8   Using Chart and Table with Power Point

Creating slide layout for table and charts

The built slide layout makes it easy to combination text with chart and table in your presentation.

Crating a new title slide

- On new slide, click OK to open Title slide.
- Click to add title, and type Congressional Information.
- Click to add sub title, press enter
- Type Based on the 105th Congress.
- On the Format menu, click Apply design.
- On the presentation design tab, click Notebook, pot, and then click apply.
- On the File menu, click save, and type House Organization.

Creating an organization chart

Using the organization chart template you can quickly and easily create one.

Creating a new slide for an organization chart
- On the insert menu, click new slide.
- Double-click the organization Chart Auto Layout.
- Click to add title.
- Type House organization Chart.

Creating an organization chart
- Double-click to add org chart.
- In the Microsoft Organization Chart window, Click the Manager button.
- Type Speaker, press enter, and type office of the Speaker.
- Click the select button.
- Click the leftmost chart box on the bottom row. The mouse pointer becomes an I-beam.
- Select the text Type name here, and press backspace.
- When <Name> appears, press enter, and type Inspector General.
- Select the text Type name here in the middle chart box on the bottom row, and press backspace.
- When <Name> appears, press enter, and type House Oversight.
- Select the text Type name here in the rightmost chart box on the bottom row, and press backspace.
- When <Name> appears, press enter, and type Cong. Compliance.
- Click the inspector General chart box, and on the styles menu, Click the Assistant option.
- Click the house Oversight chart box, and on the Styles menu, Click the Assistant option.
- Click the cong. Compliance chart box, and on the style menu, click the Assistant option.
- Click the subordinate button, and click Speaker chart box.
- Click the new box, press enter, and in the <Title> field type Parliamentarian.
- Click the Right Co-worker button, and click the Parliamentarian chart box.
- Click the new blank box, press tab, and type Chief Admin officer.
- Click the left Co-worker button, and click the chief Admin Officer chart box.
- Click the new blank box, press tab type Sergeant at Arms.
- Select Chart title and press back space.
- On the File menu, Select close and return to House Organization. (If Power point asks whether you want to up date the object, click yes.)

Changing the size of the organization chart

- Right-click one of the organization chart boxes and Click Format object on the menu, and click the size tab.

- Select Lock aspect ratio and Relative to original Picture size.

- In the Scale height window, click the up arrow to 125%, or type 125% in the box. Note that the Width value also changes.

- Click OK, and click and drag the organization chart to center the chart on the notebook page.

CHAPTER 14

Introduction to Computer Graphics

14.1 Introduction

In computer graphics, two and three-dimensional images are created by computer that are used for scientific research, artistic pursuits, and in industries to design, test market products. Computer graphics have made computer easier to use. Graphical user interfaces (GUIs) and multimedia systems such as the World Wide Web, the system of interconnected worldwide computer resources, enable computer users to select pictures to execute orders, eliminating the need to memorize complex commands. Before an image can be displayed on the screen it must be created by a computer program in a special part of the computer's memory, called a frame buffer. One method of producing an image in the frame buffer is to use a block of memory called a bitmap to store small, detailed figures such as a text character or an icon. Dividing the computer's display screen into a grid of tiny dots called pixels creates a graphical image. Frame buffer memory can also store other information, such as the colour of each pixel.

Computer graphics started with the display of data on hardcopy plotters and cathode ray tube (CRT) screen soon after the introduction of computers themselves. It has grown to include the creation, expanding set of fields, and physical, mathematical, engineering, architectural, and even conceptual structures, natural phenomena, and so on. Computer graphics today is largely interactive. The user controls the contents, structure, and appearance of objects and of their displayed images by using input devices, such as a keyboard, mouse, or touch-sensitive panel on the screen. Because of the close relationship between the input devices and the display, the handling of such devices is included in the study of computer graphics.

Until the early 1980s, computer graphics was a small, specialized field, largely because the hardware was expensive and graphics based application programs that were easy to use and cost effective were few. Then, personal computers with built-in raster graphics display such as the Xerox star and later, the mass-produced, even less expensive Apple Macintosh and IBM PC and its clones popularised the use of bitmap graphics for user-computer interaction. A bitmap is ones and zeros representation of the rectangular array of points on the screen. Once bitmap graphics is ones and zeros an explosion of easy-to-use and inexpensive graphics-based applications soon followed. Graphics-base user interfaces allowed millions of new users to control simple, low-cost application programs, such as spreadsheets, word processors, and drawing programs.

14.2 Types of Computer Graphics

There are two types of computer graphics.

Bit Mapped Graphics

In computer science, Bit mapped graphics are stored and held as collections of bits in memory locations corresponding to pixels on the screen. Bit mapped graphics are typical of paint programs, which treat images as collection of dots rather than as shapes. Within a computer's memory, a bit mapped graphics is represented as an array (group) of bits that describes the characteristics of the individual pixels making up the image. Bit mapped graphics displayed in colour require several to many bits per pixel, describing some aspect of the colour of a single spot on the screen.

Pixel. In computer graphics, short form of picture element is sometimes called a pixel. One spot in a rectilinear grid, of thousands of such spots that are individually "painted" forms an image is produced on the screen by a computer or on paper by a printer. Just as a bit is the smallest unit of information a computer can process, a pixel is the smallest elements that display or print. Hardware and software can manipulate in creating letters, numbers, or graphics. For example, the letter A is actually made up of a pattern of pixels in a grid such as the one below:

An image can also be represented in more than two colours – for example, in the shade of grays. If a pixel has only two colour values (typically black and white), it can be encoded by 1 bit of information. If more than 2 bits are used to represent a pixel, a larger range of colours or shades of gray can be represented: 2 bits for four colours or shades of gray, 4 bits for sixteen colours, and so on. Typically, an image of two colours is called a bit map, and an image of more than two colours is called a pixel map.

14.3 Vector Graphics

Vector graphics in the field of computer science, is a method of generating images that use mathematical descriptions to determine the position, length, and direction in which lines are to be drawn. In vector graphics, objects are treated as collections of lines, rather than as patterns of individual dots (pixels), as is the case with raster graphics.

14.4   Raster Graphics

The most common type of graphics monitor that employs a CRT is the raster scans display, based on television technology. In a raster scan system the electron is swept across the screen, one row at a time from top to bottom. As the electron beam moves across each row, the beam intensity which is turned on and off creates a pattern of illuminated spots. Picture definition is stored in a memory area called the refresh buffer or frame buffer. This memory area holds the set of intensity values for all the screen points. Stored intensity values are then retrieved from the refresh buffer and "painted" on the screen one row at a time. Each screen point is referred to as a pixel.

14.5   Computer Graphics

The capability of a raster scan system to store intensity information for each screen point makes it well-suited for the realistic display or scenes containing subtle shading and colour patterns. Home television sets and printers are examples of other systems using raster scan methods.

Intensity range for pixel position depends on the capability of the raster system. In a simple black and white system, each screen point is either on or off, so only one bit per pixel is needed to control other intensity of screen positions. For a bi-level system, bit value of 1 indicates that the electron beam is to be turned 'ON' at that position, and a value of 0 indicates that the beam intensity is to be 'OFF'. Additional bits are needed when colour and intensity variations can be displayed. Up to 24 bits per pixel and a screen resolution of 1024 by 1024 requires 3 megabytes of storage for the frame buffer. On a black-and-white system with one bit per pixel, the frame buffer is commonly called a bit map. For systems with multiple bits per pixel, the frame buffer is often referred to as a pixel map.

Refreshing on raster-scan displays is carried out at the rate of 60 to 80 frames per second, although some systems are designed for higher refresh rates. Sometimes, refresh rates are described in units of cycles per second, or Hertz, where a cycle corresponds to one frame. Using these units, we would describe a refresh rate of 60 frames per second as simply 60 Hz. At the end of each scan line, the electron beam returns to the left side of the screen to begin displaying the next scan line. The return to the left of the screen, after refreshing each coated onto the inside of the CRT screen, and the displayed colour depend on how far the electron beam penetrates into the phosphor layers. A beam of slow electrons excites only the outer red layer. A beam of very fast electrons penetrates through the red layer and excites the inner green layer. At intermediate beam speeds, combinations of red and green light are emitted to show two additional colours, orange and yellow. The speed of the electrons, and hence the screen colour at any point, is controlled by the beam acceleration voltage. Beam penetration has been an inexpensive way to produce colour in random-scan monitors, but only four colours are possible, and the quality of pictures is not as good as with other methods.

14.6   Uses of Computer Graphics

User Interfaces

Most of the application that run on personal computer and workstations have user interfaces that rely on desktop window systems to manage multiple simultaneous activities, clicking facilities that allow user to select menu items, icons and other objects on the window; typing is necessary to input text to be stored and manipulated. Word processing, spreadsheets, chart wizard, paint systems and desktop and commercial publishing programs are typical applications that take advantages of such user interface techniques.

14.7   Graphs Plotting in Commercial Applications and Technology

The next common use of graphics is probably to create 20 and 30 graphs of mathematical, physical and economic function, histograms, bar and pie charts, spreadsheets, task scheduling charts, inventory and production charts, and the like.

All these are used to present meaningfully and concisely the treads and patterns glanced from data, so as to clarify complex phenomena and to facilitate informed decision-making.

14.8   Desktop Publishing

The use of graphics for the creation and dissemination of information has increased enormously since the advent of desktop publishing on personal computers. Desktop publishing sets up columns for entering text and rearranges the text in the columns to fit the new size. The test runs horizontally, except when more powerful systems allow you to change the text direction. Also, we can mix graphics into the text and this is possible because the system treats text as a graphics object, knowing the precise position coordinates, rotation, size and style of every letter.

14.8.1   Electronic Publishing

Electronic publishing can produce traditional printed documents and electronic documentation that contains text, tables, graphs, and other forms of drawn or scanned graphics. Hypermedia systems that allow browsing of network of interlinked multimedia documents are proliferating.

14.8.2   Computer Aided Design (CAD)

CAD systems allow for speedy, simple design of buildings, mechanical systems, floor plans, electronic circuits boards, or engineering drawings. CAD systems save time and energy, when you are revising the original design. Sometimes, the user merely wants to produce the precise drawings of components and assemblies, as for online drafting or architectural blue prints. CAD systems aim to be user-friendly; one need not know algorithms or programming but one still must thoroughly understand the geometric and mathematical essentials that underlie objects and the special commands that manipulate drawings.

14.8.3   Simulation, Animations and Video Games

Simulation indicates a touch or visualization, which makes the process of simulation more convincing. From the synthetic visualization of a complicated chemical process to the simulation of natural phenomena like a storm or a surface cloud, cyclones, or of an engineering component assembly using CAD packages are all parts of the simulation. Computer produced animated movies and display of the time varying behavior of real and simulated objects are becoming increasingly popular for scientific and engineering visualization. We can use them to study abstract mathematical entities as well as mathematical models of such phenomena as fluid flow, relativity nuclear and chemical reactions, physiological system, organ function and deformation of mechanical structure under various loads. Another advanced technology area is interactive cartooning. The simpler kinds of systems for producing flat cartoon are becoming cost-effective key frames. Cartoon characters will increasingly be modeled in the computer as 3D shape descriptions whose movements are controlled by computer commands, rather than by the figures being drawn manually by cartoonists. Television commercials featuring flying logos and more exotic visual trickery have become common, as have elegant special effects in movies.

14.9   Types of Graphics Devices

Output or video display device

CRT or (Cathode Ray Tube)

Typically, the primary output device in a graphics system is a video monitor. The operations of most video monitor are based on the standard cathode ray tube (CRT) design.

Basic Operation of CRT : A beam of electron (cathode ray) is emitted by an electrons gun that passes through focusing and deflection system that directs the beam towards specified positions on the phosphor-coated screen. The phosphor then emits a small spot of light at each position contacted by the electron beam. The light emitted by the phosphor fades very rapidly. To maintain this screen picture, one way is to redraw the picture repeatedly by quickly directing the electron beam back over the same points. Such a type of display is called refresh CRT.

Persistence : Persistence is defined as the time it takes the emitted light from the screen to decay to one tenth of its original intensity. Lower persistence phosphors require higher refresh to maintain a picture on the screen without flicker. Such phosphors are used in animations. High persistence phosphors are useful for displaying highly complex, static picture.

Working *:* Beam passes between two pairs of metal plates, one vertical and other horizontal. A voltage difference is applied to each pair of plates according to the amount that the beam is to be deflected in each direction. As the electron beam passes between each pair of plates, it is bent towards the plate with the higher positive voltage.

The basic component of electron gun is heated metal, cathode and a control grid, heating filament supplies heat, directing a current through the filament causes electrons to be boiled "off" the hot cathode surface. In the vacuum inside the CRT envelop, the free, negatively charged electrons are then accelerated towards the phosphor coating by a high positive voltage. The accelerating voltages can be generated with a positively charged metal coating on the side of CRT envelope near the phosphor screen or an accelerating anode can be used.

Sometimes the electron gun is built to contain the accelerating anode and focusing system within the same unit.

Resolution *:* The maximum number of points that can be displayed without overlapping a CRT is referred to as the resolution. Precisely, the number of points lies per centimeter that can be plotted horizontally and vertically. This depends on the type of phosphors used and the focusing, and deflection system.

Aspect Ratio *:* This is an important property of video monitors. This number gives the ratio of vertical points to horizontal points necessary to produce equal length lines in both directions on the screen. An aspect ratio of ¾ means that a vertical line platted with three points has the some length as a horizontal line platted with four points.

Raster Scan Monitor

In a raster scan system, the electron beam is swept across the screen, one row at a time from top to bottom. As the electron beam moves across each row, the beam intensity is tuned 'ON' and 'OFF' to crate a pattern of Illuminated spots. Picture definition is stored in a memory area called the refresh buffer or frame buffer. This memory area holds the set of intensity values for all the screen points. Stored intensity values are then retrieved from the refresh buffer and "painted" on the screen one row at a time. The capability of a raster is suited for the realistic display of screen containing subtle shading and colour patterns.

Refreshing on raster scan is done at the rate of 60 to 80 frames per second, some systems are designed for higher refresh rates. Refresh rate are sometimes described in units of cycles per second, or hertz (Hz), where a cycle corresponds to one frame. At this rate, the electron beam traces over all screen lines from top to bottom. A picture rate below this makes picture to flicker. Interlacing is often used when higher refresh rates are needed.

Colour CRT Monitor

To display colour pictures, combination of phosphorus that emits different coloured light is used. There are two different techniques for producing colour display with a CRT.

1. Beam Penetration Method.   2. Shadow Mask Method

Beam-Penetration Method

This method is used with random-scan monitors. Two layers of phosphor, (red and green) are coated onto the inside of CRT screen. Displayed colour depends on how far the electron beam penetrates into the phosphor layers. A beam of slow electrons excites only the outer red layer. A beam of very fast electrons penetrates through the red layer and excites the inner green layer. At intermediate beam speeds, combinations of red and green light are emitted to show two additional colours, orange and yellow. The beam acceleration voltages control the speed of electrons.

Beam penetration method produces only four colours, and the quality of pictures is not as good as with other methods. This method is an expensive way to produce colours in random scan monitors.

Shadow Mask Method

This method is commonly used in raster-scan system because it produces a much wider range of colours than the above method.

Shadow-mask CRT has three phosphor colour dots at each pixel position. One phosphor dot emits a red light, another emits a green light and the third emits a blue light. Such a CRT has three electron guns, one for each colour dot, and a shallow mask grid just behind the phosphor-coated holes aligned with the phosphor dot patterns.

The three beams pass through a hole activating a dot triangle, which appears as a small colour spot on the screen. Phosphor dots are arranged in a triangle so that each electron beam can activate only its corresponding colour dot when it passes through the shadow mask. Variant intensity levels of electron beam obtain different colour combinations.

Direct View Storage Tube

This is an alternative method to monitor a screen image, as it stores the picture information inside the CRT instead of refreshing the screen. A direct view storage tube (DVST) stores the picture information as a charge distributes just behind the phosphor-coated screen.

Two electron guns are used – one is primary and the second is flood gun. First one stores the picture patterns and the second one maintains picture display. The primary electron gun is used to draw the picture definition on the storage grid, a non-conducting material. High speed electron from primary gun strikes storage grid and knocks out electrons, which are attached to the collector grid. Storage grid being non-conducting, the areas where electrons have been removed will keep a net positive charge. This stored positive charge pattern on the storage grid is the picture definition. The flood gun produces a continuous stream of low-speed electrons that pass though the control grid and are attached to the positive areas of the storage grid. These low-speed electrons penetrate through the storage grid to the phosphor waiting, without affecting the charge pattern on the storage surface.

A DVST monitor has advantages and disadvantages both compared to the refresh CRT. As no refreshing is needed, very complex picture can be displayed at a very high resolutions without flicker. Disadvantages of DVST system are that they ordinarily do not display colour and that selected part of a picture cannot be erased. To eliminate a picture section, it has to be redrawn. The erasing and redrawing take several seconds for a complex picture and because of these reasons, storage displays have been largely replaced by raster system.

Flat Panel Display

The term flat display refers to a class of video devices that have reduced volume, weight and power requirement compared to a CRT. A significant feature of flat panel displays is that they are thinner than CRTs, and we can hang them on walls or wear them on our wrists. Current uses for flat panel displays include small TV monitors, calculators, pocket video games, laptop computer, arm rest viewing or movies on airlines, as advertisement boards in elevators, and as graphics display in application requiring rugged, portable monitors.

Flat panel display can be classified into two categories: emissive display and non-emissive display. The emissive displays are devices that convert electrical energy into light. Plasma panels thin film electron luminescent displays and light diodes are example of emissive displays. In flat CRTs, electron beams are accelerated parallel to the screen, and then deflected to the screen. But flat CRTs have proved to be a failure. Non-emissive displays use optical effects to convert sunlight or light from some other source into graphics patterns. LCD (Liquid Crystal Device) is an example of non-emissive flat panel display.

Plasma Panel Display

The plasma panel is an array of tiny neon bulbs. Each bulb can be put into on 'ON' (intensified) state or on 'OFF' state, and it remains in the state until explicitly changed to the other plasma panels that typically have 50 to 125 cell per inch, with a 10 to 15 inch diagonal but 40 by 40 inch panels with 50 cells per inch are sold commercially.

The neon-bulbs are not discrete units, but are rather part of single integrated panel made of three layers of glass. The inside surface of the front layer has thin vertical strips of an electrical conductor. The center layer has a number of holes (the bulbs), and the inside surface of the real layer has thin horizontal strips of an electrical conductor. Matrix addressing is used to turn bulbs 'ON' and 'OFF'. To turn 'ON' a bulb, the system adjusts the voltages on the corresponding lines such that their difference is large enough to put electrons from the neon molecules thus firing the bulbs and making it glow. Once the glow starts, a lower voltage is applied to sustain it. To turn 'OFF' a bulb, the system momentarily decreases the voltage on the appropriate lines to use the sustaining voltages. Bulbs can be turned 'ON' or 'OFF' in about 15 microseconds.

The plasma panel has the advantage of being flat, transparent and rugged and does not need a bitmap refresh buffer. It can be used with a rear projection system to mix photographic slides as static background for computer generated dynamic graphics. Its most use in military applications, where small size and rigid ness are important.

Thin-film Electro Luminescent Displays

It consists of the same grid-like structure as used in plasma display. Between the front and back panels is a thin (500 nanometer) layer of an electro luminescent material, such as zinc sulfide doped with manganese that emits light when in a high electric field (approx. 106 volts per centimeter). When a sufficiently high voltage is applied to a pair of crossing to electrodes, the phosphor becomes a conductor in the area of intersection of two electrodes. Electrical energy is then absorbed by the manganese atoms, which then release the energy as a spot of light similar to the glowing plasma effect in a plasma panel.

These displays are bright and can be switched 'ON' and 'OFF' quickly, and transistors at each pixel can be used to store the image. Major disadvantages of these displays are that their power consumption is higher than that of the LCD panel. However, their brightness has led to their use in some portable computer.

Liquid Crystal Display (LCD)

The term liquid crystal refers to the fact that these compounds have a crystalline arrangement of molecules, yet they flow like liquid. Flat panel display commonly uses threadlike liquefied crystal compounds that tend to keep the long axes of the rod-shaped molecules aligned. Rows of horizontal transparent conductors are put into the other plate. The intersection of two conductors defines a pixel position.

Normally, the molecules are aligned. Polarized light passing through the material is thrusted so that it will pass through the opposite polarization. The light is then reflected back to the viewer. To turn off the pixel, we apply a voltage to the two intersecting conductors to align the molecules so that light is not thursted. This type of flat panel device is referred to as passive matrix LCD.

Picture definitions are stored in a refresh buffer, and the screen is refreshed at the rate of 60 frames per second, as in the emissive device. Back lighting is also commonly applied using solid-state electronic device, so that the system is not completely dependent on outside light sources. Colours can be displayed by using different materials or dyes and by placing a triad of colour pixels at each screen location.

Another method of constructing LCDs is to place a transistor at each pixel location, using thin film transistor technology. The transistors are used to control the voltage at pixel locations and to prevent charge from gradually leaking out of the liquid crystal cells. These devices are called active matrix displays.

Input Device

Input device allows us to communicate with computer. Using this one can feed in the information. Most commonly used input devices are :

- Mouse
- Trackball
- Data glove
- Touch Panels
- Image Scanners
- Digitizers
- Joystick
- Keyboard.

MOUSE : Mouse is an integral part of the fancy graphical user interface of any software application. There is a cursor in the shape of an arrow or crosshair always associated with a mouse. Wheels or rollers on the bottom of the mouse can be used to record the amount and direction of movement. Another method for detecting mouse motion is with an optical sensor. For these systems, the mouse is moved over a special mouse pad that has a grid of horizontal and vertical lines. The optical sensor detects movement across the lines in the grid. The potentiometer attached to the ball estimates the relative position of the mouse. Several instructions or commands in software are activated using a mouse. In such cases, a specific action or command is associated with a particular screen location. When the coordinates of a commands screen location are equated with the current mouse cursor position, the command is executed with the press of the mouse button.

A new but different type of mouse is optical mouse. Here, two apertures – one for the optical source and the other for receiving the optical ray reflected from the metallic mouse base plate – replace the ball.

TRACKBALL : Trackball is some sort of an inverted mouse where the ball is held inside a rectangular box. In mouse, the positioning of the cursor on the screen is associated with the orientation of the track ball. A potentiometer captures the trackball orientation, which is calibrated with the translation of the cursor in the screen. In an advanced track ball version, in space ball, other than cursor position, ball orientation can be measured.

DATA GLOVE : Data glove is a device to interact with animated artificial objects. The glove is constructed with a series of sensors that detect hand and finger motions. Electromagnetic coupling between transmitting antennas and receiving antennas is used to provide information about the position and orientation of the hand. The transmitting and receiving antennas can each be structured as a set of three mutually perpendicular coils, forming a three-dimensional Cartesian coordinates system. Input from the glove can be used to position or manipulate objects in a virtual scene. A two dimensional projection of the scene can be viewed on a video monitor, or a three dimensional projection can be viewed with a headset.

TOUCH PANELS : Touch panels allow displayed objects or screen positions to be selected with a touch of a finger. A typical application of touch panels is for the selection of processing options that represent a graphical icons. Such tool is especially helpful when a user has to select one or a set of processing operations based on a number of interactive query-answer sessions. Optical touch panels employ a line of infrared light-emitting diodes (LEDs) along one vertical edge and along one horizontal edge of the frame. The opposite vertical and horizontal edge contains light detectors. These detectors are used to record which beams are interrupted when the panel is touched. The two crossing beams that are interrupted identify the horizontal and vertical coordinates of the screen position selected.

Positions can be selected with an accuracy of about ¼ inch. With closely spaced LEDs, it is possible to break two horizontal or two vertical beams simultaneously. In this case, an average position between the two-interrupt beams is recorded. The LEDs operate at infrared frequencies, so that the light is not visible to a user.

An electrical touch panel is constructed with two transparent plates separated by a small distance. One of the plates is coated with a conducting material, and the other plate is coated with a resistive material. When the outer plate is touched, it is forced into contact with the inner plate. This contact creates a voltage drop across the resistive plate that is converted to the coordinate values of the selected screen position.

In acoustical touch panels, high-frequency sound waves are generated in the horizontal and vertical directions across a glass plate. Touching the screen causes part of each wave to be reflected from the finger to the emitters. The screen position at the point of contact is calculated from a measurement of the time interval between the transmission of each wave and its reflection to the emitter.

IMAGE SCANNERS : Drawing, graphs, colour and black & white photos, or text can be stored for computer processing with an image scanner by passing an optical scanning mechanism over the information to be stored. The gradations of gray scale or colour are then recorded and stored in an array. Once we have the internal representation of a picture, we can apply transformations to rotate, scale, or crop the picture to a particular screen area. We can also apply various image-processing methods to modify the array representation of the picture. For scanned text input, various editing operation can be performed on the stored documents. Some scanners are able to scan either graphical representations or text and they come in a variety of sizes and capabilities.

DIGITIZERS : Digitizer can be used to input coordinate values in either a two-dimensional or a three-dimensional space. Typically, a digitizer is used to scan over a drawing or object and to input a set of discrete coordinate positions, which can be joined with straight-line segments to approximate the curve or surface shapes.

One type of digitizer is the graphics tablet, which is used to input two-dimensional coordinates by activating a hand cursor or stylus at selected positions on a flat surface. A hand cursor contains cross hairs for sighting positions, while a stylus is a pencil-shaped device that is pointed at positions on the tablet. Tablet size varies from 12 by 12 inches for desktop models to 44 by 60 inches or larger for floor models. Graphic tablets provide a highly accurate method for selecting coordinate positions, with an accuracy that varies from about 0.2 mm on desktop models to about 0.05 mm on larger models.

Many graphic tablets are constructed with a rectangular grid of wires embedded in the tablet surface. Electromagnetic plates are generated in sequence along the wires and an electric signal is induced in a wire coil in an activated stylus or hand cursor to record a tablet position. Depending on the technology, either signal strength, coded pulses, or phase shifts can be used to determine the position on the tablet.

Acoustic (or sonic) tablets use sound waves to detect a stylus position. Either strip microphones or point microphones can be used to detect the sound emitted by an electrical spark from a stylus strip. The position of the stylus is calculated by timing the arrival of the generated sound at the different microphone positions. An advantage of two-dimensional acoustic tablets is that the microphones can be placed on any surface to form the "tablet" work area.

JOYSTICK : A joystick consists of a small, vertical lever mounted on a base that is used to steer the screen cursor around. Most joysticks select screen positions with actual stick movement; others respond to pressure on the stick. Some joysticks are mounted on a keyboard; others function as standalone units.

The distance that the stick is moved in any direction from its center position corresponds to screen-cursor movement in that direction. Potentiometer mounted at the base of the joystick measures the amount of movement, and springs return the stick to the centre position when it is relaxed. One or more buttons can be programmed to act as input switches to signal certain actions once a screen position has been selected.

In another type of movable joystick, the stick is used to activate switches that cause the screen cursor to move at a constant rate in the direction selected. Eight switches, arranged in a circle, are sometimes provided, so that the stick can select any one of the eight directions for cursor movement. Pressure-sensitive joysticks, also called isometric joysticks, have a non-movable stick. Pressure on the stick is measured with strain gauges and converted to movement of the cursor in the direction specified.

KEYBOARD : An alphanumeric keyboard on a graphics system is used primarily as a device for entering text strings. The keyboard is an effective device for imputing such that no graphic data as picture labels associated with graphics display.

Keyboards can also be provided with features to facilitate entry of screen coordinates, menu selections, or graphics functions.

Cursor control keys and function keys are common features on general-purpose keyboards. Function keys allow users to enter frequently-used operations in a single keystroke, and cursor-control keys can be used to select displayed objects or coordinate positions by positioning the screen cursor. Additionally, a numeric keypad is often included on the keyboard for fast entry of numeric data.

HARD COPY DEVICES

The printer is an important accessory of any computing system. In a graphics system, it is the quality of printed output, which is one of the key factors necessary to convince both the user and the customer. The major factors, which control the quality of a printer, are individual dot size on the paper and the number of dots per inch (dpi)

Individual dot size on the paper : The ordered collection of dots creates a figure. The minimum the size of the dot, the better the detail of the figure reproduced. The size of dot is specified by the diameter of the dot.

Number of dots per inch (dpi) : This is a function of dot size and the inter-dot spacing. Higher dpi values increase the sharpness and detail of a figure and enhance the number of intensity levels that a printer supports. Controlling the number of dots in a given area reproduces the intensity of a point. Consider a 3 x 3 matrix on the paper. Assume that each element of the matrix is of the same size as that of a single dot. If no dot is placed in any element of this matrix, the intensity level corresponds to white, else intensity level corresponds to black. By controlling the number of dots in between the white and block limits, a whole range of intensity levels, eight levels to be precise, can be created. This process is known as half toning or dithering. The images printed in magazines and newspapers are all examples of half toning.

The dot matrix printer is a commonly used hard copier system. The printing is executed using a printer head, which contains 9-24 pins. These pins are ultrathin but stiff, which, through an ink ribbon, strike the paper. The colour supported by the printer depends on the colour of ink in the ribbon. The pins are usually arranged vertically where marginal offsets are provided between columns in order to reduce the inter dot spacing. The printer head prints along every raster row of the printer paper and sometimes the printing is repeated along the same scan line to enhance the print quality. The quality of output depends on the ribbon and the ink quality. As a whole, dot matrix printer is not recommended for a graphics system.

The laser printer employs technology similar to photocopy machine. A laser beam focuses and scans a positively charged selenium-coated rotating drum. The laser gun removes the positive charge from the drum except for the area to be printed.

The negatively charged toner first adheres to the positively charged area of the drum from where it is transferred to the white paper. The paper is then subjected to a mild heating process to fix the toner on the paper. The laser printer is mainly a bi-level printer. In the case of colour lasers, this process is repeated three times. Thermal printers also produce excellent colour graphics hardcopy. They transfer coloured wax pigments on the paper using micro nibs whose tips are rapidly heated and cooled. Some thermal printers and special quality papers are required for printing high-resolution graphics.

Postscript

Postscript is a unique concept proposed by Adobe in the early 1980s. It is the most-used page description language, which is meant for generating quality output. Almost all laser printers have postscript compilers to process documents and images.

Page description languages convert documents or images on almost machine-independent format. It defines a print area of the paper and then converts the information to be printed to a program written in a page description language. For viewing the output in the screen, compilers are available in the host computer. The postscripted document or image displayed in a screen is what-you-see-what-you get (WYSWYG) in the printer. Like any programming language, postscript language contains a set of keywords and their parameters.

CHAPTER 15

Applications of Computers in Pharmaceutical and Clinical Studies

15.1 Introduction

Now-a-days computers are used in pharmaceutical industries, hospitals and in various departments for drug information, education, evaluation, analysis, and medication history and for maintenance of financial records etc. They have become indispensable in the development of clinical pharmacy, hospital pharmacy and in pharmaceutical research. They co-ordinate effective communication and support clinical and financial management functions.

Effective functioning of any organization largely depends upon continuous flow of information, i.e., receiving the information, storing it, processing it and disseminating it. An effective management information system always provides the needed information in the right form, at the right time and at the right place. Actually each information of organization is connected with other informations through communication channels, thus making organizational entity a decision-making point.

Computers play an effective role for retrieval of information. In hospitals, data management involves creating, modifying, adding and deleting data in patient files to generate reports. Now many doctors for further investigation, as they are connected through various personal computers, share these reports. Some popular Data Base Management System (DBMS) packages for personal computer are: Dbase III+ and Fox Base +. Hence, computers help in maintaining overall health care system and this can be best-illustrated by enlisting its applications.

15.2 Patient Monitoring

Patient's monitoring includes monitoring of physiological processes in patients such as blood pressure, pulse rate, temperature, etc. This information plays special role in detection and prevention of critical conditions in patients. It helps in giving warning of critical conditions for immediate nursing attention and enables medical staff to make accurate judgments of patients' progress. It further provides data for research purpose to monitor patients under intensive care.

Hence, computers play an important role in communication by acquiring the data about patient's metabolism and then communicating the same to medical staff by displaying graphs. Detecting critical conditions and generating alarms involve both numerical and logical data processing. This processing helps in giving warning of critical conditions, enabling the medical staff for proper judgment of patients progress, and in the long-term provides a data for medical research.

Actually computers control number of equipments simultaneously to obtain samples of body fluids and then get them analyzed through auto-analyser for their physical and chemical parameters.

After analysis of parameters "AND or OR" statements indicate logical relationship where as IF...THEN mark a conditional computation. This combination of logical and conditional data processing enables the patient monitoring system as a decision-making instrument for interpretation of results.

15.3 Medication Monitoring

To meet the goal of optimum drug therapy, medication is very essential. In this case, prescription of the patient received over a period of time is entered into the computer data, which serves as a chronological drug file or the patient. It helps in suggesting number of drugs along with their dosage schedule. Computers provide two types of information.

    (a)   Pharmacokinetic   (b)   Non-Pharmacokinetic

Pharmacokinetic Information

"NONLIN" is a computer program which can predict pharmacokinetic parameters very easily. These parameters include volume of distribution, bioavailability, rate of clearance etc. It helps in maintaining dosage schedule of various drugs like antibiotics, aminoglysosides etc.

Non-Pharmacokinetic Information

It includes various allergic reactions, drug interactions, adverse drug reactions etc. For such information two computer programmes are available.

1. MEDIPHOR (Monitoring and evaluation of drug interactions by a pharmacy-oriented reporting).

2. PAD (Pharmacy Automated drug interaction screening).

15.4 Maintenance of Records

Various records like patient's medication history, current treatment and financial records etc. are maintained in computers by feeding accurate data – 'DATA' is a collection of facts and computer works as a 'DATA BASE' manager. MEDLINE is a data base package used for such purpose. It gives the current information of patients regarding their name, age, sex, room number, weight, allergic reaction etc. These records are stored in a 'FILE' like "Physician name" file, "Direction" file, "Drug Interaction" file etc. Now these files contain specific information like physician's name, registration number, phone number, address, etc. and provide such information whenever required.

15.5 Materials Management

Computers play vital role in material planning, purchasing, inventory control and forecasting prices. Inventory control is very essential because it maintains the balance between stock-in-hand and excessive capital investment. Techniques such as ABC analysis and EOQ can be easily programmed. It will eliminate the tedious and time-consuming task of calculations. Computers are used to detect the items, which had attained minimum order level. It then prepares a list and purchase orders for further supplies. Generally there are two systems for inventory control.

    (a)   Periodic inventory control   (b)   Perpetual system.

    (a)   ***Periodic Inventory Control System:*** In this system stock levels are checked manually and the amount of inventory in hand is compared with minimum and maximum stock maintained in the computers. Computers help in placement of order to different suppliers after checking their terms and conditions because all the entries of stocks are present in it.

    (b)   ***Perpetual System :*** In this system computer tells about the present position of all the drugs because when they are received, they are entered in the initial stocks to get the current stocks. When the drugs are delivered to various departments the quantities are subtracted accordingly. Such type of additions and deletions from inventory balance is done with the help of "data base" package.

The information as output from the computer may be obtained in various forms like,

- Planning of material
- Drugs formulary
- Vendor detail for procurement
- Tender rate and analysis
- Determination of EOQ
- Pending supply orders
- Inventory analysis
- Records points
- Safety stocks

- Ledger for narcotics
- Over/under stocking
- Slow moving/Fast moving items
- Expired drugs.

15.6   Data Storage and Retrieval

In hospital administration, computer helps in rapid data storage and retrieval, particularly when the data stored is subjected to frequent changes and when group of items based on the stored data need to be retrieved. Admission of in-patients and their discharge from a hospital require data, which gets changed every minute, e.g., admission of in-patient ties up resources like clinical and nursing staff, a bed, operation theatre, Intensive care unit, pharmacy department, radiological services, etc.

Hence, decision to admit a new patient is not a simple one. Even the availability of a suitable bed is difficult to determine in male and female ward, isolation ward etc. A prediction must be made that a suitable bed will be available at future date because if the estimation is over optimistic, patients who are called in may by turned away at the last minute. If the prediction is over-pessimistic expensive resources lie idle and the waiting period for treatment is extended.

Once the patient gets admitted, computer records and stores information, clinical information, catering information, diagnosis, sex, medication etc. It helps in providing detailed information about medical and paramedical staff including their duty chart. It helps the senior personnel to keep a check on ward-by-ward loading of nursing staff and to allocate additional help whenever required.

15.7   Diagnostic Laboratories

Computers meet the growing demand for testing laboratories as manual procedures are lengthy and time-consuming, whereas automated computerized instruments perform number of tasks with accuracy in diagnostic laboratories. Generally LIS (Laboratory Information System) is used to manage large amount of data. In this, instruments contain preprocessors, which convert raw data into digital format and help in transmitting numerical values for report generation. LIS also performs administrative and managerial function, including specimen tracking, product analysis and quality control. Similarly many instruments have microprocessors that facilitate all phases of testing processes, including calibration of instrument till reporting of results.

The developments of powerful computers offer opportunity for improved viewing and interpretation in radiology department. In this many of the latest imaging techniques such as Computerized Tomography (CT) and Magnetic Resonance Imaging (MRI) are inherently digital. In this, computer creates a "functional image" by performing complex calculations on measured data.

15.8   Pharmaceutical Education

Computer-aided instructions help in improving the shortcomings of traditional teaching methods. They provide a medium for interactive learning and offer immediate student-specific feedback. Support individuals tailored instructions finally form a basis for objective testing.

15.9   Hospital Pharmacy and Retail Pharmacy

Computers are used in pharmacies to maintain accessible, legible and up-to-date medication records. They help in keeping overall patient care by maintaining their records, consumption of drugs, registration numbers and detailed records of accounts and purchase section. Even for retail pharmacist, computers have been of valuable assistance in the prescription processing. It includes display of computer information about patient and drug, its adverse drug reaction, causation, duplication of orders, labeling conditions etc.

Following are the other applications in hospital and retail pharmacy :

- Calculation of monthly gross income
- Generating pay slips
- Updating the employee information
- Placement of supply order
- Keeping track of total payment and amount due to supplier
- Checking the quality and quantity of hospital supplies recorded and identifying any discrepancies.
- Recording purchases for accounting purposes.

A number of computer programs have been developed to assist physicians in dosing and scheduling drug. But there are certain drugs, which are extremely sensitive to certain patients. For such patients physicians use computer programs to forecast drug levels and to choose the amounts and schedule of drug doses that will achieve target level. Similarly 'HELP' is a system, which identifies abnormal chemistry levels, concurrent diseases and other related patient conditions.

15.10   Hospital Setting

Duties of the pharmacist have been changing tremendously and hence it has become impossible to remember and to recheck everything. Therefore, computer manages the hospital systems and allows the pharmacists to check the work. Software is available for the pharmacist to provide professional services and to automate the technical staff. This will ultimately result in efficient and cost-effective operation and will further maximize clinical and patient-oriented functions of pharmacists.

15.11   Patient Counseling

Computers play an important role in in-patient counseling. Sophisticated software is available to educate patients by giving patient education leaflets. These leaflets provide information about name of medication, its uses, side-effects, precautions, drug interactions, missed dose, storage, how to take the medication etc.

It should always be kept in mind that computer program should be an intelligent one so that it should not affect adversely by giving too much or too less of the information to patient.

15.12   Drug Interactions

Pharmacists cannot remember each and every medication, its therapeutic usage, its effects and drug interactions. Therefore computers offer knowledge base systems to extend their professional services. Computerized pharmacy can alert physician/ pharmacist for serious drug-drug, drug-food and drug-disease interactions, which are likely to occur in prescription. Examples of such database and online services are MEDLINE, IDIS and pharmline.

15.13   Community Pharmacy

Computers help in streamlining refilling of prescriptions. It has terminated the long standing problem and waiting in a queue for refilling of prescription. It has been becoming popular because it reminds the patient for refilling and compliance of medication. These systems not only help in filling of individual prescriptions but in processing the prescription in a right manner. It also enables to manage inventory, sales, accounts, etc. in community pharmacy.

15.14   Drug Information Services

Various software, Internet, Intranet and online services are available for the pharmacist to provide drug information service to medical, paramedical professionals and patients. Computer-aided drug design helps the chemist to formulate a new drug molecule possessing desired therapeutic action. These new drug entities can be generated through graphics and by changing molecular configuration. CD-ROM technology has helped a lot in the evolution of compact electronic libraries. Various software programs of different companies are listed here.

15.15   Important Pharmacy Websites

1. www.aaps.org - American Association of Pharmaceutical Scientists
2. www.abpi.org.uk/- Association of the British Pharmaceutical Industry
3. www.wizard.pharm.wayne.edu - American Chemical Society Division of Medicinal Chemistry.
4. www.who.int/dap/Word Health Organization program
5. www.accp.com American Clinical pharmacy
6. www.bpsweb.org Board of pharmaceutical Specialties
7. www.fda.gov:80/default.htm Food and Drug Administration
8. www.pharmweb.net - Guide to pharmacy and related resources on the internet
9. www_sci.lib.uci.edu~martindale/pharmacy.html- Hugesite with pharmacy, pharmacology, clinical pharmacology and toxicology information.
10. www.aegis.com- Largest AIDS/HIV database in the world
11. www.merek.com/pubs/manual-Manual of diagnosis and therapy
12. http://www.pharmweb.net/- Extensive Directory of Most Aspects of Pharmacology
13. www.medmarket.com/tenants/.-Covers regulated product industries
14. community.net/~neils-Pharmaceutical drug directory, links
15. www.bio.com/.-Directory of pharmaceutical and biotechnology companies.
16. www.lilly.com - Eli Lilly and Company
17. www.glaxowellcome.co.uk/-Glaxo wellcome
18. www.hmri.com - Hoechst Marion Roussel USA
19. www.hoechst.com/-Hoechst
20. www.jnj.com/-Johnson & Johnson
21. www.nerck.com - Merck & co.
22. www.novartis.com -Novartis
23. www.oncor.com -Organon
24. www.pg.com-P & G Global Community
25. www.parke-davis.com/varsions_1/index.html-Parke-Davis
26. www.pfizer.com/main.html-Pfizer
27. www.pnu.com/ns4index.html-Pharmacia & Upjohn
28. www.rpr.rpna.com-Rhone-Poulence Rorer
29. www.roche.com-Roche
30. www.searlehealthnet.com/searle -Searle

31. www.sb.com -Smithkline Beecham
32. www.arcwebserv.com/pharm-weekly pharmacy articles by registered pharmacist
33. http//157.142.72.143./gaps/pkbio/pkbio.html-Onlinecourse pharmacokinetics and biopharmaceutics
34. www.hmri.com/managingyourhealth/guides/tym.html-Instructions about dose, route and taking of medication-www.rxlist.com/top200.htm -List of the 200 most popular US pharmaceuticals
35. www.henryschein.com/medical.htm-Henry Schein Medical products – Online Ordering